# MANUAL OF CARDIAC ARRHYTHMIAS

# MANUAL OF CARDIAC ARRHYTHMIAS

*Edward K. Chung*, M.D., F.A.C.P., F.A.C.C.

Professor of Medicine
Jefferson Medical College of
Thomas Jefferson University
and
Director of the Heart Station and
Attending Physician (Cardiologist)
Thomas Jefferson University Hospital
Philadelphia, PA 19107

Fellow, American College of Cardiology
Former Governor for West Virginia, American College of Cardiology
Fellow, American College of Physicians
Member, American Federation for Clinical Research
Member, American Medical Association
Member, World Congress of Cardiology
Member, Asian Pacific Congress of Cardiology
Member, International Congress of Electrocardiology
Member, Pennsylvania Medical Society
Member, Philadelphia County Medical Society
Member, Korean Medical Association

Editorial Board Member for
Cardiology,
The Journal of Electrocardiology,
Heart and Lung,
Primary Cardiology,
Cardiology Clinics,
and
Hospital Physicians

**Butterworths**
Boston London Singapore Sydney Toronto Wellington

Every effort has been made to ensure the drug dosage schedules within this text are accurate and conform to standards accepted at time of publication. However, as treatment recommendations vary in the light of continuing research and clinical experience, the reader is advised to verify drug dosage schedules herein with information found on product identification sheets. This is especially true in cases of new or infrequently used drugs.

ISBN 0-409-90172-5

Library of Congress Catalog Number 85-040841

Butterworth Publishers
80 Montvale Avenue
Stoneham, MA 02180

10 9 8 7 6 5 4 3 2

Printed in the United States of America

*To My Wife, Lisa,*
*and*
*To Our Children, Linda and Christopher*

# Contents

# *Preface*

The primary intention of *Manual of Cardiac Arrhythmias* is to describe common cardiac arrhythmias that are encountered frequently in our daily practice. Thus, the purpose is not to discuss in depth every aspect of various cardiac rhythm problems, especially uncommon cardiac arrhythmias, which are considered to be beyond the scope of this publication.

The contents are intended to be clinical, concise, and practical, so that this manual will provide all readers with up-to-date materials that will assist them directly in the daily care of patients with common cardiac arrhythmias.

The format is organized to provide all necessary information in the diagnosis as well as management of common cardiac arrhythmias expeditiously. Consequently, the manual will be particularly valuable to medical house staff and all primary care physicians (e.g., family physicians, emergency room physicians, internists, and so forth). In addition, medical students (junior and senior), anesthesiologists, cardiothoracic surgeons, and cardiac care nurses will benefit greatly by reading this manual for a better understanding of various common cardiac arrhythmias.

I would like to express my appreciation to my personal secretary, Michele M. Harvey, for her valuable assistance.

Finally, I owe a deep gratitude and appreciation to my father, Dr. Il-Chun Chung, who has always offered guidance and inspiration.

Bryn Mawr, Pennsylvania

Edward K. Chung, MD

# *Terms Commonly Abbreviated*

AF: atrial fibrillation
APC: atrial premature contraction
AT: atrial tachycardia
AV: atrioventricular
AV JEB: AV junctional escape beat
AV JER: AV junctional escape rhythm
AV JPC: AV junctional premature contraction
AV JT: AV junctional tachycardia
BBBB: bilateral bundle branch block
BFB: bifascicular block
BP: blood pressure
BTS: bradytachyarrhythmia syndrome
CAD: coronary artery disease
CCU: coronary care unit
CHF: congestive heart failure
CNS: central nervous system
COPD: chronic obstructive pulmonary disease
CPR: cardiopulmonary resuscitation
CSS: carotid sinus stimulation
DC shock: direct current shock
DI: digitalis intoxication
ECG: electrocardiogram
IHSS: idiopathic hypertrophic subaortic stenosis
JEB: junctional escape beat
JER: junctional escape rhythm
JPC: junctional premature contraction
JT: junctional tachycardia
LBBB: left bundle branch block
LGL: Lown–Ganong–Levine syndrome
LVH: left ventricular hypertrophy
MAT: multifocal atrial tachycardia
MI: myocardial infarction
MVP: mitral valve prolapse
PAT: paroxysmal atrial tachycardia
PDA: patent ductus arteriosus
RBBB: right bundle branch block
RHD: rheumatic heart disease
RVH: right ventricular hypertrophy
SA: sinoatrial
SSS: sick sinus syndrome
TFB: trifascicular block
VA: ventriculoatrial
VEB: ventricular escape beat
VER: ventricular escape rhythm
VF: ventricular fibrillation
VPC: ventricular premature contraction
VT: ventricular tachycardia
WPW: Wolff–Parkinson–White syndrome

# *Suggested Readings*


CHUNG EK: Ambulatory Electrocardiography: Holter Monitor Electrocardiography. Heidelberg-New York, Springer-Verlag, 1979.

CHUNG EK: Artificial Cardiac Pacing, 2nd ed. Baltimore, Williams & Wilkins, 1984.

CHUNG EK: Cardiac Arrhythmias: Self Learning. New York, Yorke Medical Books, 1985.

CHUNG EK: A Clinical Manual of Cardiovascular Medicine. E. Norwalk, CT, Appleton-Century-Crofts, 1984.

CHUNG EK: Fundamentals of Electrocardiography. Baltimore, University Park Press, 1984.

CHUNG EK: Office Electrocardiography. Baltimore, University Park Press, 1984.

CHUNG EK: Principles of Cardiac Arrhythmias, 3rd ed. Baltimore, Williams & Wilkins, 1983.

CHUNG EK: Quick Reference To Cardiovascular Diseases, 2nd ed. Philadelphia, Harper/Lippincott, 1983.

CHUNG EK:, CHUNG LS: Introduction To Clinical Cardiology. Basel, Switzerland, Karger, 1983.

FOX W, STEIN E: Cardiac Rhythm Disturbances, A Step-By-Step Approach. Philadelphia, Lea & Febiger, 1983.

HARRISON DC: Cardiac Arrhythmias: A Decade of Progress. Boston, Hall Medical, 1981.

JOSEPHSON ME, SEIDES SF: Clinical Cardiac Electrophysiology, Techniques And Interpretations. Philadelphia, Lea & Febiger, 1979.

MARRIOTT HJL: Practical Electrocardiography, 7th ed. Baltimore, Williams & Wilkins, 1983.

MARRIOTT HJL, CONOVER MHB: Advanced Concepts in Arrhythmias. St. Louis, Mosby, 1983.

NARULA OS: Cardiac Arrhythmias: Electrophysiology, Diagnosis And Management. Baltimore, Williams & Wilkins, 1979.

SCHAMROTH L: The Disorders of Cardiac Rhythm, 2nd ed. Oxford, Blackwell Scientific, 1980.

# Chapter 1

# Introductory Remarks

Disturbances of impulse formation and conduction may occur anywhere in the human heart. Over the years, various terms, such as "arrhythmia," "dysrhythmia," "ectopic rhythm," and "disorder of heartbeat," have been used in order to describe disturbances in cardiac rhythm. Of the above terms, "arrhythmia" is the most commonly used designation and has been widely accepted by most cardiologists and electrocardiographers.

## CLINICAL SIGNIFICANCE

Some cardiac arrhythmias are benign and clinically insignificant, whereas others are truly serious and need immediate and specific therapy. The most common cardiac arrhythmia is premature beats (extrasystoles). Premature beats may be atrial, atrioventricular (AV) junctional, or ventricular in origin and may be found in apparently healthy individuals. However, premature beats may become clinically significant if they occur too frequently, originate from multiple foci, or are found in individuals with proven heart disease. Their occurrence during digitalization is certainly of clinical importance. Premature beats will usually disappear with exercise if the individual is free of significant heart disease.

The study of cardiac arrhythmias should no longer be of interest only to electrocardiographers or cardiologists. The diagnosis and treatment of cardiac arrhythmias are absolutely necessary skills for all physicians, surgeons, and nurses who participate in cardiac care. Because of the wide acceptance of coronary care units (CCUs) and artificial pacemakers, a full understanding of cardiac arrhythmias has become essential. It has become obvious that certain cardiac arrhythmias both directly and indirectly influence morbidity and mortality. The mortality rate for myocardial infarction (MI) is 2 to 3 times higher when complicated by serious arrhythmias, especially those of ventricular origin. Furthermore, the mortality rate for certain digitalis-induced arrhythmias approaches 100%. Cardiac arrhythmias may be the first objective evidence of underlying heart disease; for example, one of the earliest and most common manifestations of acute rheumatic fever is first degree AV block. The immediate and proper treatment of various ectopic tachyarrhythmias is imperative, for the arrhythmia often precipitates or may be in itself an early sign of impending heart failure. The *correct* diagnosis of various tachyarrhythmias is essential because specific therapy is dependent on correct diagnosis and interpretation. Digitalis is the drug of choice for many of the supraventricular tachyarrhythmias, particularly paroxysmal atrial fibrillation (AF) or atrial flutter (unless digitalis induced); however, digitalis may be contraindicated if the tachyarrhythmia originates from the ventricle. The differential diagnosis of supraventricular and ventricular tachyarrhythmias is discussed in detail in Chapter 10. Management of the common cardiac arrhythmias is described in Chapters 15 through 21.

## ETIOLOGY

The most common cause of cardiac arrhythmias is coronary artery disease (CAD). It has been shown that 90–95% of all patients with acute MI have some associated cardiac arrhythmia. The high incidence of arrhythmias during acute MI was observed after CCUs became widely used. The most common cardiac arrhythmia during an acute MI is ventricular premature contractions (VPCs).

Digitalis intoxication (DI) is another very common cause of arrhythmias. The most common cardiac arrhythmia induced by digitalis is VPC, particularly ventricular bigeminy. An equally common arrhythmia in this group is nonparoxysmal AV junctional tachycardia (JT), especially in the presence of preexisting AF.

The presence of cardiac arrhythmias may at times suggest a specific underlying heart disease or even a noncardiac disease. For instance, AF is commonly found in rheumatic heart disease (RHD), hyperthyroidism, and Wolff-Parkinson-White (WPW) syndrome, in addition to being a well-known manifestation of coronary heart disease. Full knowledge of WPW syndrome is important because 70–75% of subjects with this syndrome have an associated rapid supraventricular tachyarrhythmia, such as reciprocating tachycardia, atrial flutter, or AF. A detailed discussion of the WPW syndrome is found in Chapter 13. Some arrhythmias are considered almost pathognomonic of certain conditions. For example, ventricular bigeminy, nonparoxysmal AV JT, and atrial tachycardia (AT) with AV block appearing during digitalis therapy almost always indicate DI. Other heart disease, such as congenital, rheumatic, luetic, hypertensive, and traumatic, may at times produce various cardiac arrhythmias. Congenital cardiac arrhythmias, such as congenital second degree and complete AV block, have also been reported. Noncardiac conditions, which include metabolic disturbances, anemia, electrolyte imbalance, anesthesia, drug intoxication, collagen disease, central nervous system (CNS) disorders, and psychoneurogenic disorders, may be associated with a variety of cardiac arrhythmias.

## INCIDENCE

It is almost impossible to determine the exact incidence in the general population of the various cardiac arrhythmias. The incidence varies at different medical institutions depending upon the nature of the institution, the type of patients seen, and the ability and interest of the physicians interpreting the electrocardiograms. The highest incidence is usually found in large general hospitals where the elderly and known cardiac patients are usually seen. In general, premature beats—either atrial (auricular), AV junctional, or ventricular—sinus arrhythmia, sinus bradycardia, and sinus tachycardia are the most common arrhythmias. Almost as frequent are paroxysmal atrial tachycardia (PAT) or AV JT and first degree AV block. Atrial fibrillation is probably the next most frequent arrhythmia recorded. Atrial flutter, second degree AV block, and AV dissociation are relatively infrequent, and complete AV block, sinoatrial (SA) block, and ventricular tachycardia (VT) or flutter are considerably less common. The rare cardiac arrhythmias include parasystole and atrial dissociation.

## CLASSIFICATION AND GENESIS OF CARDIAC ARRHYTHMIAS

Cardiac arrhythmias have been classified in various ways, but in general they are divided into 2 major categories: (1) abnormal impulse formation and (2) abnormal conduction. A detailed classification of cardiac arrhythmias is shown in Table 1–1.

### Abnormal Impulse Formation

Active and passive impulse formations are the 2 fundamental mechanisms involved in impulse formation in the human heart.

In the normal heart, the cardiac impulse originates from the sinus (SA) node, which is called the "primary pacemaker." The impulse that originates from the sinus node spreads throughout the atria to produce atrial activation, which forms the P wave in the electrocardiogram. After the completion of atrial depolarization (activation), the impulse reaches the AV node. The time involved for the impulse formed in the sinus node to reach the AV node is, by definition, the AV conduction time (the P-R interval on the electrocardiogram). The impulse then travels through the common bundle (bundle of His), right and left bundle branches, left ante-

**TABLE 1–1. Classification of cardiac arrhythmias**

- I. Disturbances of impulse formation
  - A. Disturbance of sinus impulse formation
    - 1. Sinus premature beats (extrasystoles)
    - 2. Sinus tachycardia
    - 3. Sinus bradycardia
    - 4. Sinus arrhythmia
      - a. Respiratory
      - b. Nonrespiratory
      - c. Ventriculophasic
    - 5. Wandering pacemaker in the sinus node
    - 6. Sinus arrest (pause or standstill)
  - B. Disturbances of ectopic impulse formation
    - 1. Passive impulse formation
      - a. Atrial escape beats and rhythm
      - b. AV junctional escape beats and rhythm
      - c. Ventricular escape beats and rhythm (idioventricular beats and rhythm)
      - d. Wandering pacemaker between SA and AV nodes
    - 2. Active impulse formation
      - a. Atrial in origin
        - (1) Atrial premature beats (extrasystoles)
        - (2) Atrial tachycardia
          - (a) Paroxysmal
          - (b) Nonparoxysmal
        - (3) Atrial flutter
        - (4) Atrial impure flutter
        - (5) Atrial fibrillation
        - (6) Atrial flutter-fibrillation
        - (7) Multifocal atrial tachycardia (chaotic atrial rhythm, wandering pacemaker in the atria)
      - b. AV junctional in origin
        - (1) AV junctional premature beats (extrasystoles)
        - (2) AV junctional tachycardia
          - (a) Paroxysmal
          - (b) Nonparoxysmal
        - (3) Wandering pacemaker in the AV junction
      - c. Ventricular in origin
        - (1) Ventricular premature beats (extrasystoles)
        - (2) Ventricular tachycardia
          - (a) Paroxysmal
          - (b) Nonparoxysmal
        - (3) Ventricular flutter
        - (4) Ventricular fibrillation
        - (5) Chaotic rhythm
- II. Conduction disturbances
  - A. Sinoatrial (SA) block
    - 1. Mobitz type I (Wenckebach)
    - 2. Mobitz type II
  - B. Intraatrial block
  - C. Atrioventricular (AV) block
    - 1. First degree AV block
    - 2. Second degree AV block
      - a. Mobitz type I (Wenckebach)
      - b. Mobitz type II
    - 3. High degree (advanced) AV block
    - 4. Complete (third degree) AV block
    - 5. Dual AV conduction
    - 6. Supernormal AV conduction
  - D. Intraventricular block
    - 1. Right bundle branch block
      - a. Complete
      - b. Incomplete
    - 2. Left bundle branch block
      - a. Complete
      - b. Incomplete
      - c. Hemiblocks
        - (1) Left anterior hemiblock
        - (2) Left posterior hemiblock
    - 3. Bilateral bundle branch block (bifascicular block, trifascicular block)
    - 4. Nonspecific (diffuse) intraventricular block
  - E. Exit block
- III. Mixed disturbances of impulse formation and conduction, and ill-defined arrhythmias
  - A. Atrioventricular (AV) dissociation
    - 1. Complete
    - 2. Incomplete
  - B. Wolff-Parkinson-White syndrome (ventricular preexcitation syndrome)
  - C. Reciprocal beats and reciprocating rhythm and tachycardia
  - D. Parasystole
    - 1. Atrial
    - 2. AV junctional
    - 3. Ventricular
    - 4. Combined
  - E. Atrial dissociation
  - F. Electrical alternans
  - G. Coronary sinus rhythm
  - H. Coronary nodal rhythm
  - I. Lown-Ganong-Levine syndrome
  - J. Concealed conduction
- IV. Artificial pacemaker-induced rhythm

Reproduced with permission from Chung: *Principles of Cardiac Arrhythmias*, 3rd ed. Baltimore, Williams & Wilkins, 1983.

rior and posterior fascicles, and the Purkinje fibers to activate the ventricles and form the QRS complex. This is followed by ventricular repolarization, which produces T waves on the electrocardiogram. The wave of atrial repolarization is usually too small to be recorded by the ordinary electrocardiographic apparatus. If it were recorded, it would be superimposed on the QRS complex. The conduction system of the human heart is illustrated in Figure 1–1.

The following are criteria that should be met before the term "normal sinus rhythm" may be used: (1) P wave of sinus origin (normal mean axis of P wave), (2) constant and normal P-R interval (0.12–0.20 second), (3) constant P wave configuration in a given lead, (4) heart rate between 60 and 100/min, and (5) constant P-P (or R-R) interval.

A sinus rate above 100/min is known as "sinus tachycardia," whereas a rate slower than 60/min is called "sinus bradycardia." If the sinus node produces an impulse irregularly, this is termed "sinus arrhythmia." When sinus arrhythmia is related to respiration, it is called "respiratory sinus arrhythmia." Otherwise, it is known as "nonrespiratory sinus arrhythmia." When the sinus node fails to produce an impulse, sinus arrest or pause will result. A finding on the ECG similar to sinus arrest is SA block, in which the impulse from the sinus node is unable to spread to the atria because of a block at the SA junction.

Any cardiac impulse originating from a site other than the sinus node is termed "ectopic." When 6 or more consecutive ectopic beats appear, an ectopic rhythm is said to be present. When 2–5 ectopic beats appear consecutively, the term "group beats" or "grouped beats" may be applied. Ectopic beats or rhythm may originate from the atria, the AV junction, or the ventricles. The mechanism responsible for ectopic beats or rhythm may be active or passive.

**Passive Ectopic Rhythm:** Passive ectopic impulse formation is merely a physiologic mechanism that maintains ventricular activity. Passive AV junctional rhythm—commonly known as AV junctional escape rhythm (JER)—may appear on the electrocardiogram when the sinus node produces impulses at a slower rate than usual (sinus bradycardia). This rhythm may

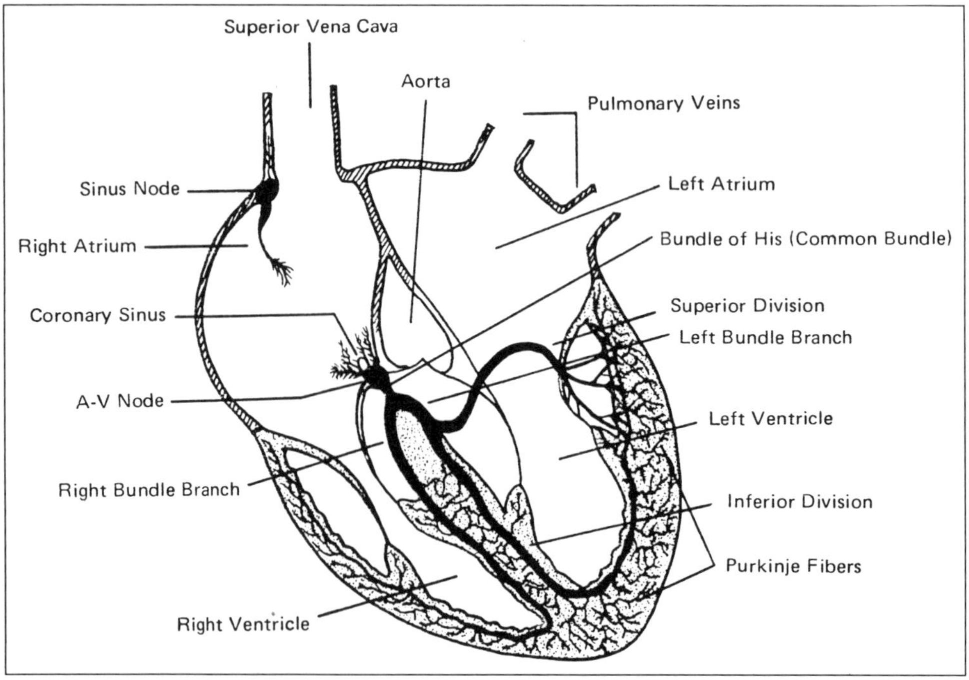


**Fig. 1–1.** Cardiac conduction system.

also occur when the sinus node is unable to generate an impulse (sinus arrest) or when the sinus impulse fails to be conducted to the AV junction. The latter may be due to either SA block or AV block. When the AV junction is unable to produce an impulse under these circumstances, the ventricles may produce a passive rhythm called "ventricular escape rhythm (VER)" or idioventricular rhythm. Conditions predisposing to VER are a severely diseased AV node and bilateral bundle branch block (BBBB). Atrioventricular junctional escape rhythm is much more common than VER, simply because the inherent rate of the former (45–60/min) is faster than the inherent rate of the latter (30–40/min). A single passive beat from the AV junction or ventricle is called an "AV junctional escape beat (JEB)" or a "ventricular escape beat (VEB)," respectively. Needless to say, a passive ectopic rhythm has a slower rate than that originating from the sinus node. Thus, ectopic escape rhythm does not appear during normal sinus rhythm or sinus tachycardia. If the impulse varies in origin from the sinus node and atria or between the sinus node and AV junction in successive cycles, a wandering atrial pacemaker is said to be present. On rare occasions, atrial escape beats or rhythm may occur.

**Active Ectopic Rhythm:** Active ectopic impulse formation is caused by augmented excitability of an ectopic focus. Ectopic foci may originate from the atria, AV junction, or ventricles. These impulses, if single, are known as atrial, AV junctional, or ventricular premature beats (extrasystoles). Six or more consecutive premature beats are termed "paroxysmal tachycardia." Active atrial impulse formation results in various atrial tachyarrhythmias, including AF, flutter, and tachycardia. Active AV junctional impulse formation results in either paroxysmal or nonparoxysmal AV JT. A detailed description of the AV JTs is given in Chapter 6. The most common rapid ventricular rhythm is paroxysmal VT. Ventricular flutter and ventricular fibrillation (VF) are less common. Occasionally, there may coexist more than one active ectopic impulse-forming center, which results in multifocal tachyarrhythmias. Atrial and AV JT, double AV JT, and bidirectional AV JT or VT are examples of multifocal tachyarrhythmias. Chaotic rhythm is usually found preceding death. These impulses often originate from multiple ventricular foci.

### Conduction Disturbances

Conduction disturbances may occur anywhere in the heart. Heart block occurring at the SA junction is termed "SA block." If the block is present in the atria, it is termed "intraatrial (intraauricular) block." The most common form of heart block is AV block of varying degree. Atrioventricular block is divided into 3 major groups: first, second, and third degree AV block. When heart block exists in the ventricles, it is known as "intraventricular block." Intraventricular block includes right and left bundle branch block (RBBB and LBBB), hemiblocks, bifascicular (BFB) and trifascicular block (TFB), and nonspecific (or diffuse) intraventricular block.

Atrioventricular dissociation may result from various combinations of abnormal impulse formation and conduction. In general, AV dissociation can be caused by 3 major disorders: (1) slowing or failure of sinus impulse formation (sinus bradycardia and/or sinus arrhythmia and sinus pause), (2) acceleration of impulse formation in the AV junction or ventricles (AV JT or VT), and (3) complete AV block and/or SA block. A detailed description of AV dissociation is found in Chapter 6.

Complex arrhythmias usually result from mixed disturbances of impulse formation and conduction. The genesis of some rare arrhythmias, such as parasystole, electrical alternans, and atrial dissociation, may not be attributable to any of the above mechanisms, and some aspects of these arrhythmias are still not clearly understood.

## BEDSIDE DIAGNOSIS OF CARDIAC ARRHYTHMIAS

From time to time, it may become necessary to diagnose a cardiac arrhythmia at the bedside. The diagnosis can at times be made by a careful history and complete physical examination. Before performing the physical examination, the physician should avail himself of all clinical information regarding previous cardiac arrhythmias or known heart disease. A detailed history should include information pertaining to the onset, frequency, and duration of the cardiac arrhythmia. Concurrent medication should, of course, be considered in the evaluation of these patients.

## Age

Age is an important consideration, since the incidence of certain arrhythmias varies among age groups. In older children and young adults, respiratory sinus arrhythmia is almost always present, whereas this arrhythmia is unusual in older people. In contrast to this, AF is relatively uncommon in children or young adults, even in the presence of the same underlying process. Children with the WPW syndrome rarely have concurrent AF, whereas AF is certainly not uncommon in elderly patients with the same syndrome. In general, AF is one of the more common arrhythmias in the older age group. When children or young adults develop rapid heart action, it is almost always a regular supraventricular tachycardia (SVT) (either PAT or AV JT). Atrioventricular block is also uncommon in younger adults or children, except during the presence of acute rheumatic fever. Needless to say, the incidence of practically any type of cardiac arrhythmia increases with age. This is primarily attributable to the increased incidence of CAD and/or hypertensive heart disease and/or the frequent occurrence of congestive heart failure (CHF). Permanent complete AV block is frequently found in elderly individuals because of long-standing degenerative changes in the conduction system. Atrial fibrillation with rapid ventricular response is extremely common in older patients with acute CHF and may persist even if the CHF resolves. Ventricular tachyarrhythmias predominantly occur in older patients with CAD.

## Rate and Regularity of Cardiac Rhythm

The rate and regularity of the apical and peripheral pulse are also of help in diagnosing cardiac arrhythmias.

**Regular Rhythm:** A heart rate below 30 beats/min is usually due to complete AV block producing idioventricular rhythm (VER). A less likely cause is second degree AV block. A heart rate between 40 and 60 beats/min may be caused by sinus bradycardia, AV JER due to complete AV block, and second degree AV block. In subjects with a heart rate between 60 and 100 beats/min, the most common rhythm is normal sinus rhythm, especially when there is no overt heart disease. On the other hand, AT with 2:1 AV block or nonparoxysmal AV JT with or without AV dissociation may also result in a heart rate between 60 and 100 beats/min, particularly when DI or acute MI is present. Sinus tachycardia is the most likely diagnosis when the heart rate is between 100 and 160 beats/min, although atrial flutter or tachycardia with 2:1 AV response and AV JT with or without AV dissociation are less likely possibilities. If the heart rate ranges from 180 to 250 beats/min, the most common rhythm is either PAT or AV JT. However, atrial flutter with 2:1 AV response or VT must also be considered. Heart rates between 250 and 350 beats/min are almost always due to atrial flutter with 1:1 AV conduction. Rarely, VT or ventricular flutter may also produce this rapid rate.

**Irregular Rhythm:** The most common cause of an irregular rhythm is premature beats (extra systoles), either atrial, AV junctional, or ventricular in origin. When an irregular and rapid rhythm (120–250 beats/min) is present, AF is almost always responsible, although other possibilities, such as AT or atrial flutter with varying AV response and multifocal atrial tachycardia (MAT), should be considered. Ventricular tachycardia may show slight irregularity on the electrocardiogram (ECG), but it does not produce any irregularity via auscultation. When the heart rate of an irregular rhythm is between 60 and 100 beats/min, this arrhythmia is often due to AF after digitalization. Less commonly, this irregularity may be due to AT or atrial flutter with varying AV block, frequent premature beats, or even sinus arrhythmia. Advanced AV block should be suspected when the ventricular rate in AF slows below 60 beats/min.

Carotid sinus pressure is a very important diagnostic and therapeutic procedure and is discussed in detail in Chapter 12.

Changing intensity of the first heart sound at the apex (cannon sound), accompanied by a regular rhythm, often indicates AV dissociation, particularly complete AV block when the atrial mechanism is sinus in origin. Careful inspection of the jugular venous pulse may be helpful in diagnosis. Without question, the precise diagnosis of cardiac arrhythmias can only be made by studying an ECG tracing.

## FUNDAMENTAL APPROACH TO INTERPRETATION OF CARDIAC ARRHYTHMIAS

The fundamental approach to interpretation of cardiac arrhythmias is presented in Chapter 3.

# Chapter 2

# Anatomy and Electrophysiology

## ANATOMY

It is essential to have a full knowledge of the anatomy of the human heart in order to understand the fundamental mechanisms responsible for a normal ECG as well as various ECG abnormalities. The human heart consists of 4 chambers, including 2 atria and 2 ventricles. Electrophysiologically, these chambers are controlled by the sinus (SA) node in healthy subjects. Anatomic structures pertinent to various ECG findings include cardiac pacemakers and conduction systems (Fig. 1–1).

### Sinus Node

Various experimental and clinical studies confirm that the sinus node is the primary pacemaker in the heart.

**Gross Anatomy:** There is considerable variation in the shape, size, and location of the sinus node. The exact location of the node depends upon the manner of encirclement of the base of the superior vena cava by the sinus node artery. In the human heart, the sinus node is generally located in the sulcus terminalis near the junction of the superior vena cava and the right atrium. The node is somewhat elongated along the axis of the sulcus terminalis, and its anterior margin is a few millimeters posterior to a crest formed by the junction of the right atrial appendage with the superior vena cava. The sinus node is located more anteriorly when the caval encirclement by the node artery is clockwise (viewed from above) than when encirclement is counterclockwise. The size of the sinus node varies considerably and is not closely proportional to the size of the heart. In general, its size is approximately 15 mm in length, 5–7 mm in width, and 1.5–2 mm in thickness. The shape of the sinus node varies, but, by and large, it resembles an extended snail with its shell, which misleads one to think of the node as having a head, body, and tail.

**Blood Vessels:** The sinus node artery in the human heart is commonly located near the center of the sinus node, but it may be eccentric. In approximately 55–60% of human hearts, the sinus node artery arises from the proximal 2–3 cm of the right coronary artery, whereas, in 40–45%, it arises from the proximal 1 cm of the left circumflex (LC) coronary artery. Other origins of the sinus node artery are rare and account for about 2% of the total. At times, there are 2 branches of the sinus node artery of equal size. The sinus node artery, regardless of whether it arises from the right or left coronary artery, courses along the anteromedial atrial wall of the base of the superior vena cava, which it encircles. This artery anastomoses with other atrial arteries of both ipsilateral and contralateral origin. Generally, the primary arterial supply of the sinus node is practically always unilateral in origin. Smaller branches of the artery are distributed throughout the sinus node.

Small veins are commonly found throughout the sinus node, whereas large veins are present infrequently.

**Nerve Supply:** The sinus node has both sympathetic and parasympathetic (vagal) innervation, but the latter is richer in the AV node. Ganglion cells are present only around the sinus node and not within the central portion of the node. The ganglion cells are commonly found at the boundary of the node and are particularly abundant at the anterior, posterior, and caval margins of the sinus node. The majority of fibers that leave the margin of the sinus node to enter the right atrium have Purkinje fiberlike features.

**Histology:** For a comparison of the sinus nodal cell with an ordinary cardiac muscle cell, a description of the latter is in order. The ordinary muscle cells of the atria and ventricles consist of a special type of cross-striated fiber with nuclei and intercalated discs. They are surrounded by a sarcolemma and contain sarcoplasm and myofibrils. The cells of the sinus node have all of these findings except for the intercalated discs. The sinus node cells are more slender and their nuclei are smaller than those of atrial muscle cells. The individual fibers of the sinus node cells contain relatively small numbers of myofibrils, and the cross-striation is less prominent than in atrial muscle cells. There is a fine reticular pattern of the sinus node cells in all age groups, in contrast to the coarse network of reticular fibers found in atrial muscles. The sinus node cells are arranged in an interlacing network, in comparison to the more regular arrangement of the atrial muscle fibers. Characteristically, the sinus node has a more abundant supply of dense collagenous and elastic fibers than have atrial muscle fibers. The sinus node fibers communicate with the musculature of the superior vena cava, the confluence of the right anterior crest and the interatrial band, the intercaval band, and the right atrial appendage. Purkinje fibers are not involved in these communications. With advancing age, there is a progressive increment of elastic and collagenous fibers, associated with an accentuation of the reticular network and an infiltration of fat.

## Atrioventricular Node (Junction)

A study of the AV node and its junctional tissue is very important if one intends to accurately interpret various cardiac arrhythmias. Not only does the AV node (junction) function as a pacemaker (1) when the sinus node fails to produce an impulse (sinus arrest), (2) when the sinus node produces an impulse slower than usual (sinus bradycardia), or (3) when the sinus impulse is not conducted to the AV node (SA and/or AV block), but it also has an important role as a conduction system. Furthermore, most of the complicated rhythm disturbances are almost always related to the function and conductivity of the AV node. For example, supernormal AV conduction, concealed conduction, unidirectional block, reciprocal beats, and so on, are intimately related to abnormal conductivity of the AV junction.

Since the discovery of the conducting tissue (common bundle, AV bundle), connecting the atria and ventricles was made by His in 1892, it now bears his name (bundle of His).

**Gross Anatomy:** The AV node lies in the lower posterior portion of the interatrial septum on the right side. The AV node is bounded by the opening of the coronary sinus, the opening of the inferior vena cava, the base of the inferior vena cava, and the base of the septal leaflet of the tricuspid valve. The AV node is only a few millimeters to the right of the coronary sinus vein and is directed toward the septal cusp of the tricuspid valve. The lower margin of the AV node is situated on the right side of the root of the ascending aorta and above the septum membranaceum. It lies between the limbus of the fossa ovalis and the tricuspid valve. The right upper side of the AV node is bordered by a prolongation of the eustachian valve (so-called sinusband). A grayish white endocardial thickening (so-called tendon of Todaro), directed medially toward the AV node and often found between the lower border of the eustachian valve and the upper border of the thebesian valve, was frequently used to localize the AV node. From the beginning of the AV node to the terminal branches of the Purkinje fibers, the entire conduction system is an anatomically continuous structure. Thus, the AV conduction system and ventricular myocardium are practically one large conduction network. The AV node is connected inferiorly to the common bundle and then right and left bundle branches with terminal Purkinje fibers (Fig. 1–1).

The shape of the AV node is that of a flattened oval structure resembling a tiny spleen. The size of the AV node varies, as does that of the sinus node, but, in general, it is approximately 5–6 mm in length, 2–3 mm in width, and 0.5–1 mm in thickness. Its yellowish color has been described by various investigators.

**Blood Vessels:** The AV node (junction) receives a disproportionally large arterial blood supply for the relatively small size of its surface.

Haas identified an artery to the membranous septum and the AV node, termed "ramus septi fibrosi" (artery of the ventriculonecteur). This artery courses the atrial septum, traverses the membranous septum, and irrigates the AV node, the bundle of His, and its bifurcation. The existence of the ramus septi fibrosi was confirmed by many early workers. This vessel is the first posterior branch arising from the posterior interventricular artery (ramus descendens posterior). In 90–94% of human hearts, the ramus septi fibrosi originates from the right coronary artery, whereas in 6–10%, it arises from the left circumflex branch of the left coronary artery. The ramus septi fibrosi divides into many branches after reaching the AV node, and one of the branches penetrates the node. Histologically, in most cases, a large artery runs along the vertical axis of the AV node without a change in the lumen of the vessel. It is not uncommon to observe several branches of the artery penetrating the AV node. In rare cases, 2 arterial branches of similar size, 1 from the left and 1 from the right coronary arteries, supply the AV node (junction). It has been pointed out that the myocardial veins and sinusoids at the AV junction influence conductivity in the AV node and common bundle.

**Nerve Supply:** It has been shown that the AV node (junction) has a rich nerve supply from both sympathetic and parasympathetic (vagal) fibers. The latter (notably the left vagus) supply most innervation to the node. As early as 1906, Tawara pointed out that there were numerous ganglion cells around the coronary sinus and in the nerve fibers of the AV node of hoofed animals. Abundant ganglia are present near the artery supplying the AV node, but only small groups of ganglion cells are present within the superficial areas of the AV node. It has been noted that the AV node possesses more abundant nerve terminals than the sinus node and that these nerve fibers arise from intrinsic parasympathetic ganglia. It is of interest that ganglion cells are found to be more abundant in the hearts of dogs than of humans.

**Histology:** The AV node consists of atypical cardiac muscle fibers in the form of a dense connective tissue network. The muscle fibers of the AV node have a structure similar to those of the sinus node, but the fibers of the AV node are smaller than those of the sinus node, atrial, or ventricular fibers. The sizes of the AV node fibers vary from 3 to 11 $\mu$m in diameter, in comparison with the ordinary ventricular myocardial fibers of 12 $\mu$m. It has been shown that the fibers of the AV node are more cylindrical, more branched, and wider in appearance than those of the sinus node. The AV node, as well as the common bundle, possesses more elastic fibers when compared with the atrial or ventricular myocardium. Each AV nodal fiber has 1 or, at times, 2 round or oval nuclei that are centrally situated. The fibers of the AV node spread without order in every direction and anastomose freely, leading to a tangled appearance. Because of this appearance, it was termed a "Knoten" (node) by Tawara. The AV nodal fibers contain a paler cytoplasm than ordinary cardiac muscle and have less cross striations. These fibers contain relatively fewer myofibrils and are, therefore, less eosinophilic than ordinary cardiac muscle fibers. Recently, accessory fibers connecting the AV node and the endocardium of the right atrium were studied by James. It was suggested that these accessory fibers may function as conduction pathways that bypass from the sinus node to the ventricles.

## Common Bundle (Atrioventricular Bundle of His), Right and Left Bundle Branches, and Purkinje Fibers

As described previously, the uninterrupted conduction system of the heart includes the AV node, the common bundle, RBBB, LBBB, and Purkinje fibers in downward order (Fig. 1–1). Therefore, destruction of the AV node or common bundle or bilateral bundle branches produces complete AV block, although the clinical significance of each lesion is significantly different (Chapters 8 and 9).

**Common Bundle (Atrioventricular Bundle or Bundle of His):** The common bundle, which is a continuous downward structure from the AV node, penetrates into the central fibrous body. This penetrating portion of the common bundle is traced into the branching portion of the bundle, which traverses the crest of the muscular interventricular septum. The size of the common bundle is much larger than the AV node, and it is 10–20 mm in length and 1–4 mm in width.

**Right Bundle Branch:** The right bundle branch is the more direct continuation of the AV node and runs along the inferior aspect of the septal band of the crista supraventricularis between the conus and the sinus of the right ventricle. The first third of the right bundle branch is subendocardial or relatively superficial in location, up to the level of the muscle of Lancisi. It then penetrates the septal musculature, becomes superficial again in the terminal third, submerges at the moderator band, and continues as Purkinje fibers into the anterior papillary muscle and other structures. The color of the right bundle branch is the same as ordinary muscle, in contrast to the paler color of the AV node and the penetrating portion of the common bundle.

Variations in the structure of the right bundle branch have been described. At times, 2 right bundle branches may be present in 1 heart. One of the branches may end blindly, or a single right bundle branch may bifurcate initially and then the 2 branches become 1 branch distally.

**Left Bundle Branch:** The left bundle branch is situated beneath the endocardium and divides into an anterior and posterior ramus descending toward the apex of the heart. The main left bundle branch is again divided into 2 divisions, including anterior and posterior fascicles (Fig. 1–1). The left bundle branch fibers become progressively larger toward the apex. The terminal fibers end in the anterior and posterior papillary muscles and also course toward the apex of the heart. The left bundle branch is usually larger than the right bundle branch, and its width is approximately 3–6 mm.

**Purkinje Fibers:** The terminal conduction system of the heart is a complex of Purkinje fibers, which are continuous structures from the right and left bundle branches (Fig. 1–1). This terminal conduction network was described as early as 1845 by Purkinje. Purkinje fibers are distributed diffusely in every portion of the ventricles except for the central upper portion of the ventricular septum. This terminal network connects fibers together and leads to countless loops in the ventricular septum. Purkinje fibers are distributed in both subendocardial and subepicardial myocardium, although they are more abundant in the former. The general directions of the terminal Purkinje fibers are at an oblique angle directed from the apex to the base of the right ventricle and at a right angle to the inner surface of the left ventricle. The typical Purkinje muscle fibers are larger in diameter than ordinary cardiac muscle fibers and contain abundant glycogen.

**Blood Vessels:** The common bundle and right and left bundle branches are supplied by the ramus septi fibrosis, as is the AV node. The conduction tissues immediately distal to the common bundle, except for the first portion of the right bundle branch, are supplied by vessels nourishing the adjacent tissues. The branches of the left coronary artery supply the anterior portion of the ventricular septum, whereas the descending branches of the right circumflex supply the posterior portion of the septum. The middle portion of the ventricular septum is supplied by the branches of both vessels.

**Nerve Supply:** The nerve supply of the common bundle and right and left bundle branches is similar to that of the AV node (junction). However, it is generally believed that the terminal Purkinje fibers in the human heart entirely lack a nerve supply. In general, 3 neural pathways innervate the entire myocardium. One pathway runs through the AV node, common bundle, and right and left bundle branches and myocardium. The second pathway is taken by the fibers from the epicardial plexus, which penetrate directly into the myocardium. The third pathway is carried by fibers that accompany the arterial system and then branch into the syncytial mass.

## Accessory Pathways

Various accessory pathways other than the normal AV conduction system have been described by various investigators, beginning with the discovery of the bundle of Kent in 1893.

Accessory pathways include the bundle of Kent, Mahaim's fibers, internodal pathways proposed by James, preferential pathways responsible for the WPW syndrome, and dual AV conduction. It should be pointed out that the anatomic presence of any accessory pathway is not necessarily indicative of physiologic function. These pathways may function under a certain circumstance, particularly when normal AV conduction is impaired.

## ELECTROPHYSIOLOGY

It is well documented that the ECG is an important tool in the study of the electrophysiology of the heart and for diagnosing various heart diseases. Curiously, however, the ECG is unable to supply direct information concerning the electrical activity of certain portions of the heart. This is particularly true with regard to the activities of the sinus and AV nodes, since no ECG deflection corresponds to the activation of the sinus or AV node. In addition, it is, at times, impossible to determine the exact site of the origin of the P wave or the QRS complex. Furthermore, the atrial repolarization wave is usually not recorded by an ordinary ECG because its deflection is often too small to be recorded or because it is superimposed on the QRS complex or other segments of the ECG. It is also known that no ECG deflection corresponds to the depolarization or repolarization of the common bundle. The exact site of a conduction block is difficult to determine, when dealing with complete AV block, because a block at the AV junction in the bundle or BBBB may produce similar ECG patterns. Thus, at times, one only infers the cardiac electrical events from available findings. Otherwise, His bundle ECG enables confirmation of the exact site of impulse formation or a block.

Electrophysiologic studies of the heart have been carried out extensively since the late 18th century. The use of microelectrodes in the past 25 years has enabled cardiologists to appreciate cardiac arrhythmias more easily. The electrophysiologic properties of the heart include cardiac impulse formation and conduction, namely, rhythmicity (automaticity), excitability, and conductivity. Cardiac arrhythmias may result from the alteration of any of the above properties, which are closely interrelated. Clinically, cardiac arrhythmias are commonly due to an alteration in 2 or 3 electrophysiologic properties. Cardiac cells may be divided into 2 groups: automatic and nonautomatic cells. Automatic cells are able to initiate cardiac impulses without extrinsic stimuli, whereas nonautomatic cells are excited by impulses generated by automatic cells or other stimuli. Most specialized cardiac fibers contain a large number of automatic cells, whereas atrial and ventricular muscle fibers, under normal conditions, are not automatic.

His bundle electrocardiography is discussed briefly later in this chapter.

### Rhythmicity (Automaticity)

Rhythmicity or automaticity is the capacity to produce spontaneous cardiac impulses. Such impulses may activate a portion of or the entire heart. Specialized cardiac fibers, which contain automatic cells, are capable of producing automaticity. Among the various specialized cardiac fibers, the sinus node possesses the most automatic cells, which function as a primary (natural) pacemaker under normal conditions. Under normal conditions, the sinus node produces cardiac impulses at a rate ranging between 60 and 100/min in adults. The sinus node controls the entire heart under normal conditions because the node possesses the fastest automatic rhythmicity of all cardiac fibers. This automaticity of the sinus node begins as soon as the embryo becomes viable, and it continues until death unless a given individual develops significant cardiac rhythm disturbances from any cause. It is of interest that the automaticity continues even when the heart is removed from the body.

Cardiac arrhythmias may result from an alteration of the automaticity of the sinus node or from an abnormal impulse formation from ectopic automatic tissue (cells). Clinically, an alteration of automaticity is often associated with altered conductivity and excitability. Sinus tachycardia or bradycardia results from acceleration or slowing of the automaticity of the sinus node, respectively. It has been suggested that an alteration of sinus nodal automaticity may result from a slowing of the impulse formation of the initial pacemaker fibers, leading to an escape mechanism of some other sinus nodal fibers, rather than from a change in the impulse formation rate in a single pacemaker cell.

When the automaticity of the sinus node slows significantly and is slower than the rate of the secondary pacemaker, an ectopic pacemaker (usually the AV node), which was latent, may manifest its automaticity, leading to AV JER. This may result in sinus bradycardia with AV JER producing AV dissociation, AV JER without sinus activity, or a wandering pacemaker between the sinus and AV nodes. In this circumstance, the AV JER is called "passive" ectopic rhythm.

Acceleration of the ectopic automaticity, such as AV JT, may result even when the sinus node produces a normal heart rate. This may lead to AV dissociation or an ectopic rhythm, such as AV JT without sinus activity. In this circumstance, the rhythm is a manifestation of an active ectopic rhythm. Occasionally, competition between the automaticity of 2 or more ectopic pacemakers may lead to complex arrhythmias, such as double or triple AV junctional rhythm or tachycardia.

Subsidiary pacemakers, under normal conditions, remain latent because the sinus node produces cardiac impulses faster than any subsidiary pacemakers. This results in an inhibitory mechanism that acts on the subsidiary pacemakers and leads to the prevention of their spontaneous automaticity. The inhibitory mechanism may be effective on the sinus node by rapid ectopic automaticity (active rhythm). This is evident because the sinus node requires a warming-up period until its usual rate of automaticity is reestablished following a bout of rapid ectopic automaticity. This effect is termed the "postdrive inhibition phenomenon" and is more pronounced in ectopic pacemakers. It is more evident for ventricular ectopic rhythm, particularly ventricular escape (idioventricular) rhythm. It is often observed that the rate of a VER is slow initially and gradually becomes faster, approaching its inherent rate. The use of an artificial pacemaker for the treatment of drug-resistant ventricular (occasionally supraventricular) tachyarrhythmias has been well established in the past decade by applying the postdrive inhibition phenomenon in many cases.

The sinus node, as well as other special cardiac fibers, is influenced by various factors, including the actions of vagal and sympathetic nerves, chemical mediators (acetylcholine, catecholamines, and others), cardiac and noncardiac diseases, and various drugs (digitalis, quinidine, procainamide, beta-adrenergic blocking agents, and so on), and electrolytes.

## Excitability

Excitability is that property of living tissue that allows it to respond to a given stimulation. Thus, the heartbeat will not be formed, even if the pacemaker produces an impulse, unless the heart possesses excitability. In the normal heart, excitability varies significantly in the different periods of the cardiac cycle. For example, a stimulus of minimal intensity may produce a greater-than-usual response in certain periods, whereas a stimulus of great intensity may evoke a smaller-than-usual response or even fail to evoke a response during certain periods of the cycle. In other words, the more excitable the cardiac tissue, the weaker the stimulus required to induce a given response and the greater is the response to a given stimulus. Alteration in the normal excitability pattern is one of the important causes of various cardiac arrhythmias. The strength of stimulation required to induce a response is increased when the heart is depressed, and the heart's response is decreased. When the heart is more excitable, the reverse phenomenon is observed. Aside from the different periods of the cardiac cycle, the degree of excitability depends upon the intensity and duration of the stimulus required to induce a certain response or the magnitude of the response induced by a given stimulus.

It is of interest that heart muscles obey the all-or-none law; they respond either maximally or not at all to a given stimulus. Therefore, a subthreshold stimulus is unable to produce a response, whereas a stimulus with threshold strength produces a maximum response. Increasing the strength of the stimulus fails to increase the degree of response.

It is known that the excitability varies in different periods of the cardiac cycle. The magnitude of the response of the first few heartbeats increases when a series of cardiac impulses is evoked following a long pause. This is termed the "staircase (Treppe) phenomenon" and is due to an alteration of excitability. In contrast to this, the magnitude of the response decreases, or there may be no response after a critical rate is reached, if the rate of a series of impulses is progressively increased. The response depends upon the degree of refractoriness in different portions of the heart. The refractory period is divided into absolute and relative refractory phases (Fig. 2–1). During the absolute refractory phase, which has a duration approximating that of systole, the heart is unable to respond to a stimulus regardless of its strength. During the relative refractory phase, especially in its initial period, the strength of stimulus required to evoke a response is above normal, whereas the magnitude of response produced by such a stimulus is below normal. It is noteworthy that the absolute refractory phase is

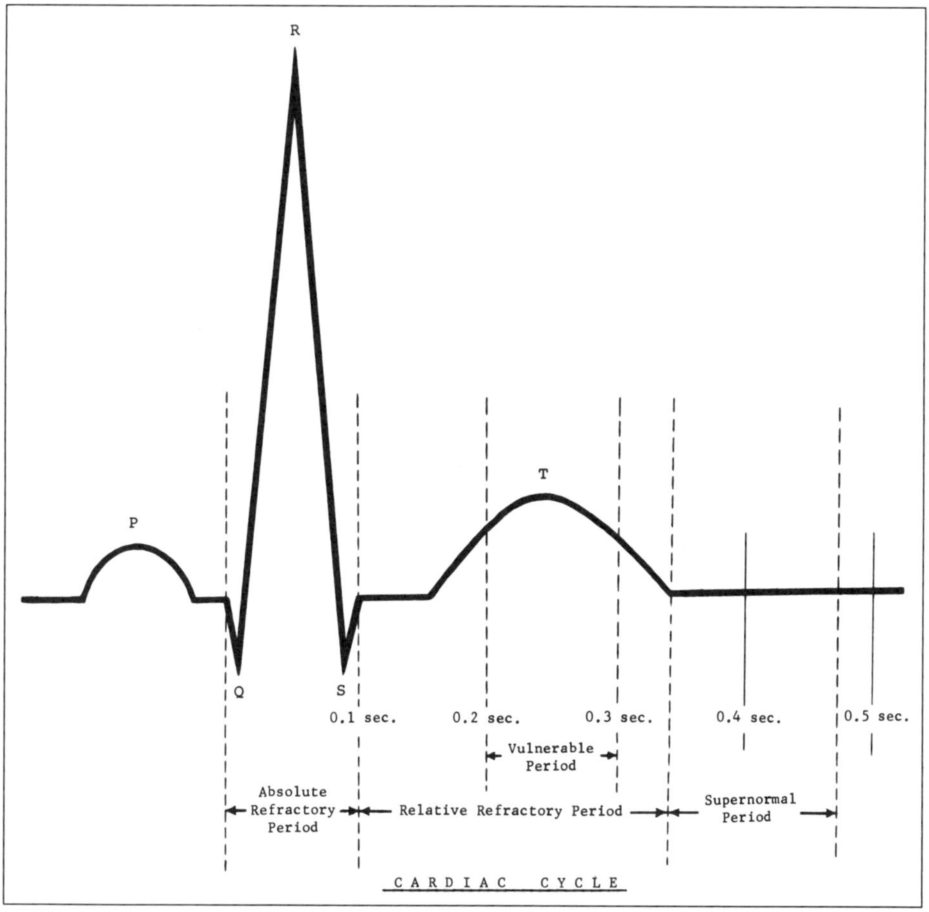


Fig. 2–1. Absolute refractory period, relative refractory period, and supernormal period are shown in relation to the P, QRS, and T complexes of the electrocardiogram. The vulnerable period is approximately coincident with the top of the T wave.

markedly shortened by an enhanced heart rate, while the duration of the relative refractory phase is not significantly altered. It has been shown that the refractory phase is shortest in atrial tissue, longest in AV junctional tissue, and intermediate in ventricular tissue. Atrial flutter with 2:1 AV response and AF with varying AV response are good examples that show the long refractory phase of the AV junctional tissue.

During a short period of the relative refractory phase, the heart is prone to develop fibrillation even with low magnitude stimuli. This portion of the cardiac cycle is termed the "vulnerable period" and corresponds approximately with the top of the T wave on the ECG. Recognition of the vulnerable period is important clinically, because VF may be produced when the electrical discharge of a direct current (DC) shock or an artificial pacemaker is superimposed on this period.

It has been demonstrated that during or immediately following the relative refractory phase, the response is greater and the strength of stimulus required to evoke the response is less than normally expected. This period is termed the "supernormal phase" (Fig. 2–1) and is only found in the depressed heart. Supernormal conduction is frequently responsible for the genesis of complex cardiac arrhythmias.

The term "latency" of heart muscle is defined as the time interval elapsing from the application of the stimulus to the production of the response. It has been shown that the refractory period and latency have different functions in heart muscle, although they have been occasionally considered to be synonymous. The refractory period and latency are approximately equal when the cardiac rate is faster than 100 beats/min, under normal conditions, whereas the refractory period is much longer and latency is relatively shorter when the rate is slower than 60 beats/min.

## Conductivity

The conductivity of the heart is intimately related to rhythmicity and excitability. The speed of the conductivity varies markedly in different portions of the normal heart. Alteration of normal speed of conductivity is one of the important causes of various cardiac arrhythmias. It has been demonstrated that the Purkinje fibers transmit impulses the fastest, at a rate of 4,000 mm/sec, atrial muscle transmits impulses at a rate of 800–1,000 mm/sec, and the ventricular muscle transmits impulses at a rate of 400 mm/sec. The AV node (junction) transmits impulses slowest, at a rate of 200 mm/sec. The slow conductivity of the AV junctional tissue is an important protective physiologic property, which prevents the conduction of an extremely rapid atrial rhythm, such as AF or atrial flutter.

The cardiac impulse may be conducted in a normal fashion, but it may propagate in an abnormal fashion, or it may not be conducted, depending upon the degree of depressed excitability.

When there is an ectopic pacemaker that produces an impulse in addition to the primary pacemaker, there will be a collision between the 2 impulses of different origin. Two different impulses may traverse in opposite directions, and in this circumstance, both impulses will be extinguished when they meet, since momentarily there exists no tissue available for further conduction. This phenomenon, called "interference," is the result of the normal, physiologic refractory phase. At times, 2 impulses from different origins may traverse in similar directions, and the second impulse will be delayed, since it transmits when the tissue is in a refractory phase resulting from transmission of the first impulse. This delayed conduction of the second impulse is another form of interference. Two impulses from opposite directions may meet within the atria or ventricles, and activation may occur. The resulting beat will show a configuration intermediate between the 2 impulses. This produces atrial or ventricular fusion (summation) beats, respectively. When an atrial and an AV nodal or ventricular pacemaker activate the atria and ventricles independently, AV dissociation results. Interference, which is a physiologic phenomenon, should be distinguished from block, which is clearly abnormal. In block, the transmission of the impulse is slower than usual, or it is completely halted, at a time when the involved area is normally receptive to conductivity. Therefore, block represents an abnormally long refractory phase due to depressed conduction.

Impairments of conductivity are manifested by prolongation of the P wave, the P-R interval, and the QRS complex (Fig. 2–2) and an unexpected absence of the P wave or QRS, T complexes or a combination of the above. Impairment of conduction is responsible for the development of various arrhythmias, including intraatrial block, SA block, AV block, intraventricular block, reciprocal beat, concealed conduction, supernormal conduction, dual AV conduction, and unidirectional block. Abnormal conduction via an accessory pathway is responsible for the WPW syndrome.

## His Bundle Electrocardiography

Since a routine 12-lead (surface) ECG is unable to provide every detail of the electrical events of the heart, these can be recorded by inserting the electrodes into the cardiac chambers. This intracardiac ECG is commonly called "His bundle ECG" because various intervals and the conduction time of the cardiac impulses between various locations can be easily and precisely measured by recognizing the His bundle potential (Fig. 2–3). As shown in the conduction system of the heart (Fig. 1–1), the His bundle (common bundle or AV bundle) is a segment of the conduction pathway located just below the AV node, connecting the atria and the ventricles, so that, in a way, it functions as a bridge

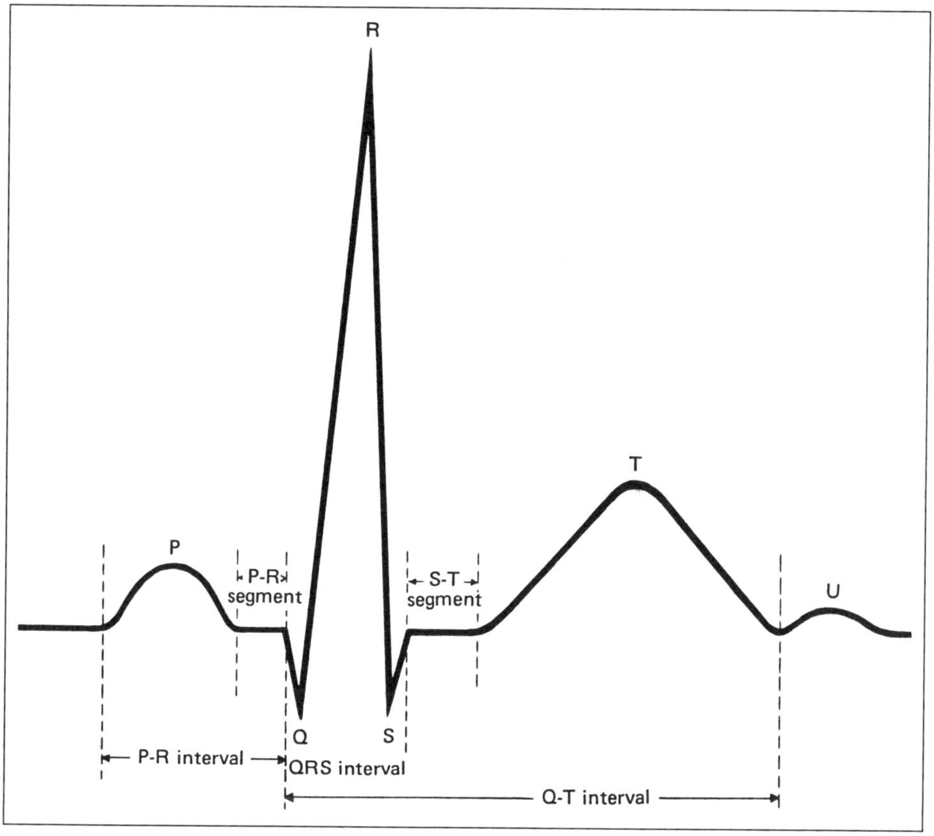


Fig. 2–2. Diagram showing normal sinus beat (lead II). Detailed explanation is given in text.

to transmit electrical impulses from atria to ventricles.

The basic technique of inserting an electrode catheter and the equipment used are essentially the same as those of cardiac catheterization, and the His bundle ECG is usually performed in the cardiac catheterization laboratory. A small risk (as with cardiac catheterization) is involved. A consent form is required before performing the test, and detailed procedures should be explained to the patient. The His bundle ECG is recorded on a photographic paper using a special recorder.

Various electrical events shown in the His bundle ECG enable physicians to understand the exact mechanism of cardiac arrhythmias, the exact site(s) of heart block (Fig. 2–4), and the exact origin of any cardiac impulse formation (Fig. 2–5). When these parameters are available, the proper therapeutic approach (e.g., determination of indication vs nonindication for artificial pacemaker, the best suitable antiarrhythmic drug(s), and so on) can be provided. For example, when the refractory VT cannot be provoked by the electrical stimuli following administration of any particular antiarrhythmic agent (e.g., lidocaine or procainamide), that particular agent will be the drug of choice for a given patient (Chapters 15 and 18). Besides the His bundle ECG, there are many other types of electrophysiologic studies that can be performed in modern medical centers, but discussion regarding them is beyond the scope of this manual.

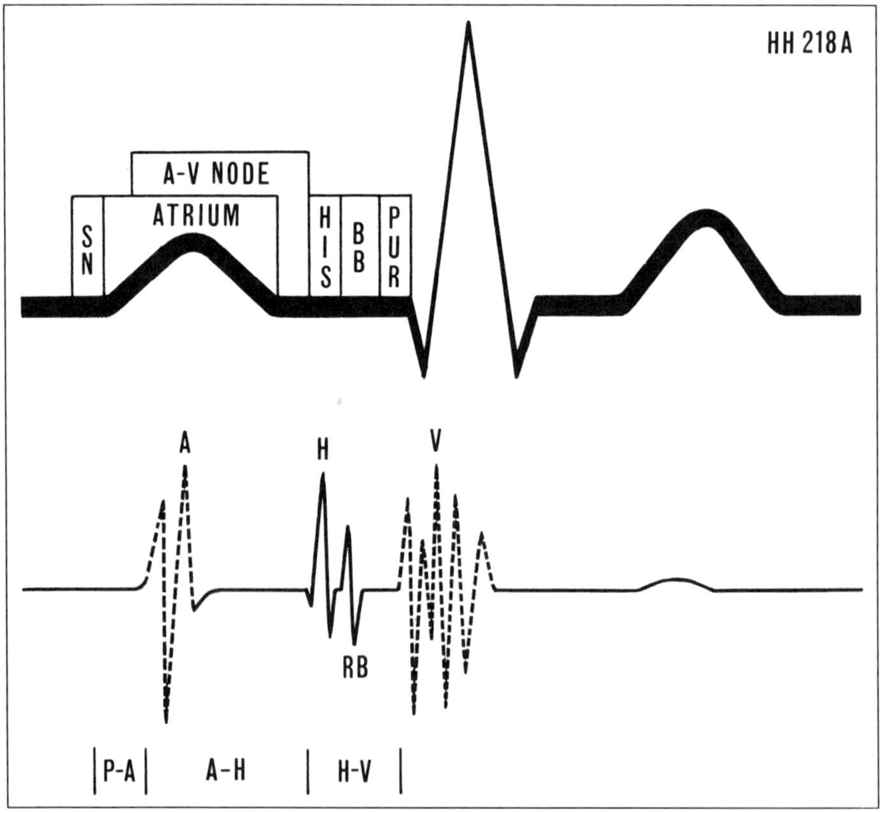


**Fig. 2–3. A.** Schematic illustration of His bundle ECG indicating conduction through the various portions of the heart during 1 cardiac cycle. Note that the impulse has reached the Purkinje fibers prior to the inscription of the QRS complex. It is important to remember that with surface ECG, only atrial depolarization (and sometimes atrial repolarization), ventricular depolarization, and ventricular repolarization are recorded. SN = sinus node; BB = bundle branches; Pur = Purkinje fibers.

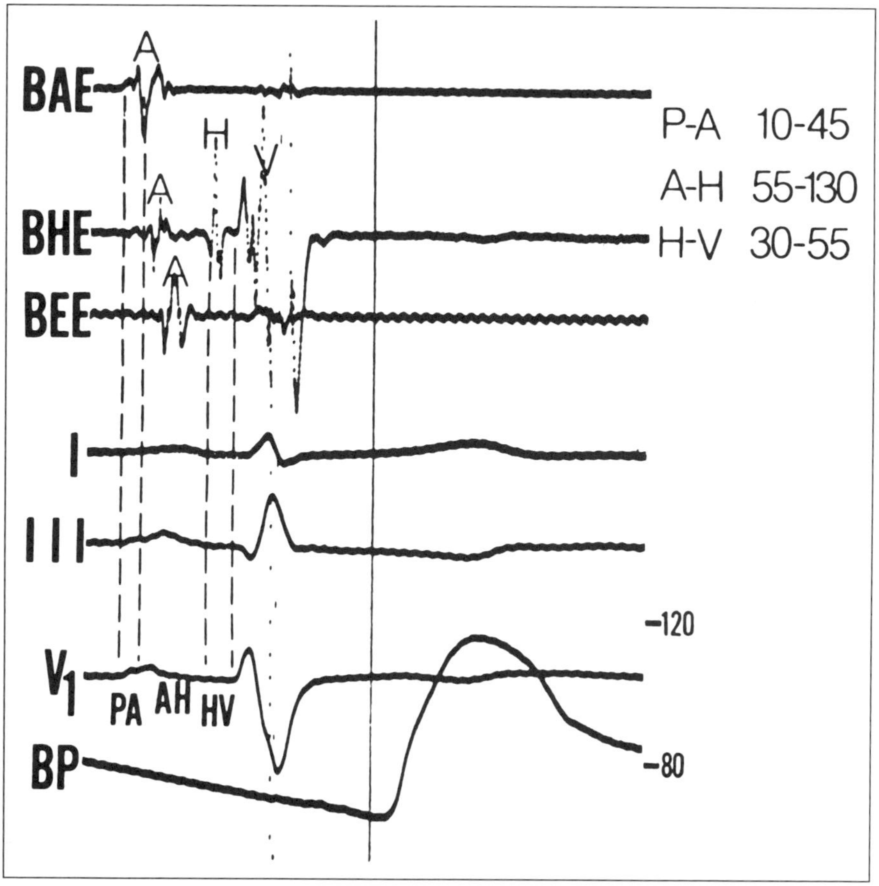


**B.** Single cardiac cycle illustrating the intervals measured during His bundle ECG. In this and all subsequent figures, the following abbreviations are used: BAE = bipolar atrial electrogram representing high right atrial activity; BHE = bipolar His electrogram representing low right atrial activity (A), His bundle activity (H), and ventricular septal activity (V); BEE = bipolar esophageal electrogram representing primarily left atrial activity; I = lead I; II = lead 2; III = lead 3; $V_1$ = lead $V_1$; P-A = P-A interval representing intraatrial conduction; A-H = A-H interval representing AV nodal conduction; H-V = H-V interval representing His-Purkinje conduction. All numbers are given in milliseconds. The paper speed is 100 mm/sec unless otherwise stated. Interrupted lines demarcate the various intervals. Note the normal sequence of atrial activation recorded with this technique: high right atrial activity precedes low right atrial activity, recorded in the BHE lead, and this precedes left atrial activity, recorded in the BEE lead.

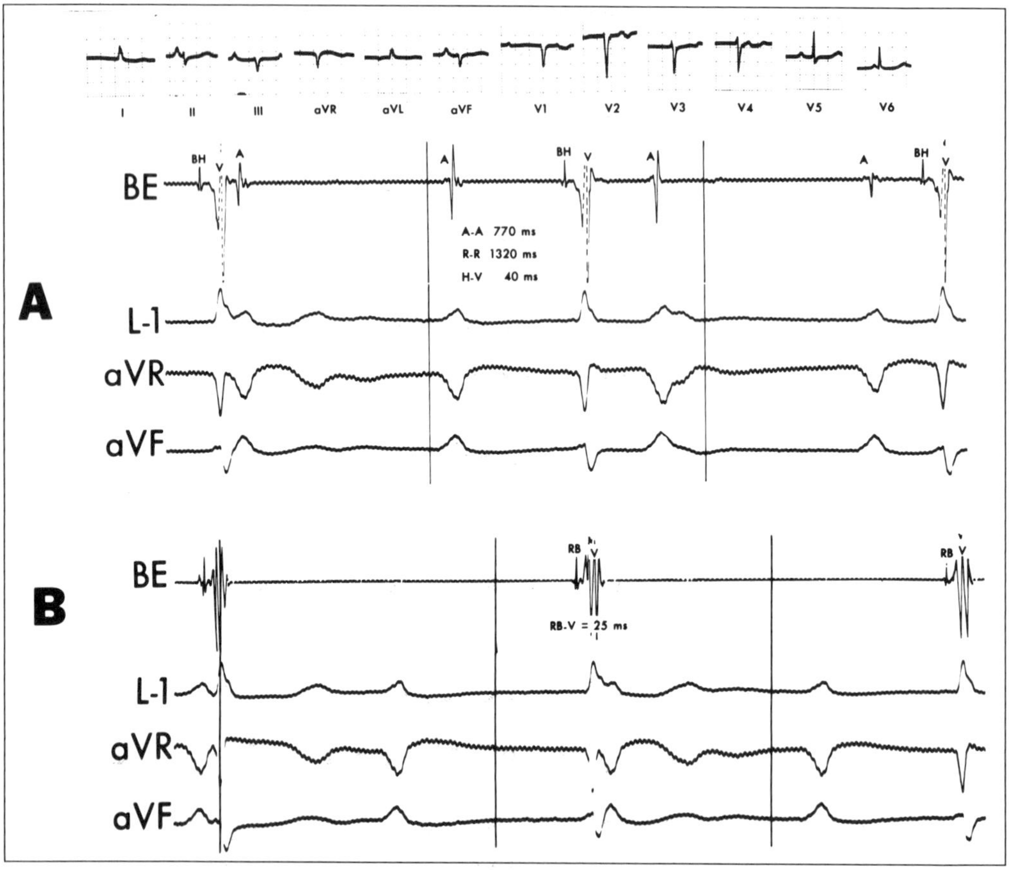


**Fig. 2–4. A.** His bundle recordings from a patient with complete AV block proximal to the His bundle. The 12 standard ECG leads show narrow QRS complexes. Simultaneous recordings of UE, BE, and 3 standard leads (L-1, aVR, aVF). Each ventricular (V) complex is preceded by a BH deflection with an interval (H-V) of 40 msec. The dissociated atrial (panel A) activity occurs at a cycle length of 770 msec and is not followed by a BH deflection.

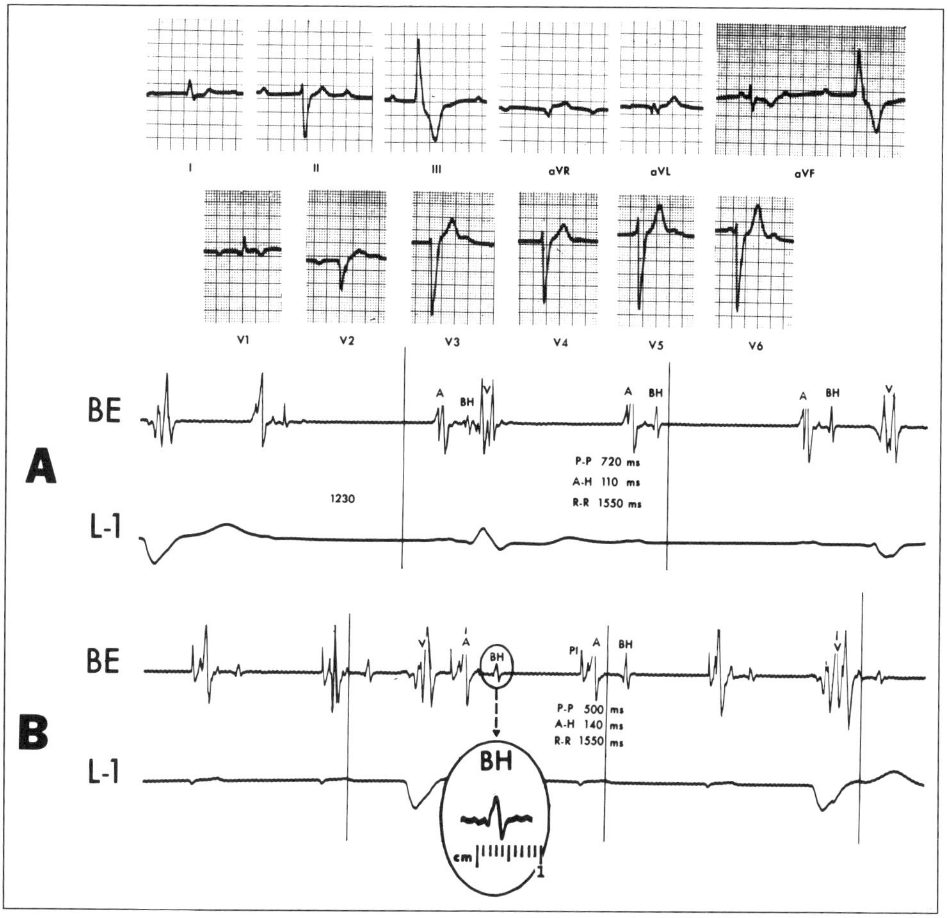


B. A typical recording from a patient with complete AV block distal to the His bundle. The 12 standard ECG leads show complete AV block. Note the 2 different types of ventricular complexes in lead aVF. *Panel A:* Simultaneous recording of bipolar electrogram (BE) and standard lead I (L-1). The A and BH deflections are temporarily coupled with an A-H time of 110 msec but are dissociated from ventricular (V) activity. R-R = 1,550 msec. Note the 2 different types of QRS complexes in lead I. *Panel B:* As the atrium was paced (PI) and the P-P interval was shortened from 720 msec *(panel A)* to 500 msec, the A-H time lengthened to 140 msec. The inset depicts the magnified BH deflection, which measures 30 msec.

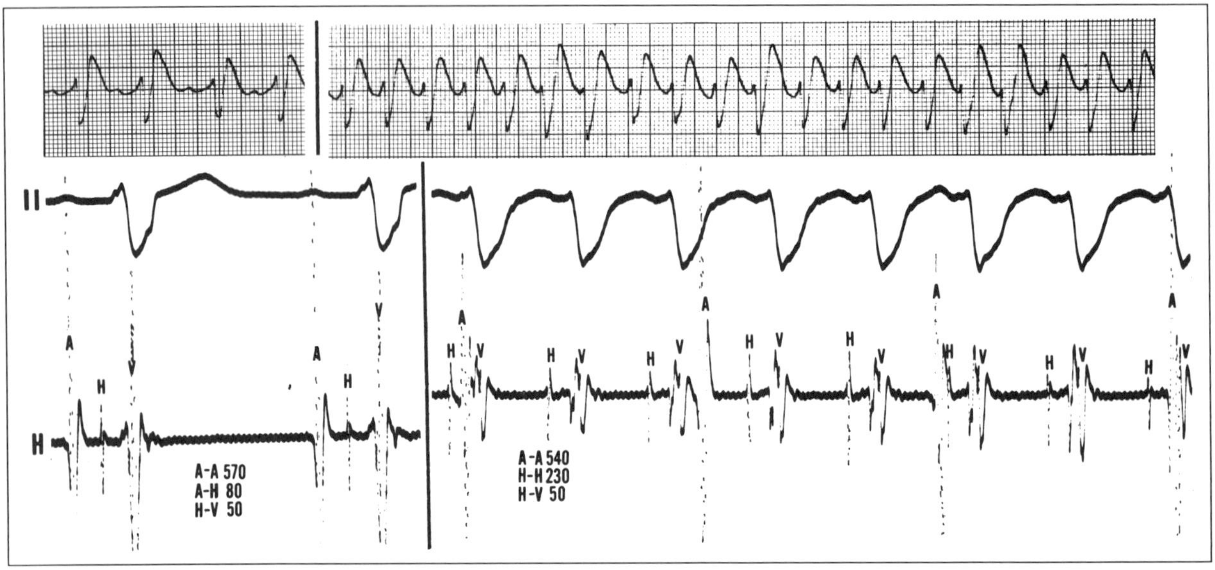


**Fig. 2–5. A.** Sinus rhythm (A) with AV JT (H-V) producing AV dissociation. Note that every ventricular deflection (V) is preceded by H potential yet is independent of the atrial deflection (A). In the panels on the left, sinus rhythm is present.

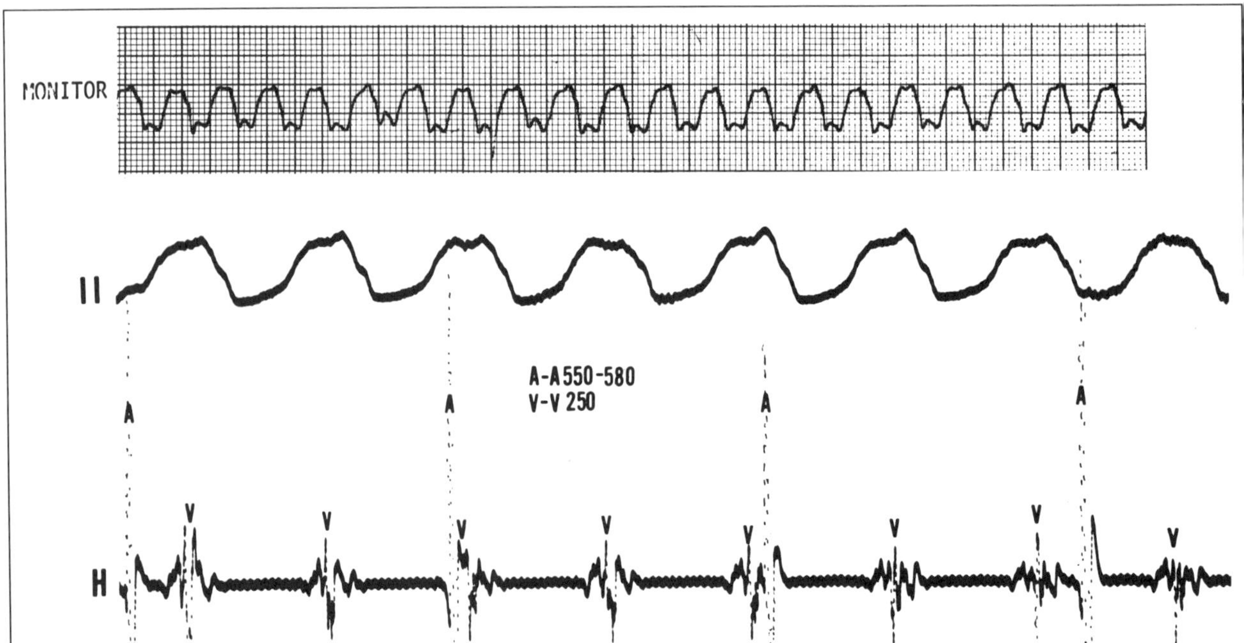


**Fig. 2–5. B.** Sinus rhythm (A) with VT (indicated by V) producing AV dissociation.

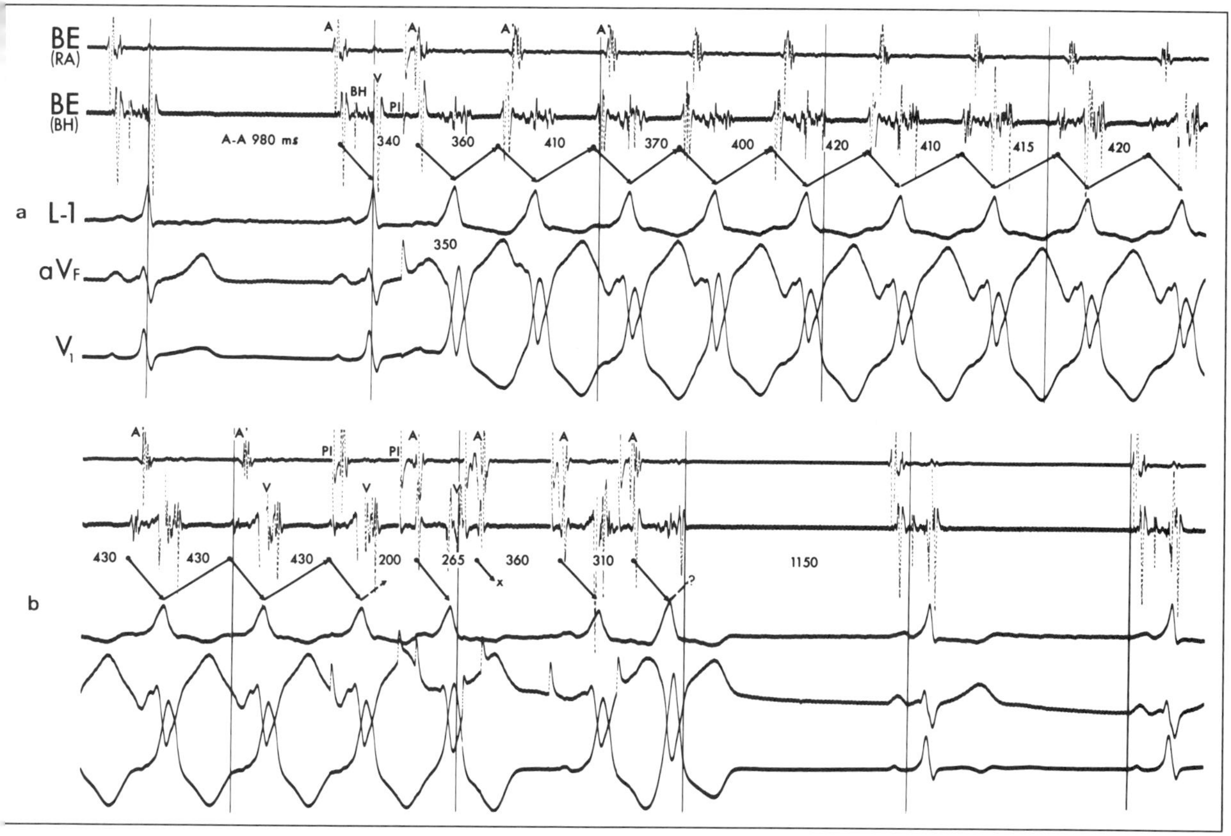


Fig. 2–5. C. Atrial tachycardia in a patient with the WPW syndrome simulating VT. *Panel A*: Simultaneous bipolar recordings from the right atrium (RA) and the His bundle region (BH) along with 3 ECG leads, L-1, aVF and $V_1$. The first two QRS complexes show His bundle recordings during normal sinus rhythm. As the premature atrial beat is induced at a coupling interval of 340 msec, reciprocating tachycardia is induced with atrial activation from low to high right atrium. In addition, the QRS complexes are more aberrant and show an RBBB pattern. The right half of the tracing closely simulates VT. *Panel B*: Atrial pacing at a cycle length of 300 msec and a successful termination of the reciprocating tachycardia.

**Fig. 2–5. C.** Atrial tachycardia in a patient with the WPW syndrome simulating VT. *Panel A*: Simultaneous bipolar recordings from the right atrium (RA) and the His bundle region (BH) along with 3 ECG leads, L-1, aVF and $V_1$. The first two QRS complexes show His bundle recordings during normal sinus rhythm. As the premature atrial beat is induced at a coupling interval of 340 msec, reciprocating tachycardia is induced with atrial activation from low to high right atrium. In addition, the QRS complexes are more aberrant and show an RBBB pattern. The right half of the tracing closely simulates VT. *Panel B*: Atrial pacing at a cycle length of 300 msec and a successful termination of the reciprocating tachycardia.

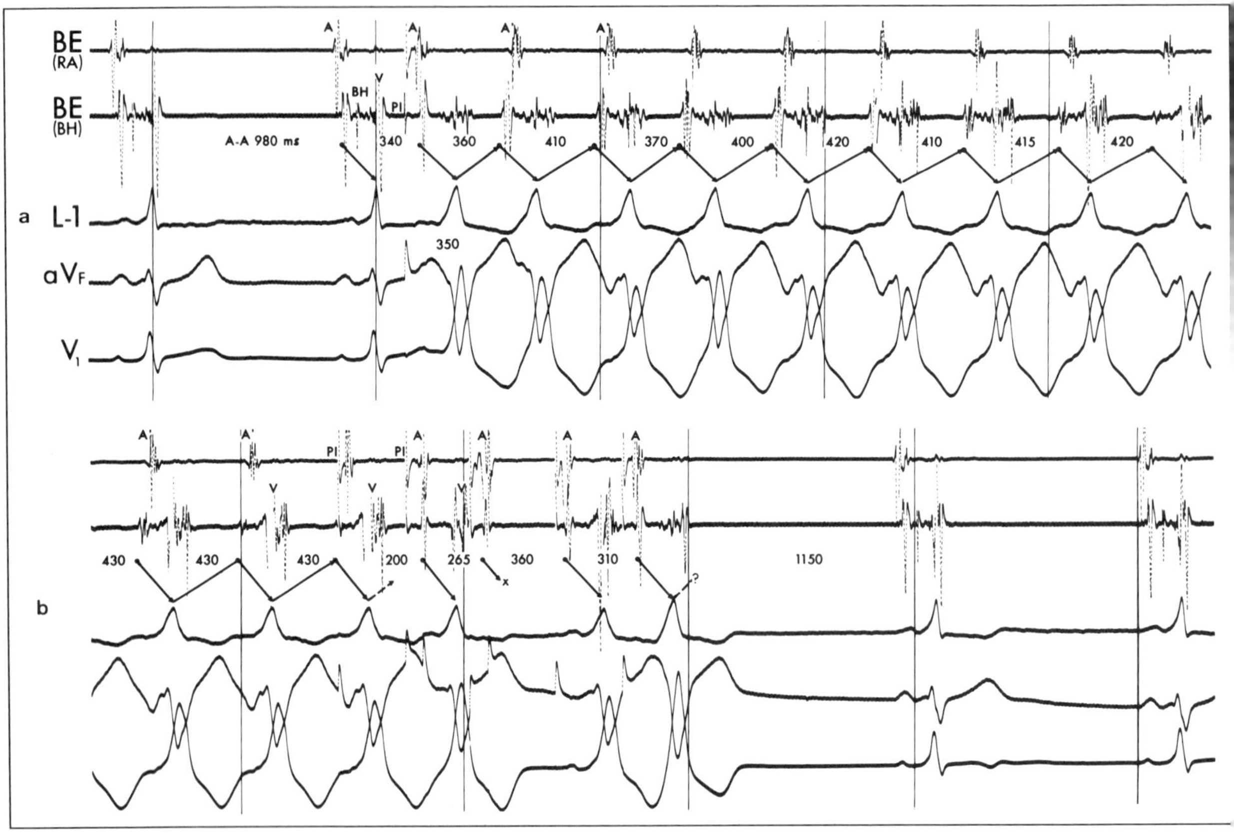

# Chapter 3

# Diagnostic Approach to Cardiac Arrhythmias

In the analysis of cardiac rhythm disturbances, it is essential to use well-designed ECG calipers. The calipers should be of such construction that the 2 legs can be set in any position, and the opposing surfaces of the 2 legs should be flat so that any rapid or slow rate may be measured. The end of each leg should be sharply pointed.

For a detailed analysis of cardiac arrhythmias, it is preferable to have a long rhythm strip of lead II, or sometimes leads III or aVF, because these leads show the P wave most clearly. Occasionally, lead $V_1$ shows the P wave more clearly than do the above-mentioned leads. Ideally, long rhythm strips of leads II and $V_1$ should be used for detailed analysis. A rhythm strip should be taken immediately following the original 12-lead ECG when any cardiac arrhythmia is suspected or found because certain arrhythmias are very transient in nature and may change within a few seconds or minutes. When the cardiac arrhythmia is rapid, long strips should be obtained during various procedures, such as carotid sinus massage, in order to clarify the fundamental mechanism involved. At times, it is necessary to take a long rhythm strip with double speed and/or double standardization in order to magnify the P waves if they are believed to be present. Rarely, esophageal leads or even atrial intracavitary leads may be obtained for further clarification of the P wave. In addition, His bundle ECG has been widely used for the interpretation of various arrhythmias, particularly in the differential diagnosis between supraventricular and ventricular tachyarrhythmias and in the determination of a site of AV block. Classification of various cardiac arrhythmias is summarized in Table 1–1.

In general, the following process should be followed in the analysis of any cardiac arrhythmia:

1. Obtain all available clinical information.
2. Conduct a general inspection of the ECG.
3. Determine the dominant rhythm.
4. Determine the presence or absence of a P wave.
5. Determine the origin of the QRS complex when atrial and ventricular activities are independent.
6. Determine the nature and origin of beats occurring prematurely or later than usual.
7. Make a final conclusion regarding the cardiac arrhythmia.

## OBTAINING CLINICAL INFORMATION

It is of great help in interpreting cardiac arrhythmias if clinical information is available. This information should include the patient's age, presence of a previous similar arrhythmia and its onset and frequency, presence of known heart disease, previous history of CHF and such noncardiac diseases as hyperthyroidism, drug administration, particularly digitalis, and electrolyte imbalance. A detailed history of an artificial pacemaker implantation, including the approximate date of implantation, type of pacemaker, and other factors, is important because malfunction of an artificial pacemaker may produce various serious arrhythmias. In addition, one must review all available previous tracings in order to determine whether the patient had any past cardiac arrhythmia, BBB, WPW syndrome, or other condition. This information is frequently invaluable in distinguishing between supraventricular and ventricular tachyarrhythmias and enhances the accuracy of the diagnosis.

## GENERAL INSPECTION OF THE ELECTROCARDIOGRAM

By a general inspection of a given tracing, it is possible to determine whether the basic rhythm is normal sinus rhythm or a type of cardiac arrhythmia. If any arrhythmia is present, one should determine whether it occurs occasionally, frequently, continuously, regularly or irregularly, repetitively, or with various combinations. Various noncardiac artifacts (Figs. 3–1 and 3–2) that may simulate cardiac arrhythmias must be detected. It is also possible to determine whether the arrhythmia is simple or complex, clinically benign or serious.

## DETERMINATION OF DOMINANT CARDIAC RHYTHM

After a general inspection of a given ECG, a determination of the dominant cardiac rhythm is the next step. The dominant rhythm may be sinus, but it could be any type of ectopic rhythm. If an ectopic rhythm is dominant, one should determine whether the ectopic rhythm is due to active or passive impulse formation. However, in most common and simple arrhythmias, the dominant rhythm is of sinus origin. The second most common dominant rhythm is AF and, less commonly, atrial flutter. Occasionally, the dominant rhythm may change from one mechanism to another (from sinus to ectopic or vice versa or even from ectopic to ectopic) on the same ECG. At times, it is difficult to determine the dominant rhythm, particularly when dealing with complex arrhythmias. Even if the dominant rhythm is ectopic in origin, as a rule, it begins with sinus beats, if they are present even occasionally. It is immensely helpful to determine whether sinus beats are present.

## DETERMINATION OF PRESENCE OR ABSENCE OF P WAVES

By knowing whether a P wave is present or absent, one can narrow the differential diagnosis significantly. When a P wave seems to be present, one should be certain that the P wave is a true P wave and not other various waves, such as AF or atrial flutter, T wave, U wave, or even artifacts that look like P waves. If a true P wave is definitely present, one should determine whether the P wave and QRS complex are related or independent. The P-R interval (AV conduction time) is, by definition, the interval from the onset of the P wave to the onset of the QRS complex. It is usually constant in a single lead, but it may differ slightly in other leads because a portion of the P wave or QRS complex may be isoelectrical. Therefore, it is ordinarily recommended that the longest P-R interval in the 6 extremity leads be measured. Dual AV conduction or any other type of AV conduction defect should be suspected when the P-R intervals in different leads vary significantly.

### Presence of P Wave

When a P wave is present, one should determine whether the P wave is of sinus or ectopic origin. In order to reach a conclusion, the following steps should be carried out:

1. Determine the origin of the P wave (mean axis of P wave).
2. Inspect the P wave configuration.
3. Inspect the regularity of the P-P cycle.
4. Measure the P wave rate.
5. Determine the relationship between P wave and QRS complex.

By the above process, if the P wave is found to be of sinus origin, one has reached a conclusion as to whether normal sinus rhythm, sinus tachycardia, sinus bradycardia, and so on are present. If the P wave is not of sinus origin, it must be originating from an ectopic focus in the atria or AV junction or, rarely, in the ventricles. When the P wave originates in the atria, the P

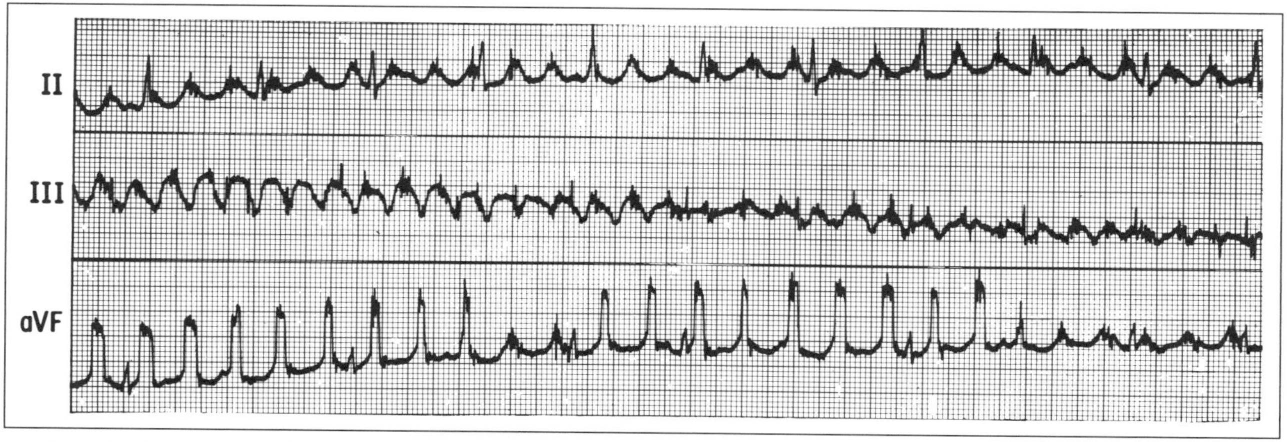


**Fig. 3–1.** Marked artifacts due to muscle tremors that closely simulate atrial flutter (lead III) and ventricular tachycardia (lead aVF) in a patient with Parkinson's disease.

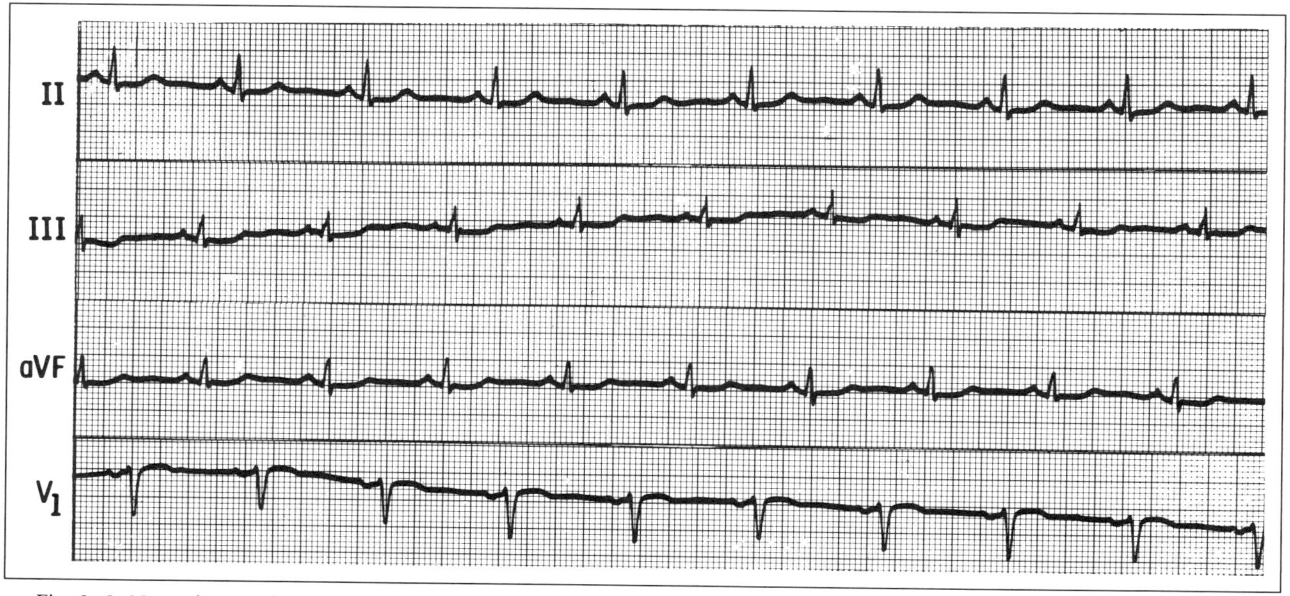


**Fig. 3–2.** Normal sinus rhythm without any artifact when the muscle tremors are eliminated after treatment in same patient as in Figure 3–1.

wave may resemble or at times be almost identical to the sinus P wave, but the rate is usually faster when impulses originate in the atria. The P wave may be conducted in a retrograde fashion if it originates from either the AV junction or ventricles. If this occurs, the P wave will be inverted in lead II but upright in lead aVR and thus have a direction almost opposite to that of a sinus P wave. When the atria are activated in a retrograde fashion from the AV junction, the P wave may appear before or after the QRS complex, depending upon whether the atria or ventricles are activated first. If the atria and ventricles are activated simultaneously, the P wave will be superimposed on the QRS complex, leading to an absent P wave. When the P wave configuration changes from beat to beat in the presence of a constant P-R interval, a wandering pacemaker is present in the sinus node. The pacemaker may wander in the atria. This may be diagnosed when one observes a changing P-R interval with fluctuations in the P wave configuration. A wandering pacemaker is present between the sinus and AV nodes when the P wave configuration changes from upright to inverted in the same lead with or without a changing P-R interval. It should be noted that respiration may slightly change the P wave configuration in some leads, and this should be distinguished from a wandering atrial pacemaker. In addition to its influence on the P wave, respiration may also affect the QRS complex and T wave in a similar fashion. An ECG taken during sustained inspiration or expiration will eliminate this problem. On rare occasions, the P wave configuration may only change after ectopic beats. This is due to aberrant atrial conduction (Chung's phenomenon). A varying P wave configuration is also observed when atrial fusion beats of varying degree appear. This is seen with atrial parasystole or atrial dissociation (Chapter 22).

An irregular P-P cycle is usually due to sinus arrhythmia but may also occur with intermittent SA block, sinus arrest, or even sinus premature beats. Ectopic atrial beats that appear during sinus rhythm also result in an irregular P-P cycle, but the configuration of the ectopic P wave is usually different from the sinus P wave. The rate of the P wave helps us determine with relative accuracy the cardiac rhythm. A P wave rate between 60 and 100 beats/min with the P wave conducted in a forward direction is usually indicative of normal sinus rhythm. Nonparoxysmal AV JT often produces the same rate as normal sinus rhythm, but the P wave during AV JT is conducted in a retrograde fashion. In general, nonparoxysmal AV JT produces retrograde P waves with a rate between 70 and 150 beats/min. When the rate of the P wave is between 180 and 250 beats/min, the ectopic rhythm present is usually either AT or paroxysmal AV JT. The P wave is conducted in a forward fashion in the former, but in a retrograde fashion in the latter. Atrioventricular junctional escape rhythm may produce retrograde P waves but at a much slower rate (40–60 beats/min) than does AV JT. Rarely, idioventricular rhythm (VER) may show retrograde P waves. These P waves usually occur after the QRS complex. It is not uncommon to find a retrograde P wave following artificial pacemaker-induced ventricular rhythm. A retrograde P wave also can be produced in reciprocal rhythm or reciprocal tachycardia (Chapter 6).

The final step in this subgroup is to appreciate the relationship between atria and ventricles. If the P-R or R-P intervals are constant, all the above-mentioned diagnostic possibilities (normal sinus rhythm, sinus bradycardia, sinus tachycardia, AT, AV JT, AV JER, and idioventricular rhythm) should be considered. This list should be narrowed after careful observation of the direction and rate of P waves. If the P-R interval varies, one must be certain whether or not the atria and ventricles are related in the cardiac cycle. The degree and frequency of this relationship must be determined. When no relationship exists between the atria and ventricles, complete AV dissociation is the end result. The underlying disorders responsible for AV dissociation may be (1) a marked slowing of sinus impulse formation, (2) acceleration of ectopic impulse formation in the AV junction or ventricles, and (3) complete AV block (Chapter 6). Complete AV dissociation need not always be present, for the atria and ventricles may at times become related (atrial or ventricular captured beats), and this rhythm is known as "incomplete AV dissociation."

When the atrial rate is found to be a multiple of the ventricular rate, second degree or advanced (high degree) AV block, such as 2:1 or 3:1 AV block, is usually present. Wenckebach AV block (Mobitz type I AV block) is characterized by a gradual lengthening of the P-R intervals until a P wave is present without a QRS complex after it. This pattern may then repeat itself. Thus, the atrial to ventricular ratio becomes 3:2, 4:3, and so on. Mobitz type II AV block also produces a 3:2 or 4:3 or greater AV block that may resemble the Wenckebach type, but the P-R intervals remain constant except when a blocked (nonconducted) P wave occurs. It should be remembered that Mobitz type II AV block represents incomplete TFB (Chapter 9).

First degree AV block has a constant but prolonged (0.21 second or more) P-R interval. The relationship between atria and ventricles may occasionally be reversed, Wenckebach retrograde VA block being the resulting abnormality.

### Absence of P Wave

When the P wave is not discernible, one should determine whether: (1) the P wave is truly absent or (2) the P wave is falsely absent.

It is not uncommon to observe a P wave superimposed on a portion of the QRS complex, ST segment, or T wave of the preceding or subsequent cycle. This occurs frequently during AT or AV JT and may occasionally be observed during sinus tachycardia. Various maneuvers, such as carotid sinus pressure and breath-holding, may enable us to delineate the P wave from other complexes by reducing the heart rate.

If after the above techniques the P wave is still not observed, the atrial mechanism must be determined. The most common cause of an absent P wave is AF or, less commonly, atrial flutter. In these cases, an AF or flutter wave is present in place of the P wave. Untreated AF usually has a rapid ventricular rate (more than 120–160 beats/min) unless a significant AV conduction defect is present. In untreated atrial flutter, the ventricular rate is usually one-half that of the atrial rate. This block is not anatomic in nature. Its presence is due to the fact that the AV junction is unable to conduct the very rapid atrial rate. Thus, the ventricular rate is frequently around 125–175 beats/min. In AV JT or JER, the P wave may be totally superimposed on the QRS complex, leading to absent P waves. This occurs when atrial and ventricular depolarization occur simultaneously. In rare circumstances, notable in severely diseased hearts, atrial activity may be completely absent because of atrial standstill.

## DETERMINATION OF ORIGIN OF QRS COMPLEX WHEN ATRIAL AND VENTRICULAR ACTIVITIES ARE INDEPENDENT

When the P wave and QRS complex are either temporarily or continuously independent, incomplete or complete AV dissociation will be produced. When this occurs, either the atrial or ventricular mechanism may equally dominate. In other words, the atria may be controlled by the sinus node or any other atrial ectopic focus (AF, atrial flutter, or AT), whereas the ventricles may be controlled by either the AV junction or a ventricular ectopic focus.

When the QRS complex is unrelated to the P wave, the fundamental genesis of the impulse that activates the ventricles should be determined. It is essential to determine whether the QRS complex is produced by active or passive impulse formation. In addition, it should be determined whether the QRS complex originates from the AV junction or the ventricles. If there is active impulse formation in the above examples, AV JT or VT, respectively, will result. In contrast to this, passive impulse formation from the AV junction and ventricles results in either AV JER or VER, respectively. The QRS complex that originates from the AV junction is usually of normal configuration, although it may be bizarre and wider than usual because of BBB. Aberrant ventricular conduction may occur when there is an extremely rapid rate or an Ashman's phenomenon (Chapter 11). The

QRS complex that originates from the ventricles is usually wide and has a bizarre configuration.

## DETERMINATION OF NATURE AND ORIGIN OF BEATS OCCURRING PREMATURELY OR LATER THAN USUAL

Various fundamental mechanisms may produce a P wave or QRS complex that occurs prematurely. The most common example of this is the ordinary premature beat (extrasystole) that may originate from the atria, AV junction, or ventricles, and rarely from the sinus node. When a premature beat is found, one should determine its origin. The origin of a premature P wave is determined by the electrical axis and configuration of the P wave and its relationship to the QRS complex. The configuration of the P wave of a sinus premature beat is identical to the P wave of the underlying sinus rhythm, whereas the P wave of an atrial premature contraction (APC) is usually slightly different in configuration from the sinus P wave. An APC is ordinarily followed by a normal QRS complex. When the coupling interval (interval from the ectopic beat to the preceding beat of the basic rhythm) is very short or when Ashman's phenomenon is present, the QRS complex following an APC may appear bizarre due to aberrant ventricular conduction (Chapter 11). At times, a premature P wave may not be followed by a QRS complex, and this is called a "nonconducted" or "blocked" APC. When the P wave is conducted in a retrograde fashion, it should be determined whether the P wave is related to the preceding or the following QRS complex or both. The P wave of an AV junctional premature beat may be preceded or followed by the QRS complex, depending upon whether the atria or ventricles are activated first. When a retrograde P wave is related to both the preceding and the following QRS complex and becomes placed between them, a reciprocal beat is usually present (Chapter 6).

The QRS complex of AV junctional premature or reciprocal beats may show a bizarre form because of aberrant ventricular conduction. The QRS complex of a VPC is usually wide and bizarre. Rarely, as previously mentioned, a P wave may follow the QRS complex of a VPC.

Recognition of an artificial pacemaker-induced cardiac rhythm is obvious because of the presence of the artificial electrical artifact that initiates the heartbeat (Chapter 19).

Rare types of prematurely appearing P waves may be due to atrial or AV junctional parasystole and atrial dissociation (Chapter 22). Ventricular parasystole produces prematurely appearing QRS complexes with varying coupling intervals.

In the presence of AV dissociation, atrial or ventricular captured beats may produce prematurely appearing P waves or QRS complexes, respectively (Chapter 6). Fusion beats (summation beats), atrial or ventricular in origin, produce variations in the shape of the P waves and QRS complexes. Fusion beats are very common in parasystole. When a QRS complex appears later than usual in the basic cardiac rhythm, it is usually either an AV JEB or VEB. The QRS complex of AV JEBs is usually normal in appearance, but not uncommonly it is wide and bizarre because of BBB. Ventricular escape (idioventricular) beats are always wide and bizarre. Escape beats, either AV junctional or ventricular in origin, follow a long pause and are seen with various arrhythmias, including SA block, sinus arrest, marked sinus bradycardia, sinus arrhythmia, second or third degree AV block, and premature beats (extrasystoles).

## FINAL CONSIDERATION

After complete clinical and electrophysiologic impressions are made, the following questions should be asked:

1. What is the origin of the dominant rhythm?
   a. Is it normal sinus rhythm?
   b. Is it an ectopic rhythm?
2. What is the fundamental genesis of the arrhythmia?
   a. Is it abnormal impulse formation?
      i. Is it active impulse formation?

   ii. Is it passive impulse formation?
   iii. Is it atrial, AV junctional, or ventricular in origin?
  b. Is it a conduction disturbance?
  c. Is it a combination of both?
3. Is the P wave present in the dominant cardiac rhythm?
  a. What is the origin of the P wave?
  b. What is the rate of the P wave?
  c. Is the P wave related to the QRS complex?
  d. If related, what is the mode of relationship between the P wave and the QRS complex?
  e. If unrelated, what is the basic disorder producing AV dissociation?
4. What is the atrial mechanism if the P wave is absent?
  a. Is it truly absent or superimposed on a portion of the QRS complex, ST segment, T or U wave?
  b. Is it AF?
  c. Is it atrial flutter?
  d. Is it AV JER or JT?
  e. Is it atrial standstill?
5. What are the origin and nature of the QRS complex if the atrial and ventricular activities are independent?
  a. Is it active impulse formation in the AV junction?
  b. Is it passive impulse formation in the AV junction?
  c. Is it active impulse formation in the ventricles?
  d. Is it passive impulse formation in the ventricles?
  e. Is it artificial pacemaker-induced cardiac rhythm?
6. What are the nature and origin of the beats that occur prematurely?
  a. Is it atrial, AV junctional, or ventricular or perhaps sinus in origin?
  b. Is it an ordinary premature beat (extrasystole)?
  c. Is it sinus arrhythmia?
  d. Is it parasystole?
  e. Is it a reciprocal beat?
  f. Is it a captured beat (in the presence of AV dissociation)?
  g. Is the wide and bizarre QRS complex due to aberrant ventricular conduction or BBB of a supraventricular beat, or is the beat of ventricular origin?
7. Is this a simple or complex, common or uncommon cardiac arrhythmia?
  a. Are there any complex mechanisms, such as concealed conduction, unidirectional block, supernormal AV conduction, involved?
  b. Is the interpretation of the arrhythmia entirely satisfactory?
  c. Are there any alternative interpretations?
8. What is the clinical significance of the arrhythmia?
  a. Is treatment indicated?
  b. What is the treatment of choice if treatment is indicated?

# Chapter 4

# Sinus Arrhythmias

When any of the 5 criteria necessary for the diagnosis of normal sinus rhythm (normal axis of the P wave, constant and normal P-R interval, constant P wave configuration in a given lead, rate between 60 and 100 beats/min, and constant P-P or R-R cycle) is lacking, a cardiac arrhythmia of sinus origin is considered to be present. Such arrhythmias include sinus premature contraction (extrasystole), sinus bradycardia, sinus tachycardia, sinus arrhythmia, wandering pacemaker in the sinus node, sinus arrest (pause or standstill), and sinoatrial (SA) block.

## SINUS BRADYCARDIA

### Diagnostic Criteria

Sinus rhythm with a rate below 60 beats/min is termed "sinus bradycardia." The usual rate in sinus bradycardia is between 45 and 59 beats/min and occasionally may be as slow as 30–40 beats/min. Sinus bradycardia is often associated with sinus arrhythmia, and the presence of sinus arrhythmia does not preclude the diagnosis of sinus bradycardia. In this case, sinus arrhythmia and sinus bradycardia simply coexist. The diagnostic criteria of sinus bradycardia are:

1. A P wave of sinus origin (normal mean axis of the P wave)
2. Constant and normal P-R interval (0.12–0.20 second)
3. Constant P wave configuration in each given lead
4. Rate between 45 and 59 beats/min (cyclic length longer than 1.00 second)
5. Regular or slightly irregular P-P cycle

Markedly slow sinus bradycardia is often misinterpreted as SA block or sinus arrest. The differential diagnosis is important because the SA block is usually benign, whereas sinus arrest often produces serious clinical symptoms.

When the rate of a sinus bradycardia becomes equal to or slower than the subsidiary pacemaker, AV JER may appear to control the ventricles. This may lead to AV dissociation or intermittent AV JER without sinus activity. This type of AV dissociation is often associated with sinus arrhythmia and is usually clinically benign. A detailed description of AV dissociation is given in Chapter 6.

### Clinical Significance

Increased vagal tone is responsible for spontaneous sinus bradycardia that may persist for a long period of time in many individuals. Various factors that reduce vagotonia, such as exercise, excitement, and atropine, increase the sinus rate. Sinus bradycardia is common in healthy young adults, particularly in the asthenic type of person and in athletes. It is also commonly observed in elderly individuals, especially during sleep or immediately after awakening. On the other hand, sinus bradycardia may occur in various cardiac and noncardiac diseases. This arrhythmia is also found during drug therapy (e.g., digitalis, beta-blocking agents, reserpine, or guanethidine). The sudden appearance of a sinus bradycardia during digitalis therapy usually is an early sign of DI. Persisting sinus bradycardia *not* due to any drug may indicate sick sinus syndrome (SSS) (Chapter 14).

Sinus bradycardia by itself seldom produces symptoms unless the rate is extremely slow (30–40 beats/min) or unless there is serious underlying heart disease (acute MI, or severe CHF). Dizziness or lightheadedness may be observed in some cases of sinus bradycardia, but syncopal episodes are rare.

Most cases of sinus bradycardia need no specific treatment. However, some patients with a markedly slow sinus bradycardia may require treatment. Atropine is often effective for marked sinus bradycardia. When the arrhythmia is drug-induced, the given drug should be discontinued. When symptomatic, patients with a marked sinus bradycardia in SSS who fail to respond to drug therapy may need artificial pacemaker implantation.

## SINUS TACHYCARDIA

### Diagnostic Criteria

Sinus tachycardia is diagnosed when all of the 5 criteria for the diagnosis of normal sinus rhythm are present but the rate is faster than 100 beats/min. The usual rate of a sinus tachycardia is between 101 and 160 beats/min, and occasionally it may accelerate up to 180–200 beats/min, particularly in young adults during physical exercise. On rare occasions, a sinus rate as rapid as 220–230 beats/min has been reported in children. Sinus arrhythmia is not uncommonly associated with sinus tachycardia in young adults or children. The following criteria are used for the diagnosis of sinus tachycardia:

1. P wave of sinus origin (normal mean axis of P waves)
2. Constant and normal P-R interval (0.12–0.20 second)
3. Constant P wave configuration in each given lead
4. Rate between 101 and 160 (up to 180–200 in some cases) beats/min (cycle length shorter than 0.60 second)
5. Regular or slightly irregular P-P cycle

### Clinical Significance

Sinus tachycardia is frequently observed in healthy individuals, particularly during emotional excitement or physical exercise. Persistent sinus tachycardia has been reported normally as a hereditary trait in certain families. Sinus tachycardia is often a compensatory mechanism to meet any physical demand or stress and for the heart to continue increasing its minute output when the maximal stroke output has been reached. Sinus tachycardia commonly occurs in healthy individuals following drinking coffee, tea, and alcohol or smoking a cigarette. Various drugs, especially sympathomimetic catecholamines, such as epinephrine, and parasympatholytic agents, such as atropine, produce a sinus tachycardia.

On the other hand, various pathologic conditions, including a high output state due to any cause, CHF, shock, acute rheumatic fever, acute MI, pulmonary embolism, and chronic lung diseases, are frequently associated with sinus tachycardia. Thus, the clinical significance of sinus tachycardia depends upon the underlying cause. In general, sinus tachycardia per se does not produce any symptoms, although some individuals may experience palpitation, restlessness, or apprehension when the rate is very fast and the arrhythmia lasts for a long period of time. A functional systolic murmur is often heard at the base or apex of the heart during rapid sinus tachycardia, particularly when it is due to a high output state.

Treatment for sinus tachycardia is usually *not* required unless the arrhythmia is associated with cardiac or noncardiac diseases. Sinus tachycardia in healthy individuals usually terminates gradually when the causative factors are removed. In disease states, the management of sinus tachycardia depends upon the underlying process.

## SINUS ARRHYTHMIA

### Diagnostic Criteria

Sinus arrhythmia is diagnosed when the P-P cycles in sinus rhythm vary 0.16 second or more. Sinus arrhythmia is frequently associated with sinus bradycardia, particularly in children and young adults, and is occasionally associated with sinus tachycardia. In addition, the presence of sinus bradycardia or sinus tachycardia does *not* preclude the diagnosis of sinus arrhythmia. Thus, the diagnostic criteria for sinus arrhythmia are as follows:

1. P wave of sinus origin (normal mean axis of the P wave)
2. Constant and normal P-R interval (0.12–0.20 second)
3. Constant P wave configuration in each given lead
4. Rate between 45 and 100 beats/min (occasionally slower than 45 and faster than 100 beats/min)
5. Irregular P-P cycle (variation of P-P interval 0.16 second or more)

Generally, sinus arrhythmia is divided into 2 major types, respiratory and nonrespiratory. A less common and more specific type of sinus arrhythmia is ventriculophasic sinus arrhythmia. This occurs most commonly in the presence of complete AV block and less commonly in the presence of second degree AV block, VPC, and artificial pacemaker-induced ventricular rhythm. Ventriculophasic sinus arrhythmia is discussed later in this chapter.

**Respiratory Sinus Arrhythmia:** The most common type of sinus arrhythmia is the respiratory form, in which the variations of the sinus cycles vary in relation to the respiratory cycle. In this type of sinus arrhythmia, the sinus rate increases gradually with inspiration and slows with expiration.

Respiratory sinus arrhythmia is produced by variations in the vagal tone by reflex mechanisms in the pulmonary and systemic vascular system in relation to the respiratory cycle. Vagal tone is accentuated by expiration, whereas it is lowered by inspiration. It can be assumed that pacemaker fibers with a higher rate in the sinus node may be suppressed by vagal stimulation, so that the pacemaker fibers with a slower rate may escape, producing a slower sinus rhythm. Subsequently, the pacemaker fibers with the higher rate in the sinus node regain their function to produce a faster rate in the presence of lower vagal tone. This cyclic variation may continue, coinciding with the respiratory cycle.

**Nonrespiratory Sinus Arrhythmia:** This type of sinus arrhythmia is the irregular sinus cycle, which is not related to the respiratory cycle. In some cases of nonrespiratory sinus arrhythmia, an etiologic factor is not demonstrable. Thus, the term "idiopathic" sinus arrhythmia is used. On the other hand, nonrespiratory sinus arrhythmia is more commonly found in individuals with diseased hearts, and the term "pernicious" sinus arrhythmia is used.

Respiratory sinus arrhythmia is usually eliminated by breathholding. The P-P interval and the configurations of the P wave are often constant in sinus arrhythmia. However, it is not uncommon to observe a slightly taller P wave with a longer P-R interval during shorter cycles and a smaller P wave with a shorter P-R interval during longer cycles.

Sinus arrhythmia, particularly in the presence of sinus bradycardia, may be associated with AV dissociation. This occurs when the rate of the AV junction is equal to or exceeds that of the sinus node. Sinus arrhythmia often disappears when the rate is increased by physical exercise, atropine, or amyl nitrite.

Sinus arrhythmia should be distinguished from sinus arrest, SA block, AV block (especially Wenckebach AV block), and APCs.

## Clinical Significance

Respiratory sinus arrhythmia is commonly observed in healthy children and young adults and also in elderly individuals. On the other hand, this arrhythmia may occur in diseased hearts as well. Nonrespiratory sinus arrhythmia may occur in healthy subjects, but it is found more commonly in subjects with diseased hearts. A marked nonrespiratory sinus arrhythmia associated with sinus bradycardia is extremely common during the first 24–72 hours after acute diaphragmatic MI. In addition, it may be observed during convalescence from any acute illness. Increased intracranial pressure from various causes may also produce sinus arrhythmia. When a marked sinus arrhythmia and sinus bradycardia develop during digitalization, it is often due to digitalis toxicity.

Morphine and other factors that increase parasympathetic tone also produce sinus arrhythmia.

In most cases of respiratory sinus arrhythmia, there are no particular symptoms. However, in marked sinus arrhythmia with periods of extremely slow rate (slower than 40 beats/min), the patient may experience dizziness and may even faint in severe cases. In nonrespiratory sinus arrhythmia, the symptomatology depends largely upon the underlying cause. In general, symptoms more commonly occur in the nonrespiratory than in the respiratory form.

By and large, no treatment is required for sinus arrhythmia. Atropine may be used when sinus arrhythmia is associated with a marked sinus bradycardia that produces symptoms. In nonrespiratory sinus arrhythmia due to cardiac disease or drugs, treatment is directed toward the underlying cause.

## Ventriculophasic Sinus Arrhythmia

Complete (third degree) AV block is characterized by independent atrial and ventricular activities, resulting in complete AV dissociation. In spite of the independent electrical activities of the P wave and QRS complex in complete AV block, it is not uncommon to observe that the P-P interval, which includes the QRS complex is shorter than the P-P interval without a QRS complex (Fig. 4–1). This phenomenon is termed "ventriculophasic sinus arrhythmia." It has been shown that approximately 30% of patients with complete AV block have an associated ventriculophasic sinus arrhythmia. In addition, the same ECG phenomenon occasionally occurs in second degree AV block, and ventriculophasic sinus arrhythmia may occur occasionally in the presence of a VPC with a full

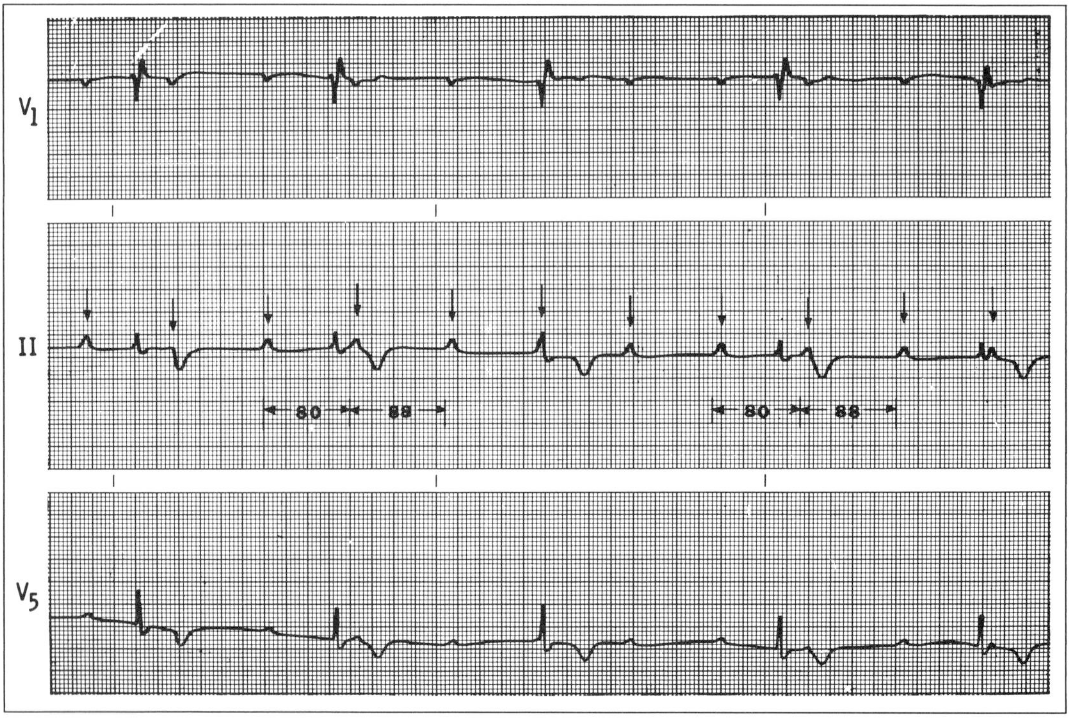


**Fig. 4–1.** Arrows indicate sinus P waves. The rhythm is ventriculophasic sinus arrhythmia with AV junctional escape rhythm due to complete AV block. Note that the P-P interval containing the QRS complex is shorter than the P-P interval without the QRS complex. (The numbers represent hundredths of a second.)

compensatory pause. That is, the P-P interval that includes the VPC is shorter than the P-P interval without a VPC. Ventriculophasic sinus arrhythmia can occur in the presence of artificial pacemaker-induced ventricular rhythm, i.e., the P-P interval that includes the artificial pacemaker-induced QRS complex is shorter than the P-P interval without the QRS complex.

The exact mechanism responsible for the development of ventriculophasic sinus arrhythmia is not clearly understood, but it seems to be caused by some mechanical or hemodynamic mechanism. Ventriculophasic sinus arrhythmia per se is insignificant clinically.

## WANDERING PACEMAKER IN THE SINUS NODE

A wandering pacemaker in the sinus node (Fig. 4–2) is frequently associated with sinus arrhythmia, and, rarely, the former exists without the latter. Thus, a wandering pacemaker in the sinus node is considered by many investigators as a variant of sinus arrhythmia or an exaggerated form of sinus arrhythmia. As in respiratory sinus arrhythmia, wandering pacemaker in the sinus node may occur in accordance with the respiratory cycle, but, at times, a wandering pacemaker occurs independent of the respiratory cycle.

The wandering pacemaker in the sinus node means that the pacemaker shifts from one part to another in the sinus node. Thus, the configuration of the P wave changes from beat to beat, but the P-R interval either remains constant or may change between 0.12 and 0.20 second (Fig. 4–2). The P wave configuration may alter slightly or markedly. In general, alteration of the P wave configuration is marked when sinus arrhythmia and wandering pacemaker coexist. The P wave is taller and the P-R interval is longer during a rapid rate, whereas the P wave is smaller and the P-R interval is shorter during a slower rate.

The fundamental mechanism involved in the genesis of wandering pacemaker in the sinus node is as follows: The location of the pacemaker shifts to a less active area of the sinus node as the more active area is suppressed. Subsequently, the active area of the pacemaker regains its function when the factors suppressing the active area (such as alteration of vagal tone and various drugs) are alleviated. In spite of a changing P wave configuration in wandering pacemaker in the sinus node, the mean axis of the P wave is generally within normal limits. This is because every impulse must originate from the sinus node. Thus, every P wave must be upright in lead II and inverted in lead aVR. The diagnostic criteria for wandering pacemaker in the sinus node are as follows:

1. P wave of sinus origin (normal mean axis of the P wave)
2. Varying P wave configuration in each given lead
3. Relatively constant P-R interval (may vary between 0.12 and 0.20 second)
4. Slightly irregular or regular P-P cycles
5. Rate between 45 and 100 beats/min (rarely slower than 45 or faster than 100 beats/min)

It should be noted that a changing P wave configuration with a precisely constant P-R interval in lead III or aVF may be due to postural changes of the heart due to respiration. This certainly may resemble a wandering pacemaker, but the respiratory variation usually influences the QRS and T complexes as well.

The clinical significance of wandering pacemaker is the same as for sinus arrhythmia. It may occur in healthy individuals, particularly when sinus arrhythmia and sinus bradycardia coexist.

## SINUS ARREST (PAUSE OR STANDSTILL)

Sinus arrest (pause or standstill) is defined as a failure of impulse formation in the sinus node. Since the impulse is not formed in the sinus node, no electrocardiographic wave is produced (Fig. 4–3). Thus, sinus arrest is manifested by absence of the P wave. In addition, there will be absence of the QRS and T complexes.

Sinus arrest may occur in normal subjects

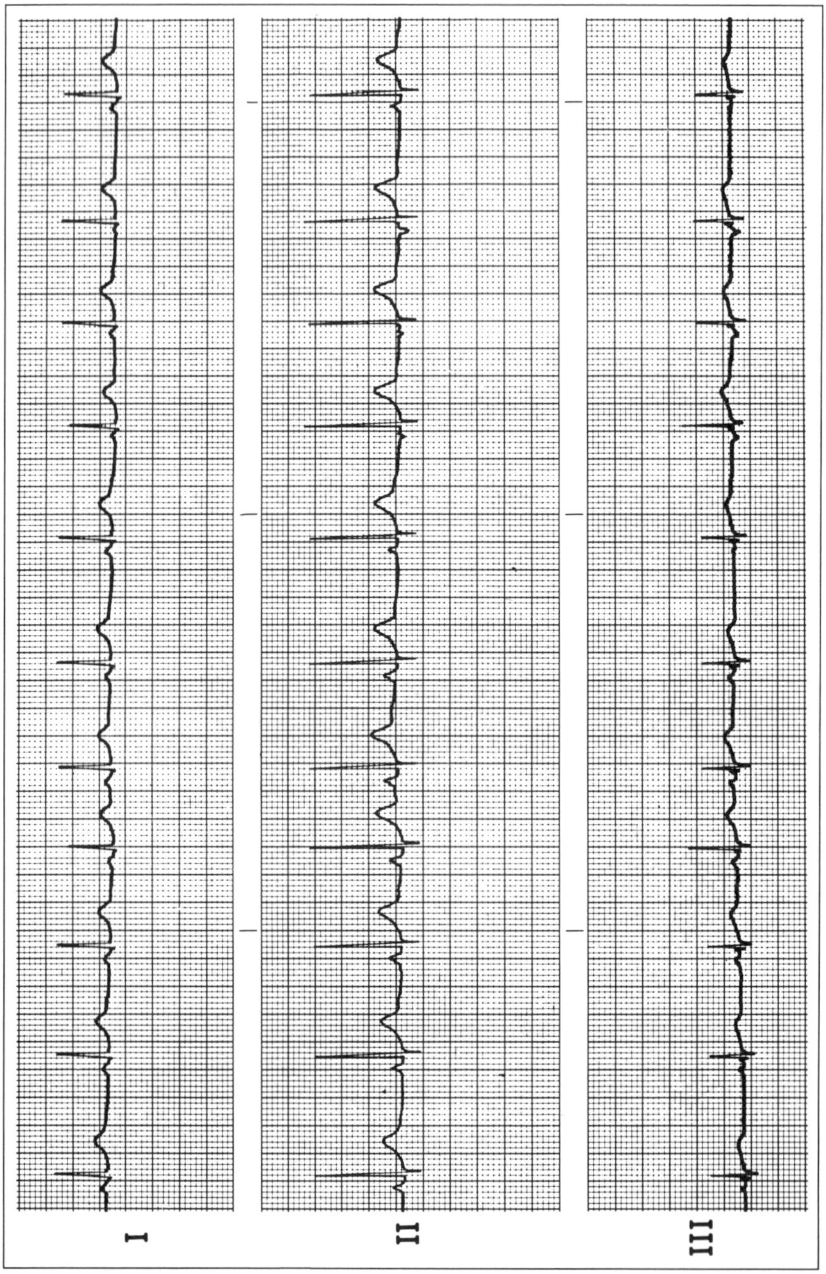


**Fig. 4–2.** Sinus arrhythmia with wandering atrial pacemaker.

with increased vagal tone or with a hypersensitive carotid sinus. Sinus arrest is commonly associated with a marked sinus arrhythmia, but it may occur without sinus arrhythmia on a reflex basis or as a result of overdosage of digitalis or other drugs (e.g., propranolol). In addition, administration of parasympathetic drugs, particularly acetylcholine, and potassium may produce sinus arrest, and heart diseases, particularly acute myocarditis or acute MI, may produce sinus arrest, especially when the sinus node is involved. It has been shown that carotid sinus stimulation (CSS) may also cause sinus arrest, particularly when DI is present. The sinus node is often suppressed by an ectopic beat or runs of ectopic tachycardia, leading to sinus arrest. This occurs because the sinus node requires a warming-up period until its usual rate of automaticity is reestablished following a bout of ectopic beats or rhythm. This effect is called the "postdrive inhibition phenomenon." The duration of the sinus arrest may be long and, at times, irreversible when the sinus node is suppressed by an ectopic tachycardia, particularly with severe underlying heart disease. Persisting sinus arrest *not* due to any drug often indicates SSS (Chapter 14).

When sinus arrest occurs, AV JEBs may appear as a physiologic mechanism to control the ventricles. In this circumstance, AV dissociation will result if the period of sinus arrest and AV JER coexist. In the presence of sinus arrest, ventricular escape (idioventricular) beat or VER may occur to control the ventricles when the AV junction is unable to produce impulses.

Sinus arrest should be distinguished from SA block because both conditions produce absence of the P, QRS, and T complexes. The P-P interval in sinus arrest is greatly variable, and the duration of the sinus arrest has no relationship to the P-P cycle of the basic rhythm. Conversely, either the P-P interval in SA block is a multiple of the basic P-P cycle or the P-P cycle shows a regular irregularity. The differential diagnosis between sinus arrest and SA block is extremely difficult or impossible when the underlying rhythm is a marked sinus arrhythmia. Sinus arrest should also be distinguished from second or third degree AV block and nonconducted APC.

The treatment and prognosis of sinus arrest depend upon the underlying cause and the underlying cardiac status. Treatment of sinus arrest may be accomplished by removal of the etiologic factor, if there is one. This is particularly true for DI. No treatment is needed when the patient is asymptomatic and the overall heart rate is faster than 45 beats/min. Sinus arrest due to SSS may require permanent artificial pacemaker (Chapter 14).

## SINOATRIAL BLOCK

Sinoatrial block may be classified into first, second, and third degree SA block analogous to AV block. However, only second degree SA block can be diagnosed with certainty. First degree SA block may occur theoretically, but it is impossible to diagnose. Likewise, third degree (complete) SA block is impossible to diagnose because there will be no P, QRS, and T complexes registered in the ECG for an indefinite period.

Second degree SA block can be divided in 2 categories: (1) Mobitz type II SA block, which is comparable to Mobitz type II AV block, and (2) Wenckebach (Mobitz type I) SA block, which is comparable to Wenckebach (Mobitz type I) AV block. It is interesting to note that Wenckebach AV block is very common, while Wenckebach SA block is uncommon compared with Mobitz type II SA block.

### Mobitz Type II SA Block

In this type of second degree SA block, there will be an occasional absence of 1 or more beats of P, QRS, and T complexes. The P-P intervals including the SA block are exactly or almost exactly multiples of P-P cycles of the basic rhythm. Thus, the long P-P interval containing the SA block will commonly be twice and less commonly 3 or 4 times the P-P cycle of the basic rhythm (Fig. 4–4). Mobitz type II SA block may occur periodically at regular or at irregular intervals. At times, 2:1 SA block may occur consecutively, leading to a slow rhythm that super-

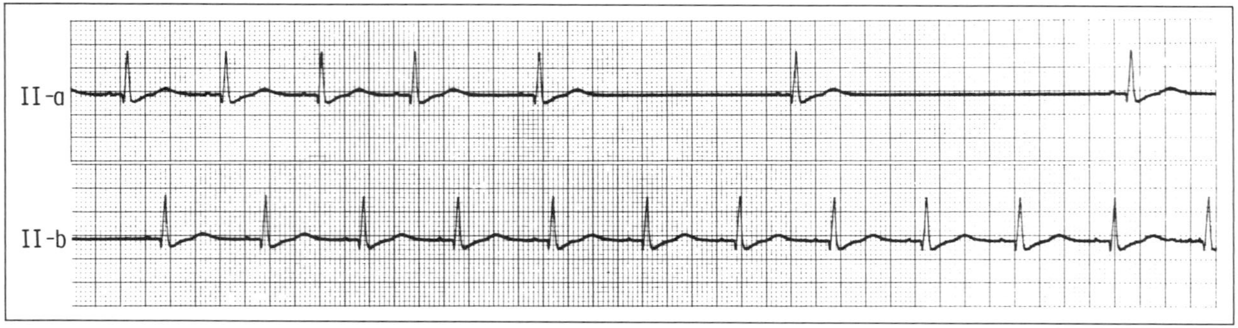


**Fig. 4–3.** Leads II-a and II-b are continuous. The rhythm is sinus arrhythmia with intermittent sinus arrest.

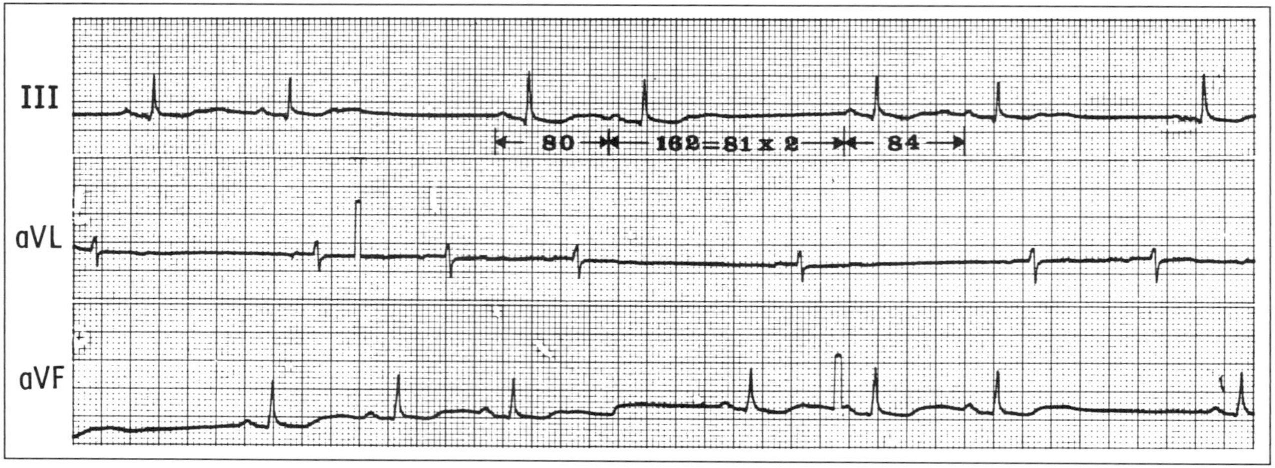


**Fig. 4–4.** Sinus rhythm with intermittent 2:1 (Mobitz type II) SA block. Note that the long P-P interval is 2 times the basic P-P cycle. (The numbers represent hundredths of a second.)

ficially resembles a markedly slow sinus bradycardia. When SA block occurs successively for 3 or more beats, this will lead to atrial standstill unless an ectopic focus takes over to activate the atria. When SA block occurs, a subsidiary pacemaker may escape to control the ventricles for 1 or more beats. In this case, AV dissociation often results.

## Wenckebach (Mobitz Type I) SA Block

In this type of SA block, the long P-P intervals due to the SA block are *not* multiples of the P-P cycles of the basic rhythm. Therefore, it is difficult to diagnose this type of SA block even for experienced cardiologists. In Wenckebach SA block, the P-P intervals due to the SA block vary; i.e., the P-P intervals preceding the longer pause become progressively shorter until a long pause occurs (Fig. 4–5). Wenckebach SA block can be diagnosed only by finding the cyclic shortening of the P-P intervals followed by a long pause. When a persisting 3:2 Wenckebach SA block occurs leading to alternating short and long P-P intervals, this produces a sinus pseudobigeminy. Wenckebach SA block often produces a regular irregularity of the P-P cycles, which superficially resembles a marked sinus arrhythmia.

The mechanism of Wenckebach SA block is analogous to Wenckebach AV block (Chapter 8) except that the conduction disturbance occurs at the SA junction in the former. In this type of SA block, measurement of the actual duration of the various cycles must be calculated because a direct measurement of the P-P intervals does *not* indicate the actual rate. In this type of SA block, the AV junction may es-

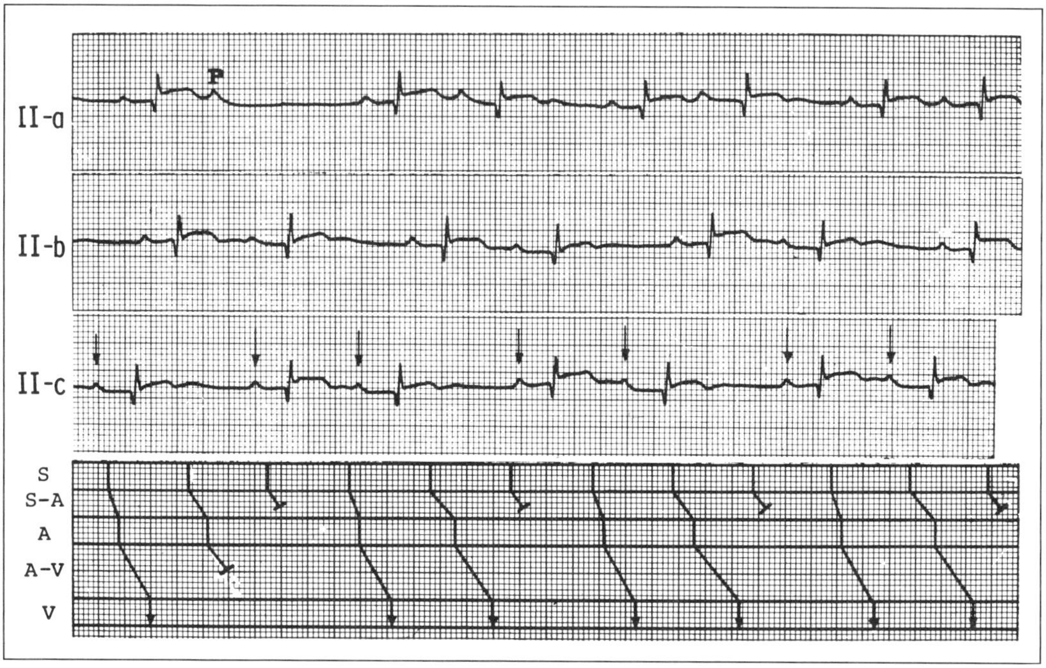


Fig. 4–5. Leads II-a, II-b, and II-c are continuous. Arrows indicate P waves. The rhythm is sinus with 3:2 Wenckebach (Mobitz type I) SA block associated with 3:2 Wenckebach (Mobitz type I) AV block in a patient with acute diaphragmatic MI. The characteristic feature of Wenckebach AV block is altered by the coexisting Wenckebach SA block. P indicates a blocked sinus P wave. Explanation is given in the diagram (S = sinus; SA = sinoatrial; A = atria; AV = atrioventricular; V = ventricles). Note that short and long P-P intervals alternate, but the long P-P interval is shorter than 2 short P-P intervals—the characteristic feature of Wenckebach SA block. Note an abnormal Q wave with ST segment elevation and T wave inversion indicative of acute diaphragmatic MI.

cape for 1 or more beats to control the ventricles, leading to intermittent AV dissociation.

Sinoatrial block should be distinguished from sinus arrest, which produces a long P-P interval unrelated to the P-P cycle of the basic rhythm. Sinoatrial block is differentiated from AV block, in which an absence of the QRS and T complexes occurs, but the sinus P waves appear regularly where expected. Sinoatrial block, particularly the Wenckebach type, should be distinguished from sinus arrhythmia.

As far as the fundamental mechanism is concerned, SA block occurs as a result of block of sinus impulse transmission in the SA junction, and the sinus node produces impulses regularly as usual.

Sinoatrial block often occurs transiently, but it may last for a long period of time. It may be found in healthy subjects with increased vagal tone or with a hypersensitive carotid sinus. This arrhythmia may also occur in acute myocarditis due to various causes and in CAD, particularly acute diaphragmatic MI. In addition, digitalis often induces SA block; in fact, DI is said to be the most common cause of SA block, particularly in children. Sick sinus syndrome should be strongly considered when persistent or recurrent SA block is *not* due to any drug (Chapter 14).

Transient SA block usually produces no symptoms. When SA block persists for longer periods, the patient may experience dizziness or even fainting episodes, particularly when a subsidiary pacemaker fails to produce an escape rhythm or when the ventricular rate of the escape rhythm is markedly slow. Continuous SA block without an ectopic escape mechanism will produce cardiac standstill and may be fatal.

Treatment of SA block depends upon the underlying cause and the underlying cardiac status. Transient SA block may not require any treatment. Drug-induced SA block is often treated by discontinuation of the drug alone (especially digitalis). In symptomatic SA block due to increased vagal tone, ephedrine sulfate, atropine, or methantheline may be given in order to diminish or abolish vagal tone. Patients with drug-resistant and symptomatic SA block due to SSS usually require permanent pacemaker implantation (Chapter 14).

# Chapter 5

# Atrial Arrhythmias

Atrial arrhythmias may originate from any portion of the atria other than the sinus node. Atrial arrhythmias are almost always generated by active impulse formation, and, therefore, some form of rapid atrial arrhythmia will result. Common atrial arrythmias include APCs, AT, atrial flutter, and AF. These arrhythmias are closely interrelated with each other in terms of mechanism and clinical significance. It has been suggested that an ectopic focus in the atria that produces an isolated APC may be capable of producing AT, atrial flutter, and AF. The relationship between atrial flutter and AF is very close, and it is common to observe that atrial flutter changes to AF, or vice versa, even on the same ECG tracing. Although atrial tachyarrhythmias are classified into AT, atrial flutter, and AF primarily on the basis of the atrial rate, it is not uncommon to observe a transitional (or intermediate) rhythm among these atrial tachyarrhythmias. This is particularly true when the atrial rate is faster than 350 beats/min and the flutter cycle is still regular. This rhythm is termed "atrial impure flutter." On the other hand, the term "atrial flutter-fibrillation" is used when the rhythm is a mixture of atrial flutter and AF. The atrial rates in AT, atrial flutter, and AF are 160–250, 250–350, and 400–650 beats/min, respectively, but these rates are arbitrarily divided. Atrial rates are often altered by various drugs, particularly quinidine and digitalis. The ventricular rates in untreated atrial tachyarrhythmias are generally between 160 and 200 beats/min simply because the AV junctional tissue is unable to conduct extremely rapid atrial impulses. This is due to the longer refractory period in the AV junction than in the atria.

Atrial tachyarrhythmias may occur in a paroxysmal or chronic form. Atrial fibrillation often persists for a long period of time when the underlying disorder is SSS or RHD, particularly mitral stenosis. Atrial tachyarrhythmias may occur in healthy subjects as well as in diseased hearts. However, AF or atrial flutter is more commonly encountered in diseased hearts. In addition, thyrotoxicosis is frequently associated with paroxysmal AF. The common occurrence of various tachyarrhythmias associated with WPW syndrome is well known. Atrial tachycardia with varying AV block occurring during digitalization almost always indicates DI.

Less common atrial arrhythmias include atrial parasystole, atrial dissociation, and slow atrial rhythm (atrial escape rhythm). Atrial standstill is rarely observed, and, if it occurs, it is almost always found in the terminal cardiac patient and in severe DI.

## ATRIAL PREMATURE CONTRACTIONS (EXTRASYSTOLES)

Atrial premature contractions (APCs) may originate from any location in the atria outside the sinus node. In most instances, the impulse from the atrial premature focus activates the entire atria, including the sinus node. The sinus node is prematurely discharged, and its inherent sinus impulse discharge will be suppressed momentarily. The propagation of the impulse in the atria from an atrial ectopic focus is usually different from that of the sinus impulse, but conduction below the AV node is identical to that in normal sinus rhythm.

### Diagnostic Criteria

Atrial premature contraction (atrial extrasystole) is diagnosed when the ectopic P wave appears earlier than the cardiac cycles of the basic rhythm (Fig. 5–1).

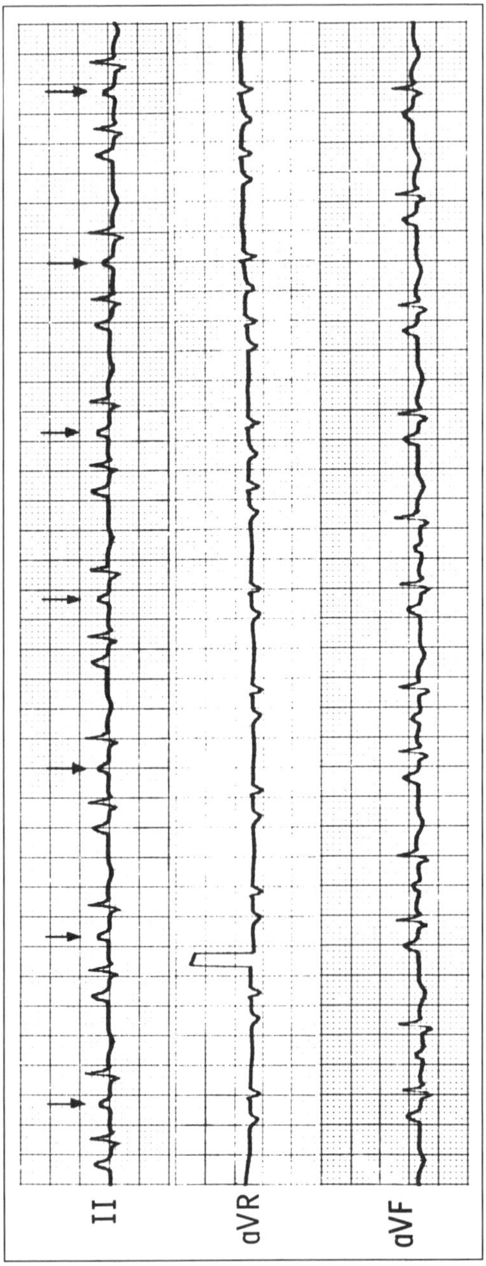


**Fig. 5–1.** Sinus rhythm with frequent APCs (indicated by arrows) producing atrial bigeminy. The diagnosis of diaphragmatic MI is made on the basis of Q waves in leads II and aVF.

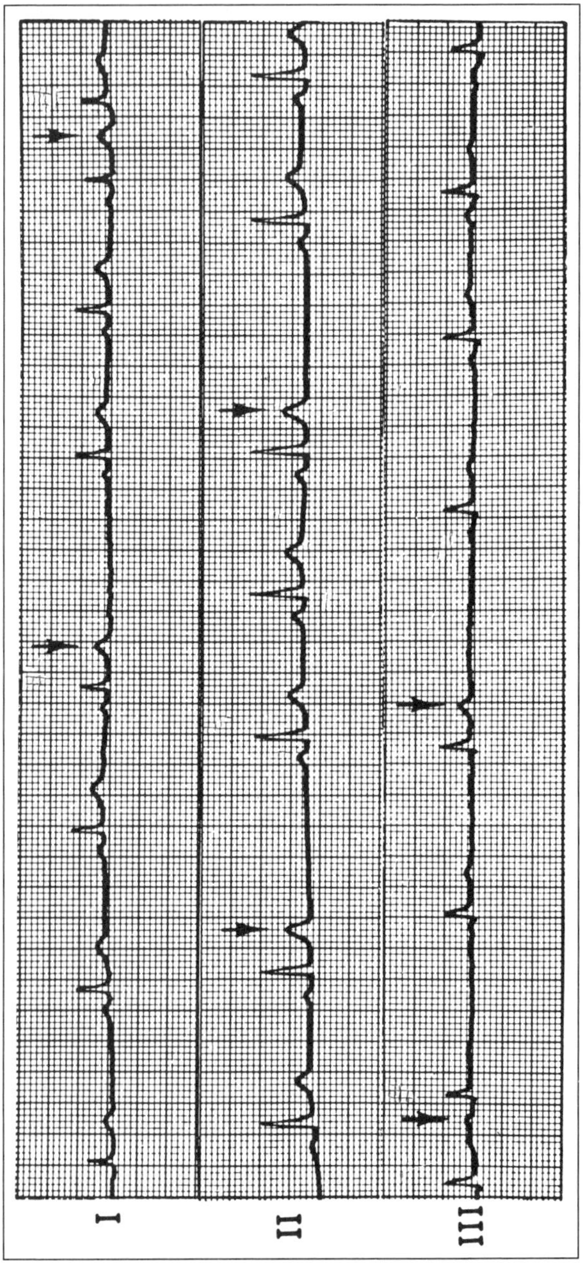


**Fig. 5–2.** Sinus rhythm with frequent APCs (indicated by arrows), and most APCs are *not* conducted to the ventricles (blocked or nonconducted APCs).

**Configuration and Mean Axis of the Ectopic P Wave:** The configuration of the P wave of the APC is usually different from that of the P wave of sinus origin. The configuration varies depending upon the location of the ectopic focus. The ectopic P wave will resemble the P wave of sinus origin when the ectopic focus is located near the sinus node. Conversely, the ectopic P wave may be conducted in a retrograde fashion when the ectopic focus is located in the posterior portion of the left atrium. In this case, differential diagnosis from AV junctional premature contraction (AV JPC) will be difficult.

**P-R Interval, and Nonconducted Atrial Premature Contraction:** The P-R interval in an APC largely depends upon the status of the AV conduction system and the degree of the prematurity. In the normal AV conduction system, the P-R interval of the APC is generally between 0.12 and 0.20 second, unless the coupling interval (the interval from the ectopic beat to the preceding beat of the basic rhythm) is very short. When there is impaired AV conduction of the basic rhythm, the P-R interval of an APC is often prolonged, and, sometimes, a nonconducted (blocked) APC may result (Fig. 5–2).

There are several other mechanisms that may be responsible for the occurrence of the prolonged P-R interval of APCs and nonconducted (blocked) APC. A prolonged P-R interval and nonconducted ectopic P wave occur when an APC appears so early during the cycle that the atrial impulse reaches the AV junction during the relative and absolute refractory periods, respectively. In addition, a prolonged P-R interval of an APC or a nonconducted APC may occur when the cardiac cyclic length immediately preceding the coupling interval is long. This occurs because the refractory phase of the AV conduction tissue is directly influenced by the duration of the cardiac cycle. This ECG finding is called "Ashman's phenomenon" (Chapter 11).

**Postectopic Pause (Returning Cycle):** It is common to observe a postectopic pause following an APC, but the pause is *not* a full compensatory pause (Fig. 5–2), which is almost the rule in a VPC. The postectopic pause following an APC occurs for the following reason. The impulse from the atrial premature focus activates the entire atria, including the sinus node. The sinus node is prematurely discharged by the ectopic atrial impulse, and the sinus node is temporarily suppressed. Consequently, the pause following the APC (returning cycle) is longer than the P-P cycle of the basic rhythm, but the sinus P-P interval including the APC is shorter than twice the P-P cycle of the basic rhythm. Thus, a full compensatory pause does not occur in this circumstance (Fig. 5–3). In addition, the postectopic pause is also due to the interference within the sinus node or the SA junction. Under these circumstances, an APC may be followed by a full compensatory pause.

Occasionally, an APC may be associated with a full compensatory pause. This is observed when the impulse from the atrial premature focus occurs late in the cycle (prematurity of the ectopic P wave is slightly earlier than the basic sinus cycle) of the basic rhythm so that the sinus node discharges the impulse as usual before the ectopic impulse reaches the sinus node (Fig. 5–3). In this case, interference between the sinus and ectopic impulses occurs near the SA junction or in the atria. This interference may produce an atrial fusion beat (Fig. 5–3). By and large, a full compensatory pause is apt to occur when the rate of the basic rhythm is rapid. From the above observations, the degree of prematurity of the APC and the rate of the basic rhythm influence greatly the postectopic pause.

On rare occasions, an APC may be interpolated. The exact mechanism for the genesis of this phenomenon is not clearly known. However, some form of protection block, which is similar to the mechanism for the production of parasystole, around the sinus node is considered to be present in order to continuously protect the sinus impulse discharge. Even in the interpolated APC, the sinus P-P interval that includes the APC is usually slightly longer than the P-P cycle of the basic rhythm.

**Constant Coupling Intervals:** The coupling interval of an APC is usually constant (Fig. 5–1). This occurs because the ectopic P wave depends upon the basic rhythm in some way that is different from atrial parasystole. In the latter case, the coupling intervals vary throughout the tracing because the parasystole produces an independent rhythm (Chapter 22). Although a constant coupling interval is a general rule in

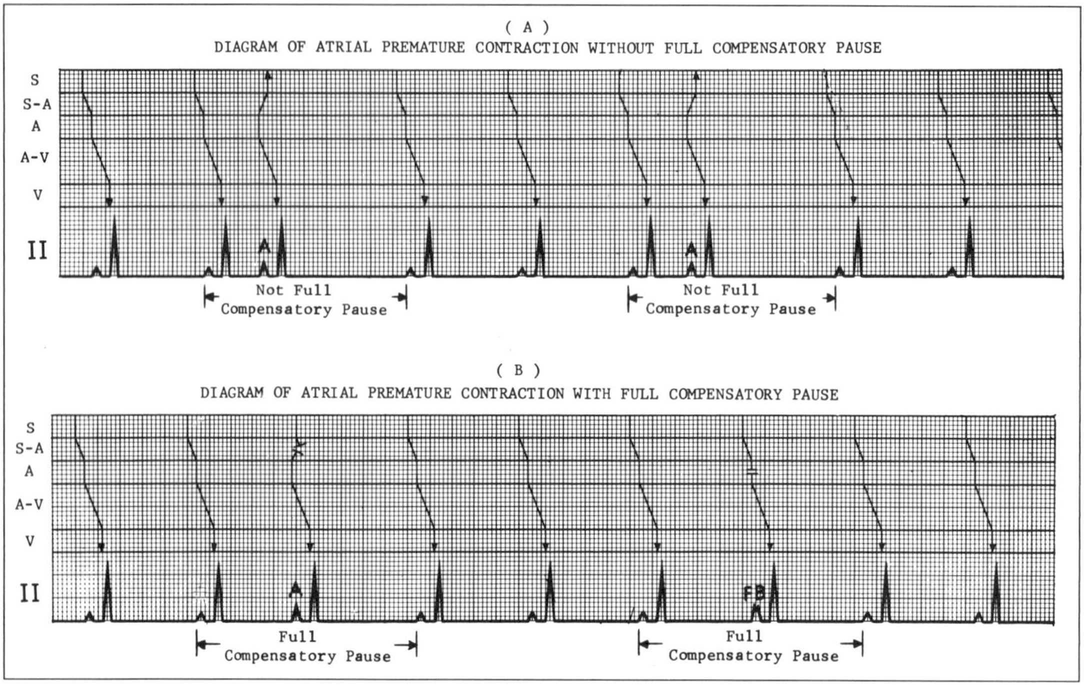


**Fig. 5–3. A.** Atrial premature contraction (A) without full compensatory pause. **B.** Atrial premature contraction (A) with full compensatory pause. Full compensatory pause is observed as long as the sinus node is not prematurely activated by the ectopic impulse. An atrial fusion beat (FB) is observed when interference between sinus and ectopic impulses occurs in the atria. S = sinus; SA = SA junction; A = atria; AV = AV junction; V = ventricles.

APC, it may vary slightly without having a parasystolic mechanism. In general, variation of the coupling interval is slightly more pronounced in APCs than in VPCs.

**Configuration of the QRS Complex:** It is known that an abnormal and wide QRS complex occurs when the impulse traverses the ventricles during a relative or nearly absolute refractory period of the intraventricular conduction system. This is termed "aberrant ventricular conduction." APC may be followed by aberrant ventricular conduction when the coupling interval is very short or when there is an Ashman's phenomenon. The degree of aberrant conduction depends upon the degree of prematurity and the status of the intraventricular conduction system. Thus, aberrant ventricular conduction may occur in a markedly impaired intraventricular conduction system even when the coupling interval is not too short. The pattern of the ventricular aberration may vary. In general, the shorter the coupling interval of an APC, the greater the tendency for aberrant ventricular conduction (Fig. 5–4). Besides the degree of prematurity of the APC and the status of the conduction system, another factor is often responsible for aberrant ventricular conduction. The longer the duration of the cardiac cyclic length immediately preceding the coupling interval, the greater is the degree of ventricular aberration (Fig. 5–5). This occurs even when the coupling intervals are precisely constant. For this reason, aberrant ventricular conduction frequently occurs after atrial bigeminy is established (Fig. 5–5). This ECG finding is Ashman's phenomenon (Chapters 10 and 11). For a similar reason, the QRS complex following an APC may show a true BBB when the bundle branch system has impaired conduction. This is a form of rate-dependent BBB. Aberrant

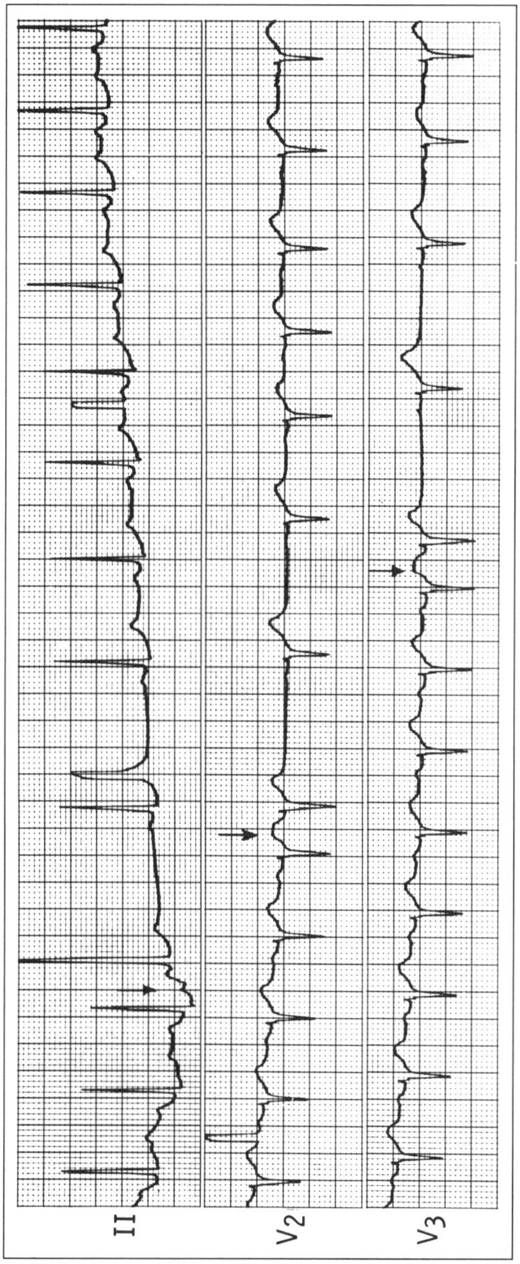


**Fig. 5–4.** Sinus rhythm and occasional APCs (indicated by arrows) with aberrant ventricular conduction because of a short coupling interval.

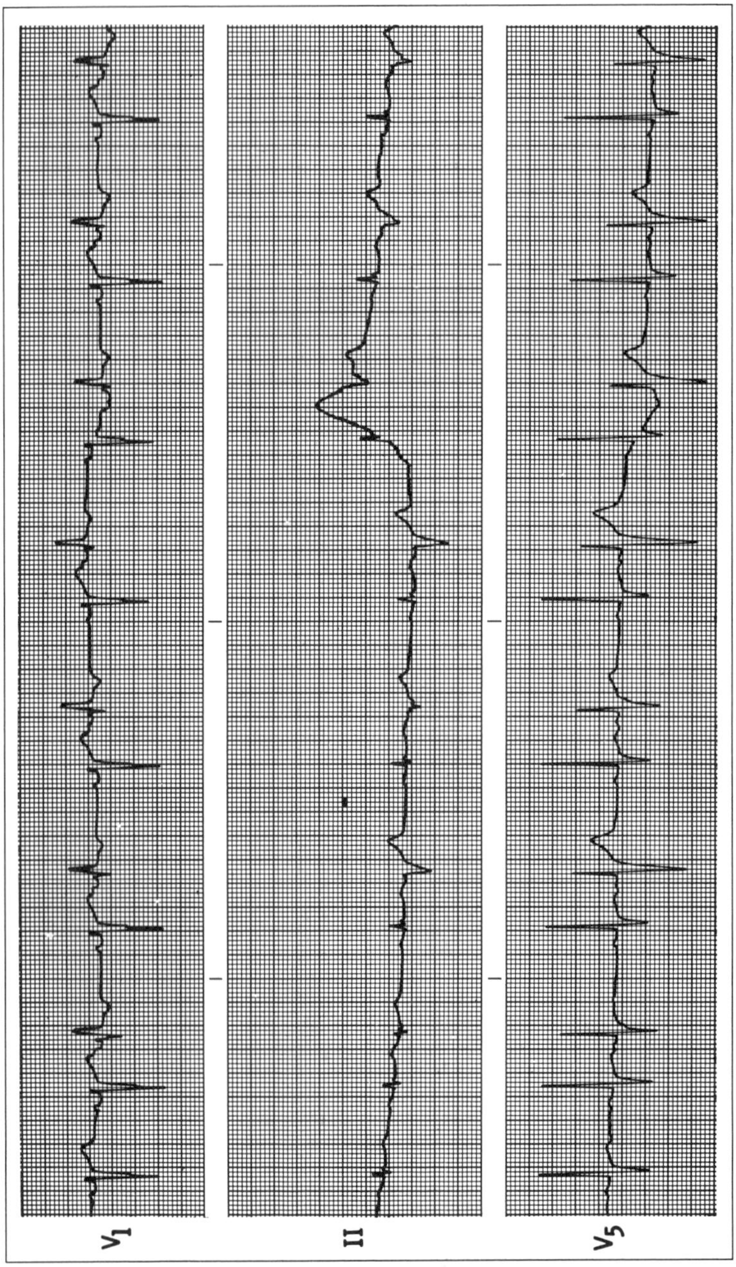


**Fig. 5–5.** Sinus rhythm and frequent APCs producing atrial bigeminy with aberrant ventricular conduction as a result of Ashman's phenomenon.

ventricular conduction in APCs closely resembles VPCs, but a prematurely appearing P wave preceding the QRS complex is a diagnostic clue for the former (Figs. 5–4 and 5–5).

**Aberrant Atrial Conduction (Chung's Phenomenon):** Not uncommonly, the P wave of the basic rhythm immediately following an APC shows a bizarre configuration that is different from the P wave of an APC or of sinus origin (Fig. 5–6). This is termed "aberrant atrial conduction" (Chung's phenomenon). Aberrant atrial conduction occurs because the refractory period in the atria is altered immediately following an APC.

**Frequency of Atrial Premature Contraction:** An APC may appear as an isolated beat, but it may appear alternatively with the basic rhythm (atrial bigeminy) (Fig. 5–5), as every third beat (atrial trigeminy), or as every fourth beat (atrial quadrigeminy). It also may appear consecutively as 2 or more beats, called group beats. When APCs appear as 3 or more consecutive beats, some authors call this a short run of AT, but, in general, AT is used when 6 or more APCs occur consecutively.

APCs may originate from more than one focus and produce an ectopic P wave of different configuration with different coupling intervals. They are termed "multifocal APCs."

## Mechanism

An APC is produced by the same mechanism as a VPC, and a detailed description is found in Chapter 7.

## Clinical Significance

Atrial premature contraction may occur in apparently healthy individuals as well as in those with diseased hearts. Occasional APCs are usually insignificant clinically. However, frequently appearing (every 6 beats or more) or group beats may lead to AT, atrial flutter, or AF. When APCs are due to CHF, they usually disappear after digitalization. It should be noted that APCs may also be induced by digitalis. By and large, no active treatment is necessary for APCs as long as the arrhythmia is asymptomatic.

APCs, particularly those multifocal in origin, are very common in chronic obstructive pulmonary disease (COPD). In addition, APCs are not uncommon in various organic heart diseases, but they may be induced by excessive consumption of coffee or alcohol and cigarette smoking.

# ATRIAL TACHYCARDIA

Atrial tachycardia (AT), like APCs, may originate from any location in the atria other than the sinus node. In uncomplicated AT, the ectopic focus activates the entire atria, including the sinus node. Thus, the sinus node is activated prematurely and loses its inherent pacemaking function as long as the AT persists. It is common to observe a long pause after termination of AT until the sinus node regains its pacemaking function. The propagation of the impulse in the atria in AT is usually different from that found in sinus rhythm, but conduction below the AV node is the same as in normal sinus rhythm. In uncomplicated AT, each ectopic P wave is followed by a QRS complex unless the atrial rate is extremely rapid. The QRS complex in AT is usually normal, but it is not uncommon to observe a wide and bizarre QRS complex either because of aberrant ventricular conduction, or preexisting BBB. Atrial tachycardia may originate from more than 1 ectopic focus and produce MAT. Atrial tachycardia frequently occurs in paroxysms but may become chronic, particularly in the presence of chronic cor pulmonale or DI.

## Diagnostic Criteria

By definition, 6 or more consecutive APCs are considered sufficient for the diagnosis of AT (Fig. 5–7), although some investigators believe that 3 or more consecutive APCs can be considered as short runs of AT.

**Configuration of the P Waves:** The configuration of the P wave in AT is usually different from that of the sinus P wave. The configura-

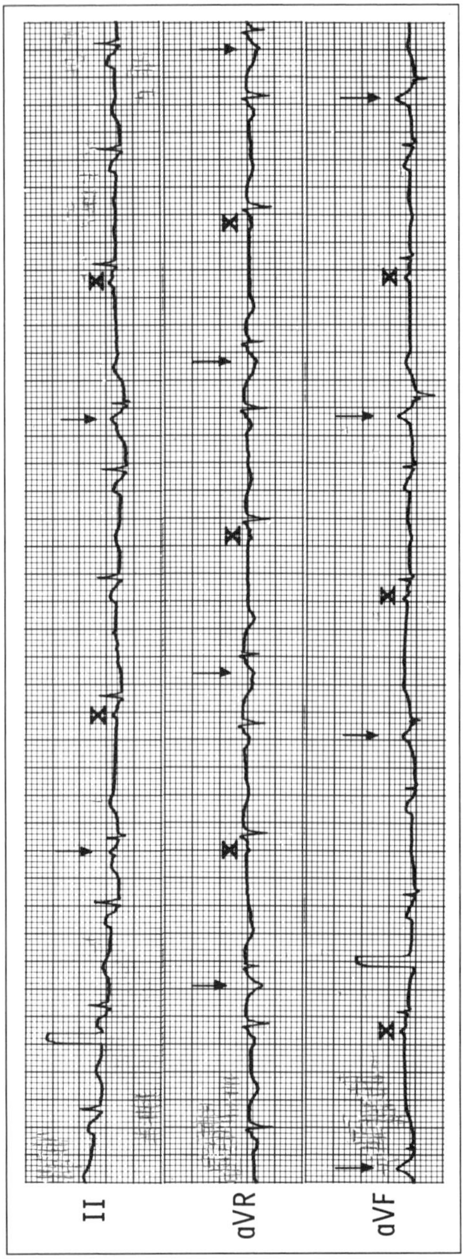


**Fig. 5–6.** Sinus rhythm with frequent APCs (indicated by arrows) followed by aberrant atrial conduction (Chung's phenomenon, marked X).

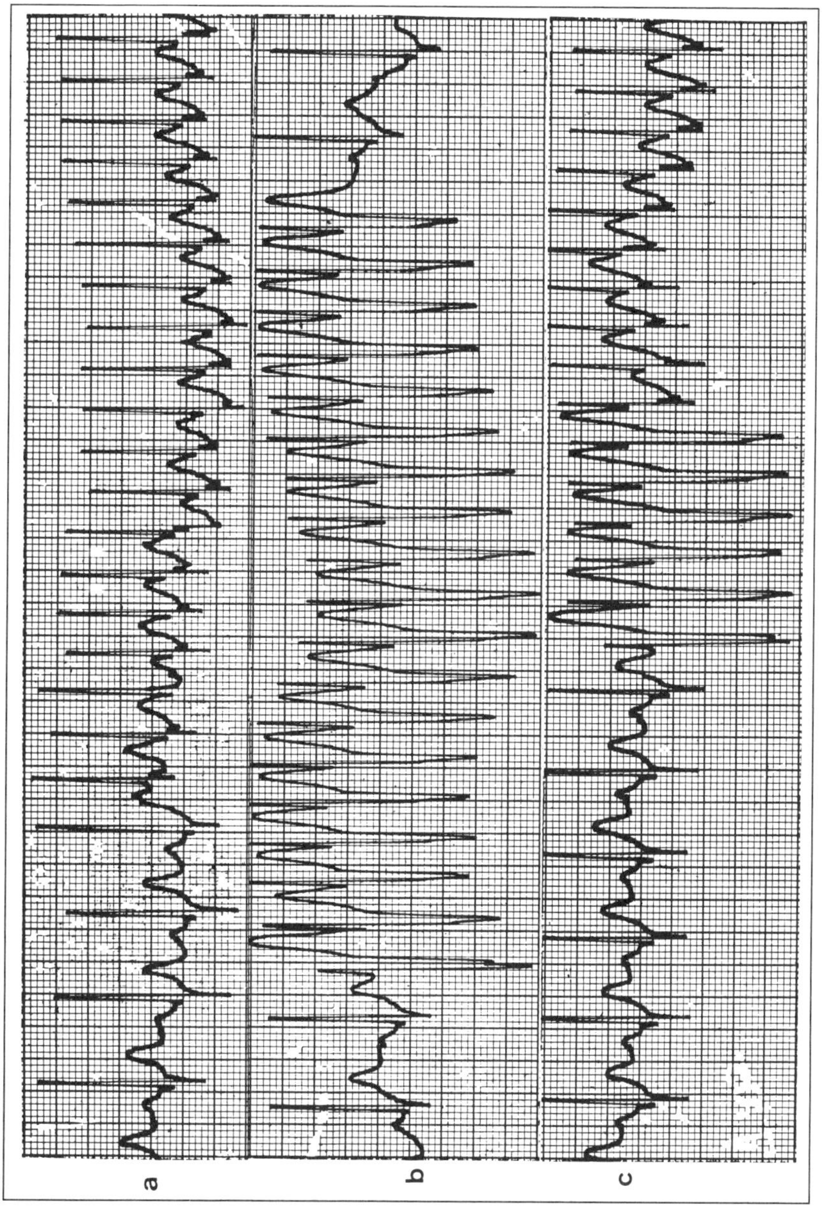


**Fig. 5–7.** The Holter monitor ECG rhythm strips a, b, and c are *not* continuous. The rhythm is sinus tachycardia and PAT (rate: 214 beats/min) with aberrant ventricular conduction of varying degree.

tion varies depending upon the location of the ectopic focus, but in most AT, the ectopic P wave is often upright in lead II and inverted in lead aVR, as in sinus rhythm. It should be pointed out that it is not unusual to observe a false absence of an ectopic P wave in AT because the P wave may be superimposed on a portion of the ST segment, the T wave, the U wave, or the QRS complex of the preceding beat. When AT originates from more than 1 focus (MAT), the configuration and the axis of the ectopic P waves vary accordingly. A detailed description of MAT is given later in this chapter.

**Rates of P Wave and QRS Complex:** In general, the atrial rates in uncomplicated AT are between 160 and 250 beats/min (Fig. 5–7), but they may be as slow as 120–140 beats/min. In addition, AT may be unusually slow when the fundamental mechanism involved is parasystole (Chapter 22). The ventricular rates depend upon the atrial rate and the status of the AV conduction system. In uncomplicated AT with an atrial rate below 200 beats/min, the ventricular rate is the same as that of the atria because of 1:1 AV conduction. However, the ventricular rate is often half the atrial rate when the atrial rate is extremely rapid (faster than 200 beats/min) because of physiologic refractoriness in the AV junction. On the other hand, the ventricular rates vary markedly when a preexisting AV conduction defect exists.

**Relationship Between the P Wave and the QRS Complex:** In most cases of uncomplicated AT, the AV conduction shows a 1:1 ratio (Fig. 5–7) unless the atrial rate is extremely rapid. When the atrial rate is extremely rapid (usually more than 200 beats/min), every other P wave is conducted to the ventricle because of the longer refractory period in the AV junctional tissue. In this case, AT with 2:1 AV response will result. On the other hand, a preexisting AV conduction disturbance will produce a true AV block in the presence of AT. This is manifested by a relatively slower atrial rate (slower than 200 beats/min) with varying degrees (often Wenckebach type) of AV block (Fig. 5–8). The latter case is often found in DI. The P-R interval in AT depends upon the status of the AV conduction system and the atrial rate. Generally, the P-R interval is between 0.12 and 0.20 second in uncomplicated AT.

**Nature of Onset and Termination:** Atrial tachycardia commonly starts and ends abruptly in paroxysmal form. It is also common to find an isolated APC preceding the onset of PAT (Fig. 5–7). Paroxysmal atrial tachycardia is frequently associated with WPW (ventricular preexcitation) syndrome, and the rate is usually very rapid (Chapter 13). When the paroxysm of AT terminates, it is often followed by a long pause (Fig. 5–7), which is usually due to suppression of the sinus node by the ectopic atrial impulses.

Atrial tachycardia often becomes chronic in diseased hearts, particularly in DI. In addition, it is common to observe a coexisting AV block of varying degree in DI (Fig. 5–8).

**Regularity of P-P and R-R Cycles:** The P-P and R-R cycles are precisely regular in most uncomplicated AT, but they may be slightly irregular. It is not uncommon to observe that the P-P intervals vary significantly in short runs of AT, particularly during the first few beats, because of irregular discharge of the ectopic impulse.

**Configuration of QRS Complex:** Just as seen in APCs, the QRS complex in AT may have a wide and bizarre configuration if there is an extremely rapid ventricular rate. This occurs because the intraventricular conduction system is partially refractory because of the consecutive rapid impulses (Fig. 5–7). For similar reasons, AT may be associated with BBB. When AT is associated with a wide QRS complex, either due to aberrant ventricular conduction or BBB, it certainly resembles VT, particularly if the P wave is not clearly discernible.

## Mechanism

The mechanism of ordinary AT is closely related to that of an isolated premature contraction, atrial bigeminy, or atrial trigeminy. There is much clinical and experimental investigative evidence to support the close relationship between paroxysmal tachycardia and isolated or coupled premature beats (Chapter 7).

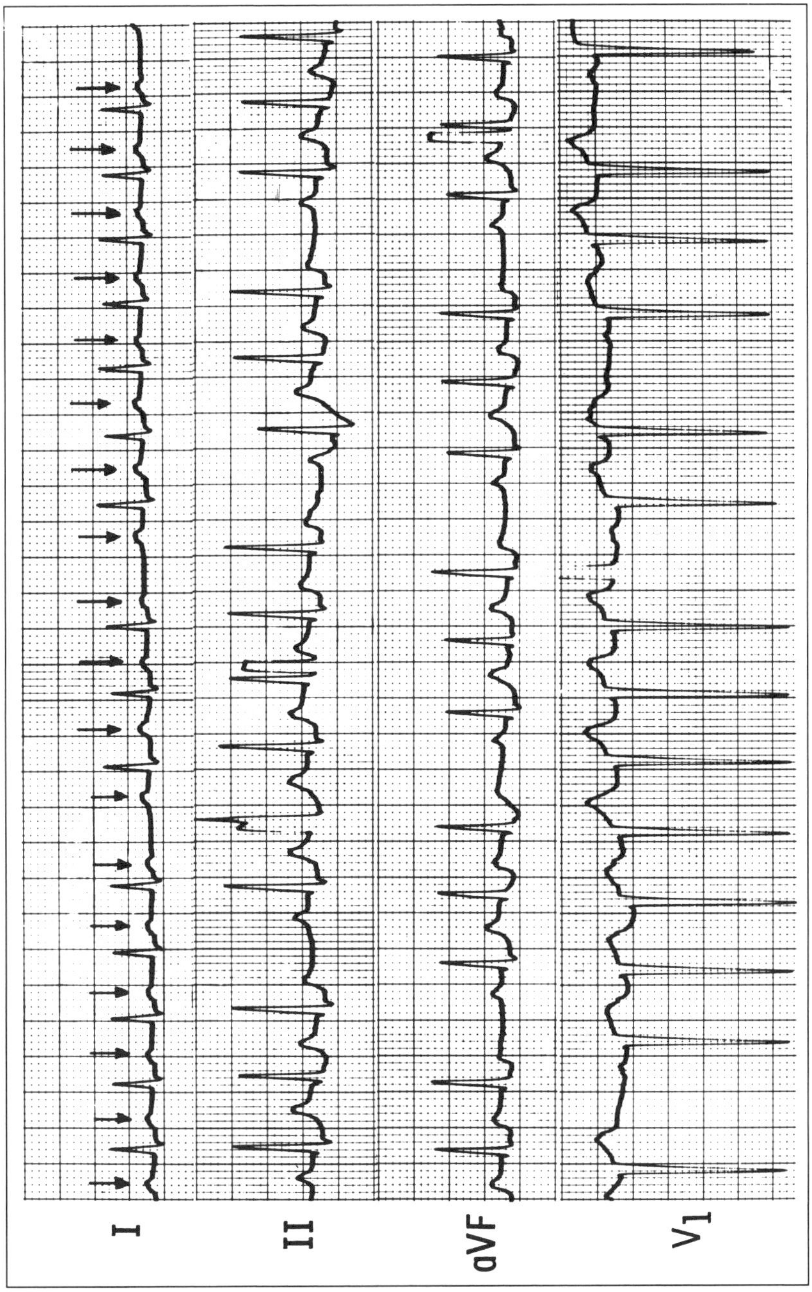


**Fig. 5–8.** Arrows indicate P waves. The rhythm is AT (atrial rate: 165 beats/min) with Wenckebach AV block induced by digitalis toxicity.

## Clinical Significance

Paroxysmal AT, as in APCs, may occur in healthy individuals as well as in those with diseased hearts. It has been shown that approximately 30% of all AT may be found in apparently healthy hearts, but the paroxysm is usually of short duration. On the other hand, the most common heart disease associated with AT is RHD, which accounts for about 30% of the total incidence of AT. The next most common heart disease associated with AT is probably mitral valve prolapse (MVP) syndrome. In addition, AT is not uncommon in CAD and DI. Atrial tachycardia comprises about 10–15% of the total digitalis-induced cardiac arrhythmias. Less commonly, AT may be associated with hypertensive heart disease, thyrotoxicosis, chronic or acute cor pulmonale, acute pericarditis, and various congenital heart diseases, such as atrial septal defect (ASD) and Eisenmenger's complex.

Most healthy subjects can tolerate PAT for long periods of time, unless the ventricular rate is very rapid. It has been shown that the cardiac output may drop when the ventricular rate is faster than 180 beats/min, even in normal individuals. Paroxysmal AT often terminates spontaneously, or otherwise, by CSS (Fig. 5–9) or the Valsalva maneuver. However, in diseased hearts, even a relatively slow ventricular rate may produce or aggravate CHF or angina pectoris because of a reduction of the cardiac output and coronary blood flow.

Various symptoms may be produced by AT, including palpitations, a tight feeling in the chest or actual chest pain, weakness, dizziness, anxiety, apprehension, or, at times, a feeling of impending death. True fainting episodes are rare. Beta-blocking agents (e.g., propranolol 10–20 mg 3–4 times daily) are often effective for PAT in various clinical circumstances.

# MULTIFOCAL ATRIAL TACHYCARDIA

Multifocal atrial tachycardia (MAT) deserves a separate discussion because of its distinctly different clinical significance in comparison with ordinary AT.

Multifocal AT has been called "repetitive multifocal paroxysmal atrial tachycardia," "chaotic atrial tachycardia or rhythm," and "wandering pacemaker in the atria" by different authors.

## Diagnostic Criteria

The ECG criteria for the diagnosis of MAT are as follows:

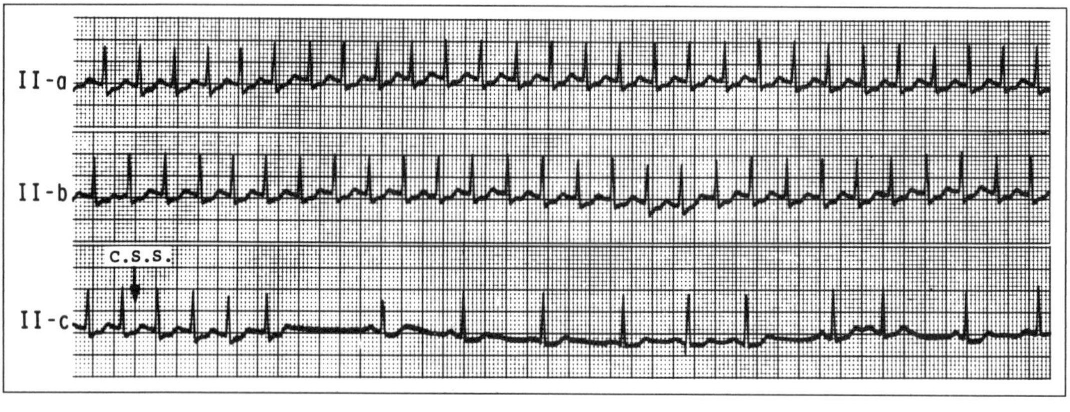


**Fig. 5–9.** Termination of supraventricular (probable atrial) tachycardia by CSS. Leads II-a, II-b, and II-c are continuous.

1. Two or more ectopic P waves with different configurations and with 2 or more different ectopic P-P cycles
2. Atrial rate between 100 and 250 beats/min (occasionally slower than 100 beats/min)
3. Isoelectrical line present between P-P intervals
4. Frequent occurrence of varying P-R intervals and AV block of varying degree (nonconducted ectopic P waves)

Multifocal AT often produces a relatively slow atrial rate and, thus, is different from an ordinary unifocal AT. The mode of the onset of MAT is usually not paroxysmal, another differential point. Similarly, the ventricular rate in MAT is often slower than in ordinary AT, probably because of the frequent association of AV block of varying degree, in addition to a slower atrial rate in the former. The ventricular rate in MAT may be as slow as 50–60 beats/min, but, in most cases, it ranges between 100 and 150 beats/min (Fig. 5–10).

The ectopic P waves in MAT are often peaked and tent-shaped because chronic pulmonary disease is a frequent underlying disorder (Fig. 5–10). Rarely, MAT may have an extremely rapid atrial rate that is slightly faster than 250 beats/min. In this case, aberrant ventricular conduction frequently occurs because of a partial refractory period in the intraventricular conduction system due to the rapid rate. Multifocal AT with aberrant ventricular conduction may resemble VT or even VF. The diagnosis of MAT can be made in this circumstance by identifying the ectopic P waves preceding the bizarre QRS complexes. Rarely, 2 atrial ectopic foci may produce a double AT, and in this case, 2 different P waves with 2 different P-P cycles occur periodically or alternately. Multifocal AT is often initiated by multifocal APCs.

### Mechanism

The mechanism of MAT is the same as that of ordinary unifocal AT except that there is more than 1 atrial ectopic focus.

### Clinical Significance

Multifocal AT is almost always found in seriously ill elderly individuals. The commonest underlying cause is COPD, which accounts for approximately 60–85%. In this circumstance, evidence of cor pulmonale is almost always present, and often intractable CHF exists. Digitalis intoxication seems to commonly coexist with MAT, but MAT is probably not digitalis-induced arrhythmia. On the other hand, digitalis often produces AV block of varying degree, leading to MAT with varying degree AV block. Coronary artery disease is an often underlying heart disease that is frequently associated with severe CHF. Multifocal AT is not uncommonly observed postoperatively after general anesthesia, and this is attributed to hypoxia. Less commonly, MAT may be observed in electrolyte imbalance, particularly hypokalemia, in pulmonary embolism, in hypertensive heart disease, valvular heart diseases, and septicemia.

Multifocal AT is often refractory to the usual management, and treatment of the underlying disease is more important than is the use of antiarrhythmic drugs. Since COPD is frequently the underlying pathology, improvement of pulmonary function and control of superimposed infection are usually more beneficial than various antiarrhythmic drugs.

## ATRIAL FLUTTER

Atrial flutter, like AT, may originate from any location in the atria outside of the sinus node. Atrial flutter may occur as a paroxysmal form, but more commonly it persists for months or years as a chronic form. Atrial flutter is less common than AF, its incidence being approximately one-tenth to one-twentieth that of AF. Most uncomplicated atrial flutters occur as a pure form and produce a characteristic flutter wave that has a sawtooth appearance. Occasionally, a form intermediate between pure atrial flutter and AF may occur, and this is termed "atrial flutter-fibrillation." It is also not uncommon to observe that atrial flutter may

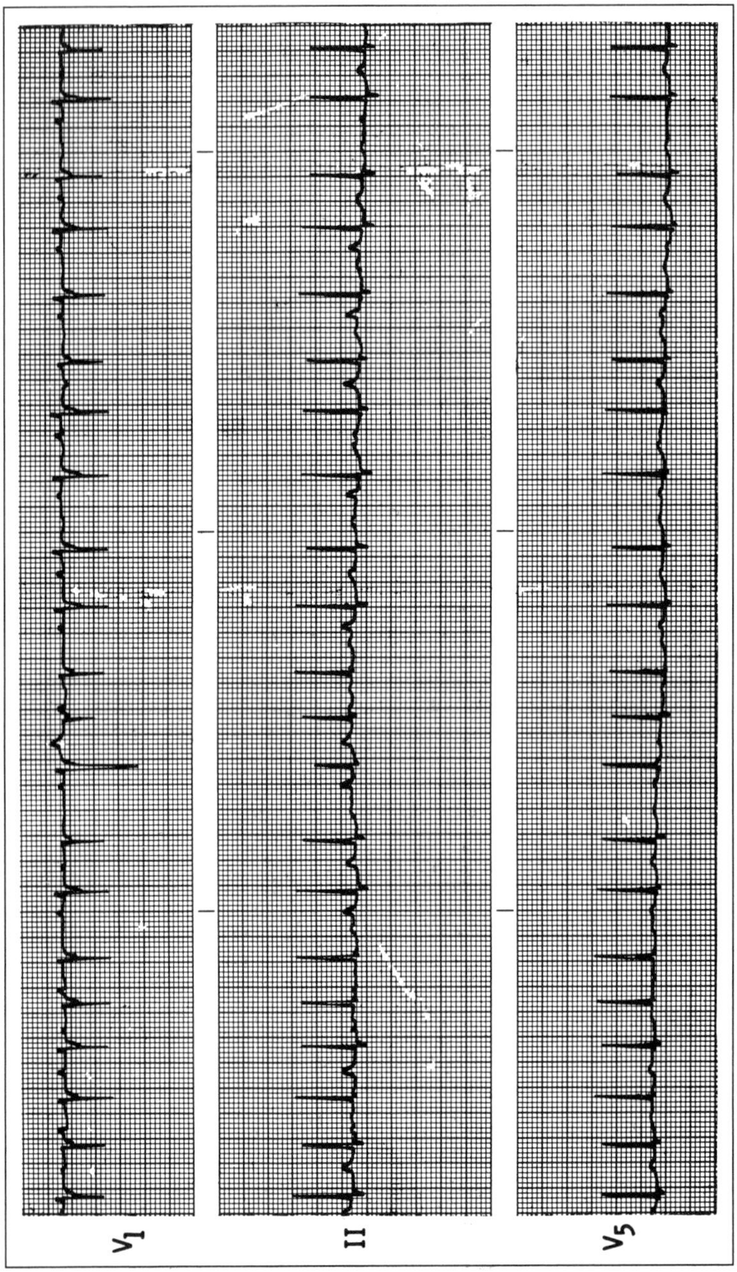


Fig. 5–10. Multifocal atrial tachycardia (MAT) with occasional aberrant ventricular conduction.

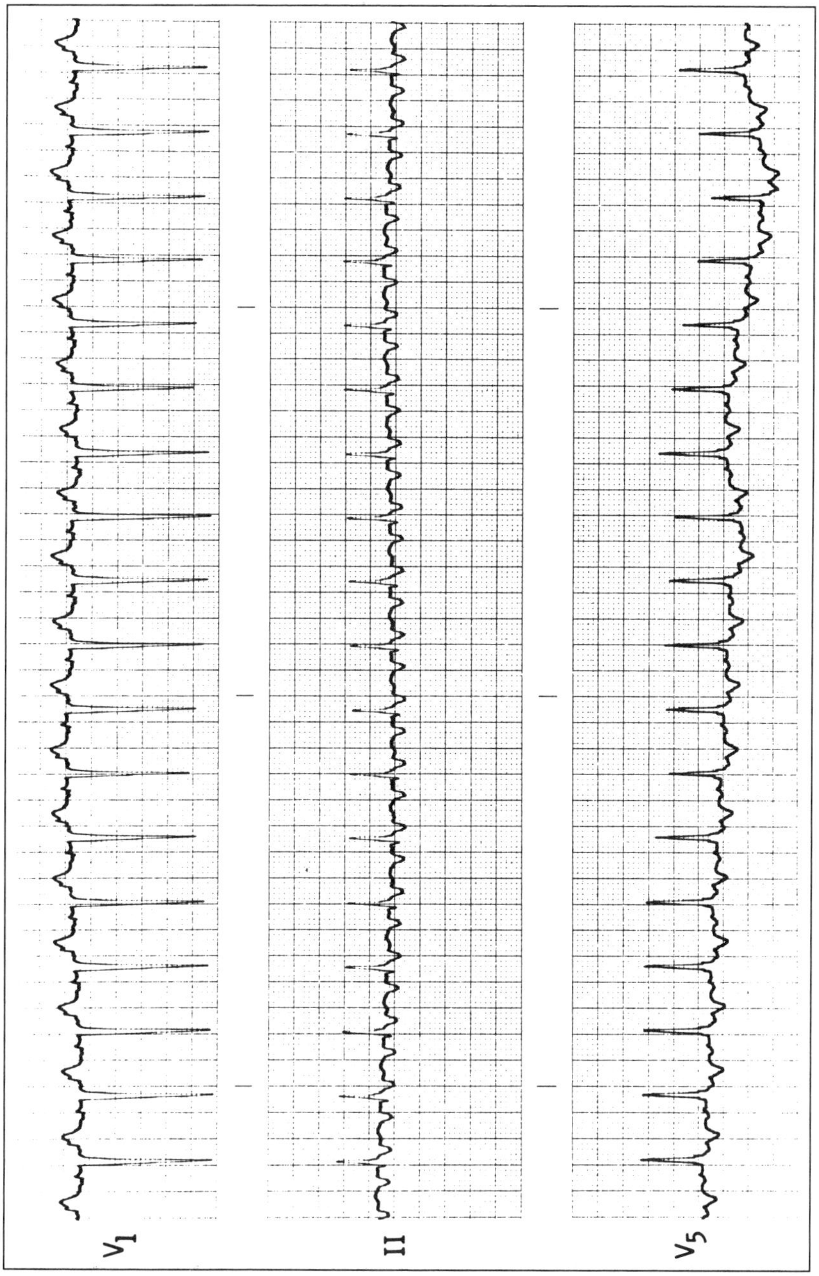


**Fig. 5–11.** Atrial flutter (atrial rate: 250 beats/min) with 2:1 AV response. The diagnosis of left ventricular hypertrophy (LVH) is obvious.

change to AF, or vice versa. This occurs either spontaneously or during the administration of digitalis or quinidine. Rarely, the direction of the atrial flutter wave may change. The atrial rate in pure atrial flutter is between 250 and 350 beats/min, but it may be slower than 200 beats/min. Rarely, the atrial rate may be as slow as 120–130 beats/min, particularly during quinidine therapy. Untreated atrial flutter almost always shows a 2:1 AV response (Fig. 5–11) because the AV junctional tissue is unable to conduct the rapid atrial rate. This occurs because of the longer refractory period in the AV junctional tissue. Thus, the ventricular rate of most untreated atrial flutters is between 150 and 175 beats/min. After treatment, particularly digitalization, the ventricular rate becomes slower because an AV block of varying degree is induced. Atrial flutter with 1:1 AV response is extremely rare.

The QRS complex in atrial flutter is usually normal in configuration, but it may have a wide and bizarre appearance because of aberrant ventricular conduction due to the rapid rate.

Atrial flutter may be initiated by an isolated APC, and it may be transformed from AF or AT.

## Diagnostic Criteria

Atrial flutter produces characteristic flutter waves, but at times it is difficult to identify them when the flutter wave is superimposed on a portion of the ST segment, T wave, or even the QRS complex.

**Configuration of the Flutter Wave:** In pure atrial flutter, the flutter wave is composed of 2 components directed in opposite directions. The first portion corresponds to the P wave of atrial depolarization, followed by the second portion, which is the Ta wave of atrial repolarization. These 2 components of the flutter wave produce the characteristic sawtooth or picket-fence appearance (Fig. 5–11). The flutter wave is not symmetric. Frequently, the negative portion of the flutter wave is more pronounced, so that it has the appearance of inverted flutter waves in leads II, III, and aVF. A typical flutter wave (sawtooth appearance) may appear in all leads, but leads II, III, aVF, and $V_{1-2}$ exhibit the most prominent flutter waves. It is not uncommon to observe that only 1 or 2 leads (usually leads II and/or $V_1$) show an atrial flutter wave and the remaining leads show a poorly defined atrial mechanism.

**Atrial and Ventricular Rates:** By definition, the atrial rates in pure atrial flutter range between 250 and 350 beats/min (Fig. 5–11), but the atrial rate may be altered by CSS or certain drugs. Quinidine or procainamide (Pronestyl) commonly produces a slowing of the flutter cycle (Fig. 5–12). Conversely, digitalization or CSS may enhance the flutter cycle. Thus, the atrial rate may be slower than 200 beats/min and faster than 350 beats/min under these circumstances.

The term "atrial impure flutter" has been used when the rate of the flutter cycle is between 350 and 400 beats/min. In this case, the flutter cycle is generally regular.

The ventricular rates in atrial flutter depend upon the rate of the atrial flutter cycle and the status of the AV conduction system. The ventricular rates in untreated atrial flutter are almost always half of the atrial rate (Fig. 5–11) unless the atrial rate is unusually slow. This occurs because the AV junctional tissue is unable to conduct every atrial impulse due to its longer refractory period. Thus, the usual ventricular rates in untreated atrial flutter range between 125 and 175 beats/min. Occasionally, the ventricular rate is the same as the atrial one, which results in a faster ventricular rate with 1:1 AV response. In this case, the ventricular rate is around 250 beats/min. In extremely rare instances, the ventricular rate may be as rapid as 300 beats/min during 1:1 AV conduction.

On the other hand, the ventricular rate may be much slower than the atrial rate in atrial flutter when there is a preexisting AV conduction disturbance or when AV block is induced by various drugs, such as digitalis. In this circumstance, the ventricular rate is usually between 65 and 85 beats/min. Rarely, the ventricular rate may become extremely slow when there is an AV block of higher degree.

**Atrial Flutter Cycles:** The flutter cycle in untreated pure atrial flutter is precisely regular

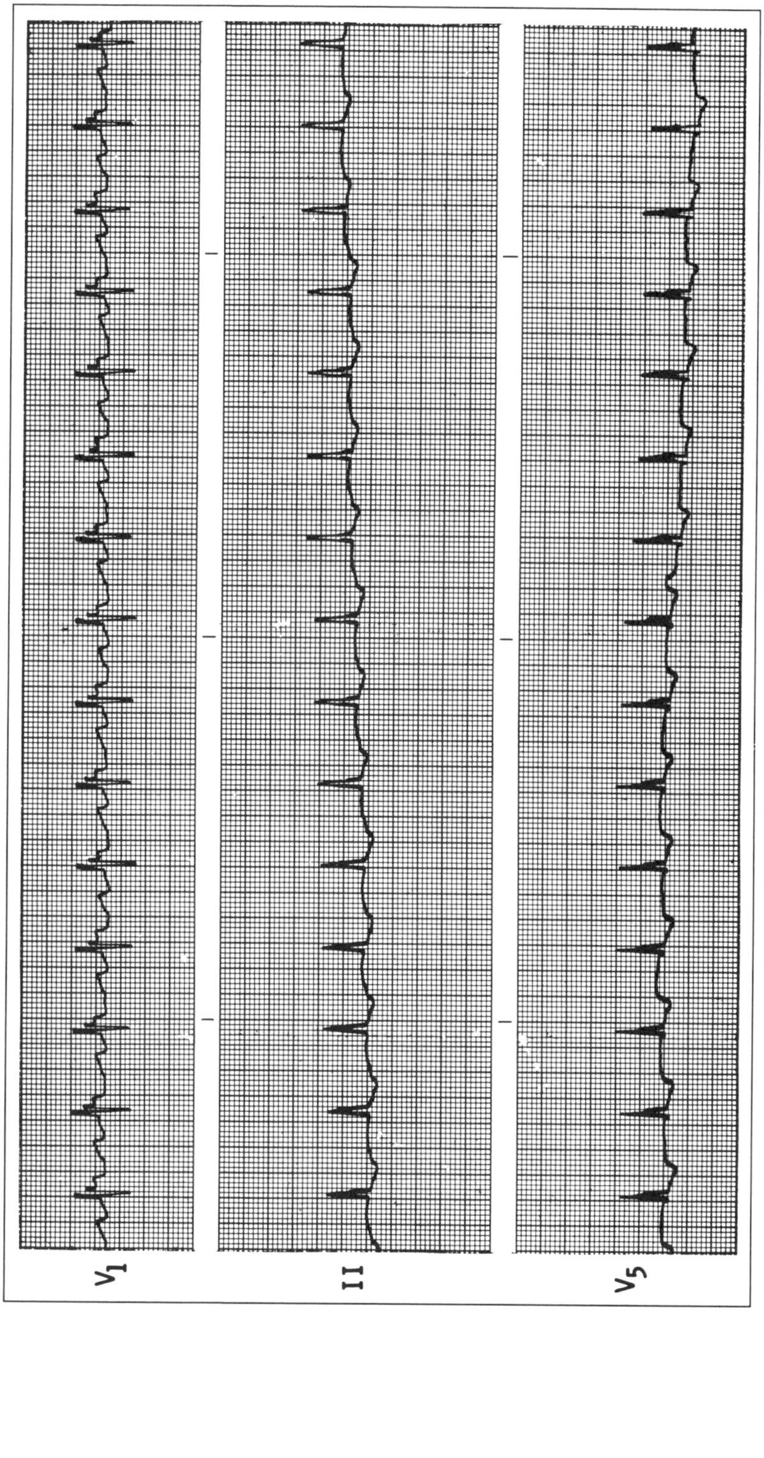


Fig. 5–12. Atrial flutter (atrial rate: 180 beats/min) with 2:1 AV conduction. Markedly slow atrial flutter cycle is due to quinidine effect.

(Fig. 5–11). Occasionally, the flutter cycle is irregular when the underlying heart disease is idiopathic cardiomyopathy, or it becomes irregular and slows during the administration of quinidine or procainamide. The flutter cycle may become slightly irregular and faster during digitalization or CSS, particularly in transition from atrial flutter to AF. An irregular flutter cycle also occurs during a short paroxysm of atrial flutter until the rhythm is well established.

**Relationship Between Atrial Flutter Wave and QRS Complex:** An exact measurement of the AV conduction time (F-R interval) in atrial flutter is difficult because the onset of the flutter wave cannot be precisely determined. However, it is possible to determine any alteration of the F-R interval in a relative way, by measuring from homologous peaks (either positive or negative) of the flutter wave to the onset of the QRS complex.

The AV ratio in most untreated flutters is usually 2:1 because of the physiologic refractory period in the AV junctional tissue (Fig. 5–11). Occasionally, the AV ratio is 1:1 in infants or during exercise, excitement, or administration of quinidine or procainamide in adults. In this case, the atrial rate is relatively slow (around 250 beats/min). On rare occasions, 1:1 AV conduction may occur in spite of an extremely rapid rate (around 300 beats/min). This is almost always associated with WPW syndrome or hyperthyroidism.

When a preexisting AV conduction disturbance is present or when AV block is induced by various drugs, such as digitalis, the AV ratio is almost always 4:1 (Fig. 5–13) and occasionally 6:1. An odd AV ratio, such as 3:1 or 5:1, in atrial flutter is extremely rare.

**Nature of Onset and Termination:** Atrial flutter may have a paroxysmal form, but it occurs much less commonly than AF or AT. Thus, atrial flutter frequently occurs as a chronic form and may last for many months or years. Atrial flutter may be initiated by an isolated APC, and it may change to AF or AT. Atrial flutter may terminate spontaneously and convert to sinus rhythm.

**Configuration of QRS Complex:** The QRS complex in uncomplicated atrial flutter is normal (Figs. 5–11, 5–12, and 5–13) unless the ventricular rate is extremely rapid. A wide and bizarre QRS complex may occur in atrial flutter when the ventricular rate is extremely rapid, particularly during 1:1 AV conduction because of aberrant ventricular conduction. This occurs when rapid atrial impulses reach the ventricles during the relative refractory period of the intraventricular conduction system. On the other hand, wide QRS complexes may be observed in atrial flutter when preexisting or rate-dependent BBB appears, and the QRS complex may be wide in atrial flutter because of WPW syndrome. Atrial flutter with a wide QRS complex often resembles VT.

## Mechanism

The fundamental mechanism responsible for the production of atrial flutter is still not settled. There are 4 theories concerning the genesis of atrial flutter, but none of them is proven or excluded at present in spite of extensive investigative works. The 4 theories are (1) the theory of circus movement, (2) the theory of multiple reentry phenomenon, (3) the theory of unifocal impulse formation, and (4) the theory of multifocal impulse formation. Detailed descriptions of these theories are given later in this chapter.

## Clinical Significance

Atrial flutter is almost always observed in diseased hearts in both the paroxysmal and chronic forms. The chronic form of atrial flutter only occurs in various organic heart diseases. However, paroxysmal atrial flutter may occur occasionally in apparently healthy subjects, particularly from emotional stress, excessive consumption of coffee or alcohol, and so on.

Atrial flutter may occur transiently for only a few seconds or minutes, but it may last for many months or even years.

Atrial flutter is most commonly encountered in rheumatic (particularly mitral stenosis), coronary, and hypertensive heart disease. Less commonly, atrial flutter may be associated with

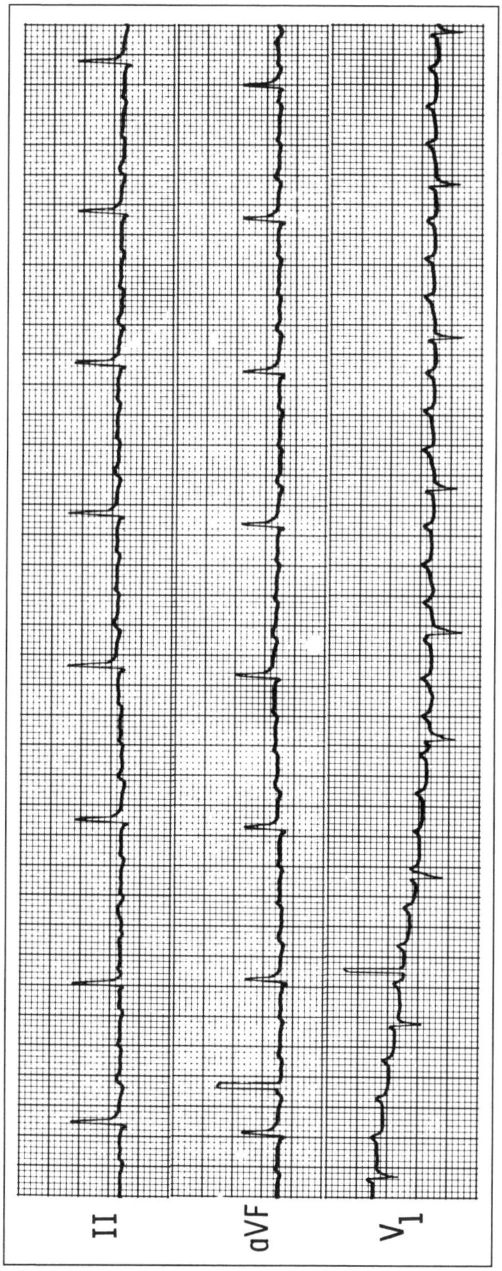


**Fig. 5–13.** Atrial flutter (atrial rate: 230 beats/min) with predominantly 4:1 AV block. This is slower than the usual atrial flutter cycle because of quinidine effect.

thyrotoxicosis, WPW syndrome, and cardiomyopathy, and rarely it may be associated with pulmonary embolism, chest trauma, pericarditis, myocarditis, congenital heart disease, and diphtheria. Atrial flutter may be induced by DI, but this is very rare. It has been reported that atrial flutter may develop during the administration of quinidine or procainamide in the treatment of AF. This is considered to be a result of a prolongation of the effective refractory period in the atria, leading to slower atrial conduction. The atrial flutter may continue when the effect of the quinidine or procainamide subsides, but continuous administration of these drugs frequently converts atrial flutter to sinus rhythm.

Untreated atrial flutter nearly always has a rapid ventricular rate in both healthy and diseased hearts. However, the ventricular rate in atrial flutter may be slow in elderly individuals even without any treatment. A rapid ventricular rate in atrial flutter is very common during acute CHF and/or acute MI.

The symptoms and signs in atrial flutter depend upon the presence or absence of heart disease, the nature of the heart disease, and the ventricular rate and duration of the atrial flutter. When the ventricular rate is relatively slow, the patient may not be aware of the presence of atrial flutter because symptoms are absent.

There is a great tendency to develop CHF because atrial flutter frequently occurs in elderly individuals with advanced heart disease, and the ventricular rate is usually rapid. When there is 1:1 AV conduction in atrial flutter, acute CHF almost always develops because of the extremely rapid ventricular rate. It has been shown that CHF occurs in one third to one half of patients with atrial flutter.

Palpitation is nearly always present, and various signs and symptoms of CHF develop. Angina pectoris is not uncommon in atrial flutter because of the reduced coronary blood flow due to a low cardiac output. For a similar reason, mental disturbances, including confusion, psychosis, and fainting, may occur in atrial flutter because of a reduction in the cerebral blood flow.

The treatment of atrial flutter depends upon the underlying etiologic factors, including the nature of the heart disease, the presence or absence of CHF, metabolic abnormalities, and drug toxicity. When atrial flutter occurs transiently with a very short duration, specific therapy is not indicated. In general, digitalis is considered to be the drug of choice for atrial flutter with rapid ventricular response. In urgent or refractory atrial flutter, DC shock should be applied immediately, and DC shock is almost 100% effective for atrial flutter.

## ATRIAL FIBRILLATION

Atrial fibrillation (AF) is intimately related to atrial flutter in terms of the fundamental mechanism involved in its genesis, the underlying heart diseases, and the therapeutic response to various drugs and DC shock. Atrial fibrillation may change to atrial flutter, or vice versa, spontaneously. Digitalis often changes atrial flutter to AF, whereas quinidine frequently changes AF to atrial flutter shortly before conversion to sinus rhythm.

Atrial fibrillation, like AT or flutter, may originate from any location in the atria outside of the sinus node. It may occur as a paroxysmal form initially, but it often persists for many months or years.

The incidence of AF is 10–20 times higher than that of atrial flutter. In fact, AF is one of the most common cardiac arrhythmias encountered in adult life, and it is the most common underlying ectopic rhythm in humans.

Atrial fibrillation shows a characteristic grossly irregular ventricular rhythm with irregular and rapid atrial waves that replace the P waves. Thus, AF is the most common cause of absent P waves. The atrial rate in AF is usually impossible to count accurately on the ordinary ECG, but it is generally between 400 and 650 beats/min. Untreated AF almost always has a rapid ventricular rate (between 120 and 180 beats/min), and the ventricular rate usually slows with digitalization. The most remarkable response to digitalis is observed when AF with rapid ventricular response is treated. This is particularly true when AF is associated with acute CHF.

## Diagnostic Criteria

Characteristically, AF shows absence of the P wave on the ECG, and the irregular atrial oscillation waves replace the P waves (Fig. 5–14). Untreated AF always has an irregular ventricular rhythm, and in most cases, the ventricular rate is rapid (Fig. 5–14). The following features are considered necessary for the diagnosis of AF.

**Configuration of Fibrillation Wave and QRS Complex:** An AF wave has a varying configuration with a varying amplitude. In addition to the actual variation in configuration and amplitude, its variation becomes more exaggerated by the superimposition of the fibrillation wave on a portion of the ST segment, T wave, or U wave and QRS complex. The amplitude of the AF wave is usually smaller than that of an atrial flutter wave. The AF wave may be more prominent in some leads, and it may not be discernible in some leads. In general, leads II and $V_1$ show the most prominent AF wave. It has been shown that coarse AF (the amplitude of the fibrillation wave is more than 1 mm) tends to have a slower atrial rate (Fig. 5–15), whereas fine AF tends to have a faster atrial rate (Fig. 5–14).

The contour of the QRS complex also often varies from beat to beat because a portion of the AF wave may be superimposed. In addition, the configuration of the QRS complex further alters because of aberrant ventricular conduction of varying degree due to the irregular and rapid ventricular rate. Most commonly, aberrant ventricular conduction occurs in AF as a result of Ashman's phenomenon (Fig. 5–16) (Chapters 10 and 11). Consecutively occurring aberrant ventricular conduction closely simulates VT (Fig. 5–16). The QRS complex is obviously wide when there is preexisting BBB (Fig. 5–17).

**Atrial and Ventricular Rates:** In most instances of AF, the actual atrial rate is nearly impossible to determine. When the atrial rate is relatively slow, as in coarse AF or atrial flutter-fibrillation, it is possible to measure the atrial rate. Nevertheless, it is said that the atrial rate in AF is between 400 and 650 beats/min. The atrial rate tends to be slower in coarse AF, and it is faster in fine AF.

Untreated AF almost always has a rapid ventricular rate (Figs. 5–14 and 5–16) unless a preexisting AV block is present. Therefore, the average ventricular rate in AF ranges from 120 to 200 beats/min, and it may be as rapid as 250 beats/min.

**Relationship Between Atrial Fibrillation Wave and QRS Complex:** A grossly irregular ventricular cycle is one of the most characteristic features of uncomplicated AF (Figs. 5–14, 5–15, 5–16, and 5–17). The ventricles are under the control of rapid impulses generated by 1 or more ectopic foci in the atria. The ventricular response is always grossly irregular in AF unless AV dissociation exists.

**Nature of Onset and Termination:** Atrial fibrillation may occur in a paroxysmal form, but it frequently becomes a chronic form and lasts for many months or years. It may be initiated by an isolated APC, or it may be transformed from or to atrial flutter or AT. Atrial fibrillation may occur spontaneously during sinus rhythm and may terminate spontaneously.

**Aberrant Ventricular Conduction:** When the ventricular rate is rapid in AF, the QRS complex has a varying configuration because of aberrant ventricular conduction of varying degrees. When the aberrant ventricular conduction is marked, it may resemble VPCs or even VT (Fig. 5–16). Aberrant ventricular conduction is prone to develop when the ventricular rate is extremely rapid because the rapidly transmitting atrial impulses find the ventricles in the relatively refractory state. In addition, the aberrant ventricular conduction tends to occur and the degree of the aberration is more pronounced in ventricular complexes following a longer R-R interval, just before the appearance of a short R-R interval. In other words, the R-R interval immediately preceding a bout of rapid ventricular rhythm with aberrant ventricular conduction in AF is often long (Fig. 5–16). This occurs because the variability of the refractory period in the ventricles depends upon the irregularity of the cyclic length. It can be said that the longer the ventricular cycle (R-R interval), the longer the refractory period following it; the shorter the pause, the shorter the refractory period (Ashman's phenomenon; Chapters 10 and 11).

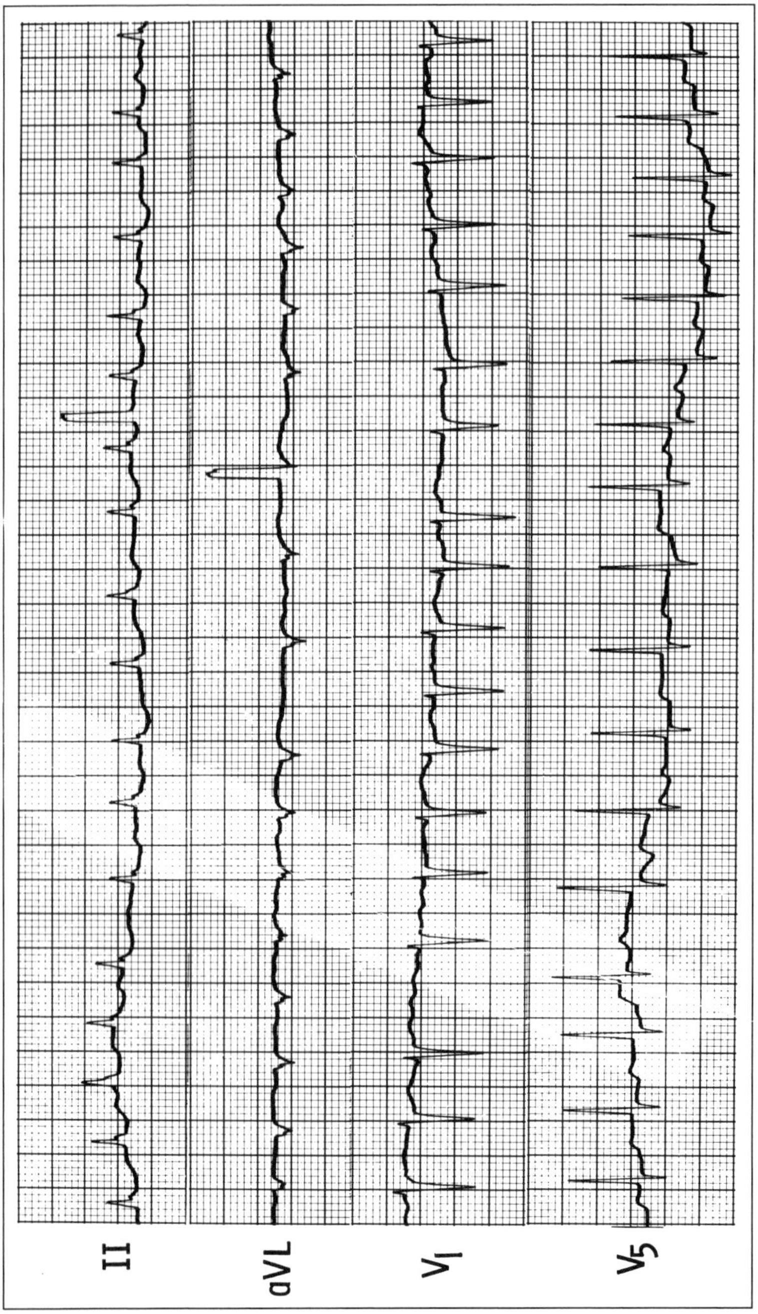


**Fig. 5–14.** Atrial fibrillation with rapid ventricular response (ventricular rate: 120–165 beats/min).

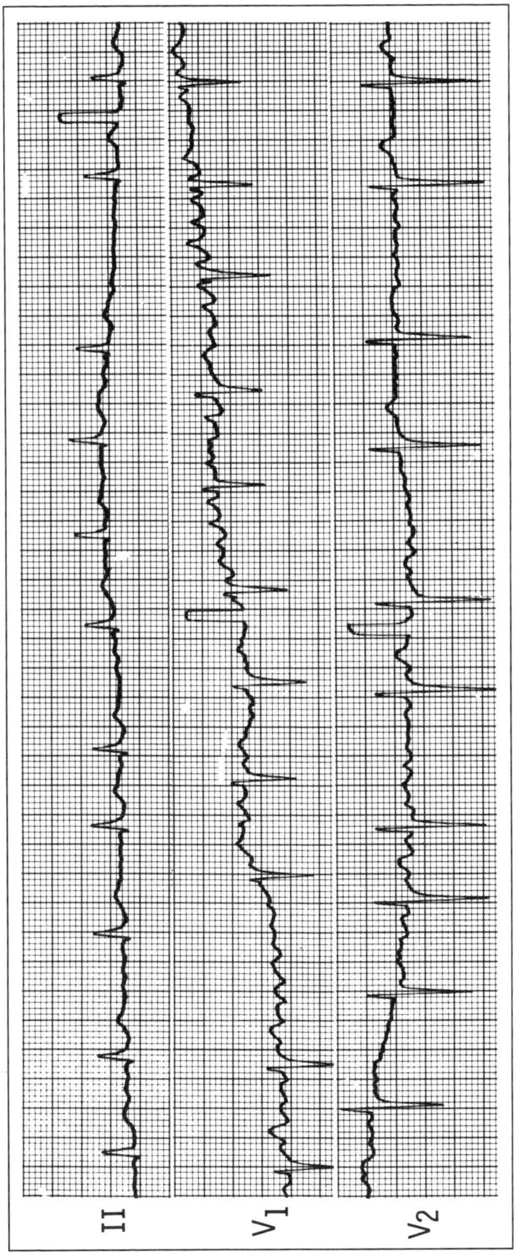


**Fig. 5–15.** Coarse AF indicative of left atrial enlargement (commonly due to mitral stenosis).

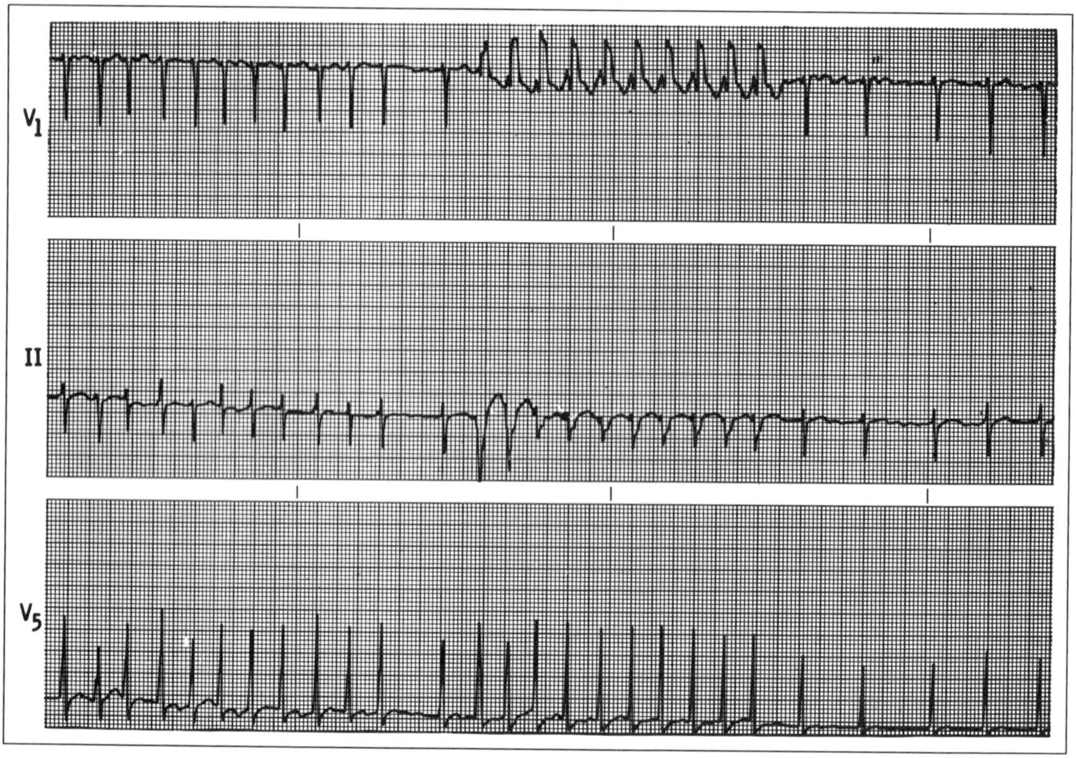


**Fig. 5–16.** Atrial fibrillation with consecutive aberrant ventricular conduction due to very rapid ventricular response (rate: 190–215 beats/min), initiated by Ashman's phenomenon.

The configuration of the QRS complex with aberrant ventricular conduction almost always shows RBBB pattern (Fig. 5–16). This occurs because the right bundle branch is more susceptible to a sudden variation of conductivity than is the left bundle branch.

## Mechanism

The fundamental mechanisms responsible for the production of AF and atrial flutter are intimately related. Therefore, the mechanisms of both AF and atrial flutter are discussed together at this time. In spite of extensive investigative studies regarding the genesis of AF and atrial flutter, the fundamental mechanism is still controversial. It is quite possible that a combination of various theories may be responsible for the production of these arrhythmias. Many theories have been proposed to explain the genesis of AF and atrial flutter, but among them, 4 theories are still considered to be strong possibilities. Nevertheless, none of these theories has been proven or excluded at the present time. The 4 theories are (1) the theory of circus movement, (2) the theory of multiple reentry phenomenon, (3) the theory of unifocal atrial impulse formation, and (4) the theory of multifocal atrial impulse formation.

**Theory of Circus Movement:** The theory of circus movement has been widely accepted as the mechanism responsible for AF and atrial flutter for many years.

The circus movement theory supposes that a primary impulse that activates the atria traverses a unidirectional, circular, and narrow path around the ostia of the superior and inferior venae cavae. This is called the "mother circus ring" (Fig. 5–18). Other atrial waves, which are centrifugally directed and which tra-

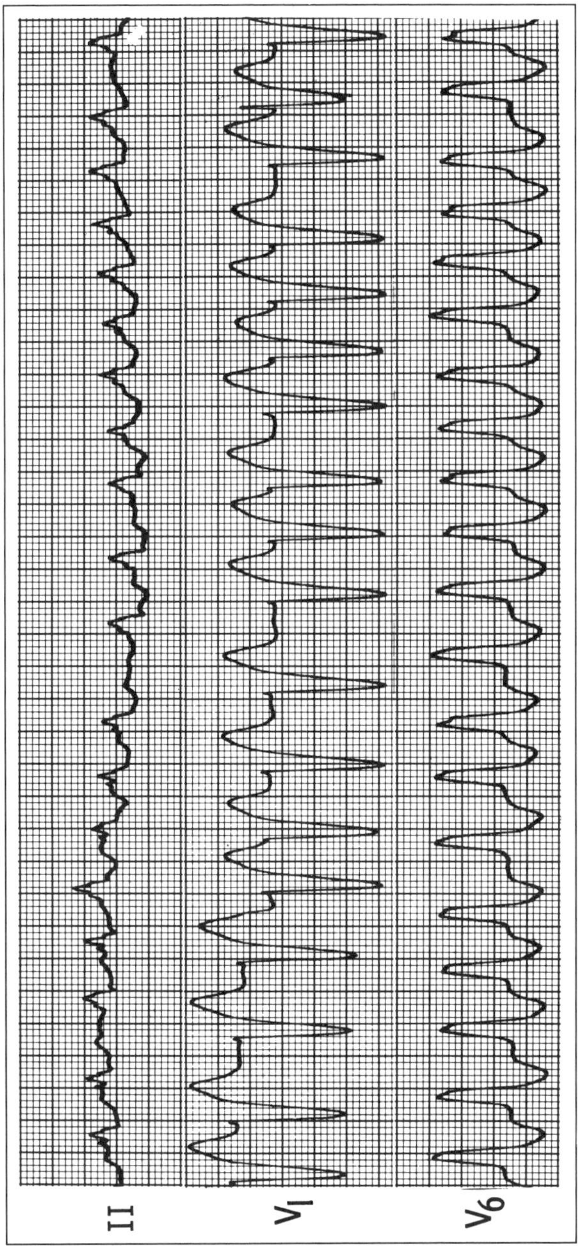


Fig. 5–17. Atrial fibrillation with LBBB.

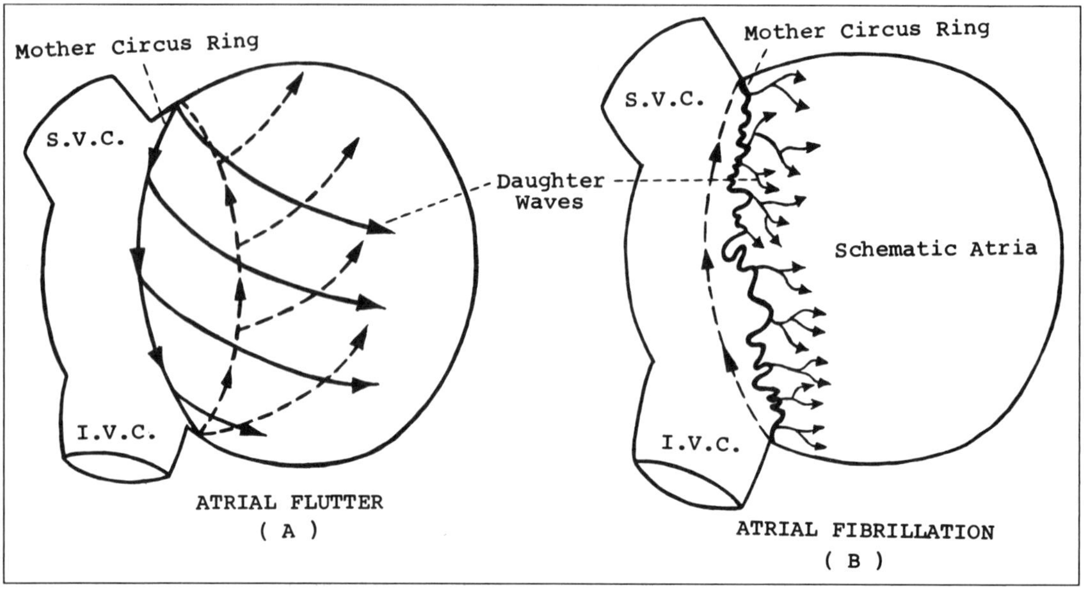


**Fig. 5–18.** The circus movement theory of atrial flutter (**A**) and AF (**B**). A detailed description of the circus movement is given in the text. S.V.C. = superior vena cava; I.V.C. = inferior vena cava.

verse the entire atria, arise from the path of the mother circus ring (Fig. 5–18). These are called "daughter waves." When 1 cycle of the mother circus ring is ended, it immediately reenters the same pathway to produce a new cycle. The circus movement will continue indefinitely as long as the atrial muscle immediately preceding the area just activated is in the nonrefractory state. Therefore, a gap of muscle in the nonrefractory state in the atria, which separates the head of the mother circus ring from its tail, is essential in order to continue the circus movement. The fundamental mechanism by which quinidine terminates AF and atrial flutter is its prolongation of the refractory period of the atrial muscle, leading to the disappearance of the gap of muscle in the nonrefractory state preceding the front of the mother circus ring.

In pure atrial flutter, the pathway traversed by the mother circus ring is thought to be longer than that in AF, leading to a slower atrial rate in the former. In addition, the atria recover more rapidly in atrial flutter than in AF, so that mother circus waves and daughter waves tend to traverse a relatively constant pathway, leading to a regular flutter cycle. In atrial impure flutter, mother circus waves are considered to traverse a constant pathway, but daughter wave impulses are believed to traverse an irregular pattern, so that a slightly irregular flutter cycle results. In AF, both mother circus waves and daughter waves traverse a grossly irregular pathway with a variable speed from cycle to cycle, leading to grossly irregular fibrillatory oscillations (Fig. 5–18). The development of atrial flutter, impure flutter and fibrillation, or conversion from one to another depends upon the regularity and diameter of the pathway and/or the speeds of the impulse traveling in the mother circus ring and the daughter wave ring.

**Theory of Multiple Reentry:** The mechanism of reentry is considered to be the genesis of most ordinary premature beats and of paroxysmal ectopic tachycardias. This theory assumes that AF and atrial flutter may be initiated by an impulse, either sinus or ectopic, that produces numerous daughter impulses of varying degrees. This occurs because many regions of the atria have local interference due to the uneven refractory period, which is an ideal ground for the development of multiple reentry. The reentry mechanism may be initiated by a single early impulse occurring during the vulnerable period of the atria. The degree of prematurity of the impulse that is sufficient to initiate the reentry phenomenon varies markedly and depends upon the electrophysiologic status of the given heart. In general, less prematurity is often sufficient to initiate reentry when the heart is markedly depressed due either to drugs or organic heart disease. Each atrial impulse traverses the syncytium whenever it finds nonrefractory muscle that is not yet stimulated by its sister impulses, and each, in its turn, results in new points of reentry. Atrial fibrillation results when the pattern of reentry is grossly irregular and when multiple impulse propagation occurs rapidly. On the other hand, atrial flutter results when the propagation of impulses and reentry follow a regular pattern. In atrial flutter-fibrillation, the pattern of impulse propagation and reentry will be more regular than in AF and less regular than in atrial flutter.

Atrial fibrillation or atrial flutter will be terminated when the multiple reentry phenomenon cannot occur. This occurs due to (1) a prolongation of the refractory phase or the fact that these impulses cannot find any atrial muscle responsive or (2) an enhancement of the speed of these impulses traveling so that they arrive in those parts of the atrial muscle that are still in the absolute refractory phase. Therefore, conversion of AF and atrial flutter from one to another or termination of these arrhythmias depends upon the speed of the impulse transmission and the duration of the refractory period in the atria.

**Theory of Unifocal Impulse Formation:** The theory of circus movement had been well accepted as a mechanism of AF and atrial flutter until recently when Scherf et al. proposed the theory of unifocal impulse formation. Scherf et al. produced AF and atrial flutter by focal application of aconitine on the atria of a dog. Atrial fibrillation and flutter were terminated immediately by cooling of the focus and reappeared when the cooling was stopped. Atrial flutter was also produced by the application of aconitine on the appendices of the right or left atrium, and the arrhythmia was stopped when the tip of the appendix was clamped off. The same authors were able to transform atrial flutter to AF by touching the area where aconitine had been applied with a probe.

Brown and Acheson proposed 2 forms of atrial flutter generated by 2 different mechanisms. One form was produced by the focal application of aconitine, and the other form was produced by a faradic stimulation after crushing. The latter was considered to be reentry flutter, which was terminated immediately by administration of quinidine or procainamide. On the other hand, aconitine-induced flutter disappeared gradually while using the same drugs. In addition, flutter induced by a faradic stimulation did not reappear once terminated, whereas aconitine-induced flutter terminated by quinidine or procainamide reappeared.

Prinzmetal et al. recorded atrial activity in dogs with high speed cinematographs during normal sinus rhythm, AF, AT, and atrial flutter. They produced atrial flutter either by direct application of aconitine to the heart or by electrical stimulation. By using direct multiple leads, it was demonstrated that an atrial flutter wave originating from anywhere in the atria is transmitted to both atria simultaneously until it reaches the extremities of the atria. The course of the atrial flutter wave is similar to that of AT, that is, the flutter wave spreads outward from its focus of stimulation in all available directions. No circus movement was demonstrated by this study.

Prinzmetal et al. also studied atrial flutter in human hearts by using esophageal leads with various positions. They observed a varying flutter wave configuration when recordings were made from different levels of the esophagus and, thus, concluded that this finding is against the circus movement theory.

Clinically, it is very common to observe that AF or atrial flutter is initiated by an isolated APC or transformed from AT. This observation strongly favors the theory of unifocal impulse formation in many cases with various atrial tachyarrhythmias.

**Theory of Multifocal Impulse Formation:** This theory is essentially the same as the theory of unifocal impulse formation except that there are believed to be multiple ectopic foci. As described previously in the chapter, APCs or AT frequently originates from a single focus, but they may be of multifocal origin. Similarly, it is logical to assume that AF or atrial flutter may be produced by a single focus or by multiple foci. It is also common to observe clinically atrial rhythms transitional between AT, particularly MAT, AF, and atrial flutter.

**Conclusion:** The fundamental mechanism responsible for the production of AF or atrial flutter is still not settled. It is quite possible that more than one mechanism may be responsible for the genesis of clinical AF or atrial flutter. This author believes that AF or atrial flutter may originate from a single focus or multiple foci, as seen in APCs and AT. In addition, from an electrophysiologic viewpoint, a reentry phenomenon is responsible for the production of clinical AF and atrial flutter in many cases.

## Clinical Significance

Atrial fibrillation is one of the most common arrhythmias, and it is certainly the most common underlying cardiac rhythm other than sinus rhythm. The incidence of AF is approximately 10–20 times higher than that of atrial flutter. It has been said that about 70% of patients with CHF have AF. Atrial fibrillation is rare in infants or children, but if it occurs, congenital heart disease is almost always present, particularly atrial septal defect, Ebstein's disease, and transposition of the great vessels. The incidence of AF markedly increases after age 40. It is not uncommonly associated with WPW syndrome in adults but is extremely rare in children with the same syndrome.

Atrial fibrillation may occur in a paroxysmal form, but it often becomes chronic, particularly when underlying heart disease is present, even after various treatments. It may last a few seconds or minutes, but it may persist for many years. As in atrial flutter, AF is commonly associated with RHD, CAD, hypertensive heart disease, hyperthyroidism, and WPW syndrome. Sick sinus syndrome is a strong possibility when dealing with chronic AF with advanced AV block (Fig. 5–19) (Chapter 14).

The clinical significance of fine and coarse AF is quite different. It has been shown that the most common cause of coarse AF (Fig. 5–15) is RHD, particularly mitral stenosis, and this is attributed to enlargement of the left atrium (Fig. 5–15). Less commonly, coarse AF may be found in thyrotoxicosis. In contrast to this, fine AF is almost always found in coronary and/or hypertensive heart disease (Fig. 5–14).

Less commonly, AF may be observed in cardiomyopathy, acute myocarditis, or pericarditis of various causes and trauma to the chest. Atrial fibrillation is rarely observed in DI, and it is unusual in congenital heart disease, luetic heart disease, and chronic cor pulmonale. Approximately 6% of AF occurs in apparently healthy individuals. Atrial fibrillation may be observed as a result of heavy smoking, excessive ingestion of alcohol, coffee, and tea, and sudden emotional excitement. The term "holiday heart syndrome" is used when various paroxysmal tachyarrhythmias, such as AF, occur following excessive consumption of alcohol. At times, AF is found in tense individuals, and it may be familial. When an underlying cause for the AF is not found, it has been called "idiopathic" or "benign" AF.

Symptoms vary depending upon the presence or absence and nature of the heart disease, the presence or absence and degree of CHF, the ventricular rate, and the duration of the AF. Transient AF may not produce any symptoms. Because of the high incidence of AF in CHF, the symptoms primarily depend upon the severity of the CHF. Mild symptoms may include palpitations, anxiety, a fluttering or pounding sensation, and skipping of the heartbeats. Serious symptoms include full-blown CHF, syncope, and a feeling of impending death. Angina may be produced by or exaggerated by AF.

Digitalis is the drug of choice for the treatment of AF with rapid ventricular response (Fig. 5–14), regardless of whether it is associated with CHF. The drug is most effective when significant CHF is present. When chronic AF with advanced AV block is considered to be due to SSS, a permanent artificial pacemaker is usually indicated (Chapter 14).

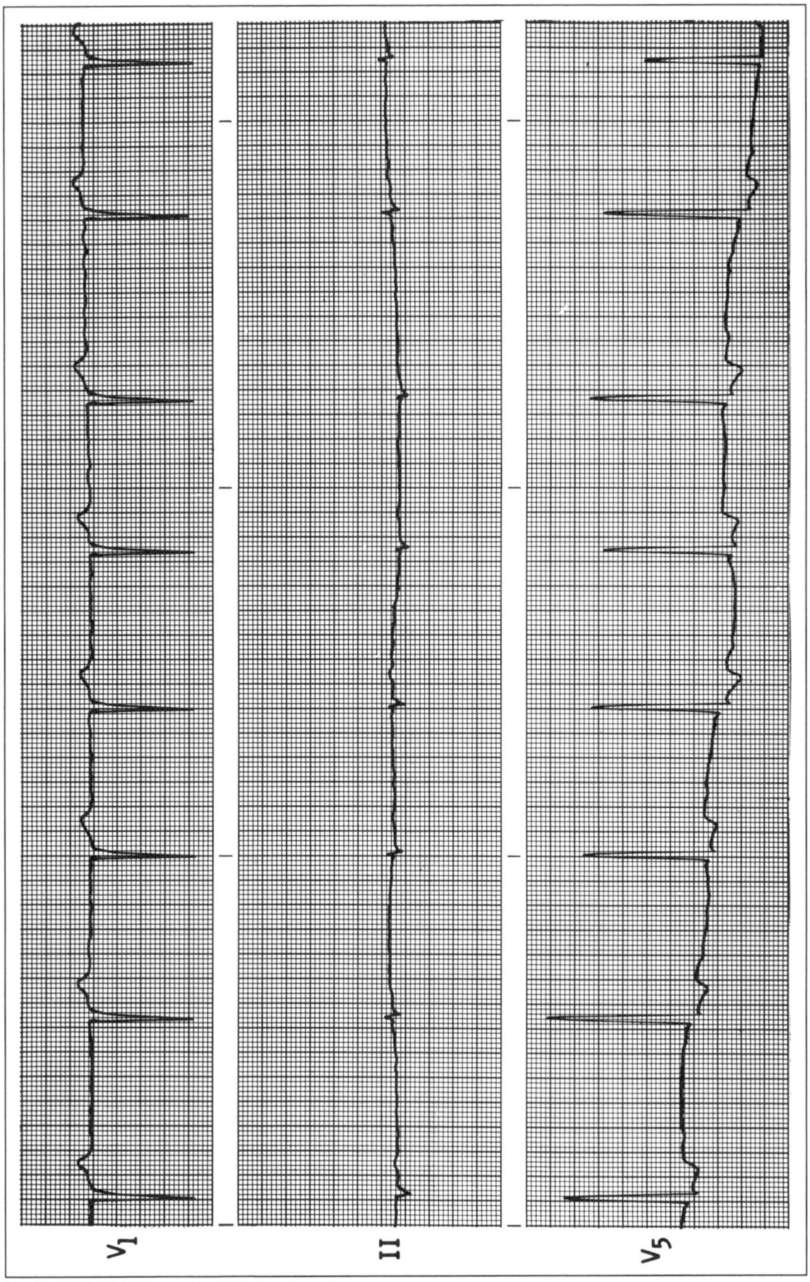


Fig. 5–19. Atrial fibrillation with advanced AV block producing slow ventricular response (rate: 40–50 beats/min) and occasional AV JEBs. The underlying process is most likely advanced SSS. Note the evidence of LVH.

## ATRIAL STANDSTILL

Atrial standstill may occur transiently for a short period and at times it may last for months or years. Atrial standstill is often the result of other primary cardiac rhythm disorders. For example, a temporary and short atrial standstill commonly occurs in marked sinus arrhythmia with sinus bradycardia, sinus arrest, and SA block. In fact, sinus arrest and SA block are the commonest causes of atrial standstill. Permanent atrial standstill may result when there is a complete SA block or a long sinus arrest, unless the atria are activated by other ectopic pacemaker(s). Atrial standstill may occur when the sinus node is suppressed by an ectopic rhythm or tachycardia because of the postectopic inhibition phenomenon.

### Diagnostic Criteria

Diagnosis of a temporary atrial standstill is always obvious because the primary rhythm disorder (e.g., SA block, sinus arrest) can be diagnosed readily in most instances. However, permanent or long-standing atrial standstill is not always easy to diagnose.

The following criteria may be used in the diagnosis of permanent atrial standstill:

1. No atrial activity (either sinus or ectopic) in any lead of the conventional or intracardiac ECG
2. No "a" wave in the neck veins or in the intraatrial pressure tracing
3. Immobile atria on fluoroscopy and cineangiocardiography
4. A regular and slow ventricular rhythm

Nevertheless, in permanent atrial standstill, it is not uncommon to observe 1 or 2 P waves occurring very slowly and irregularly in the presence of an independent regular ventricular rhythm.

### Clinical Significance

Clinically, a temporary atrial standstill may occur during carotid sinus massage or pressure on the eyeball in healthy individuals, as well as in patients with diseased hearts. The most common cause of either temporary or permanent atrial standstill is DI, and the next most common cause is quinidine toxicity. Permanent atrial standstill not uncommonly develops during the terminal stage of an acute MI, particularly when the atria are infarcted. Less commonly, atrial standstill may be observed in hyperkalemia, carbon dioxide toxicity, and hypoxia.

For the treatment of atrial standstill, removal of the underlying cause is the most important step, particularly when drug toxicity is present.

## ATRIAL PARASYSTOLE

Atrial parasystole is discussed in Chapter 22.

# Chapter 6

# Atrioventricular Junctional Arrhythmias

Atrioventricular junctional arrhythmias may originate from any location in the AV junctional tissue. Generally, there are 2 major fundamental mechanisms responsible for the production of various AV junctional arrhythmias: active impulse formation and passive impulse formation. Active impulse formation in the AV junction may produce AV JPCs and AV JT, whereas passive impulse formation results in AV JEBs or JER. Active impulse formation occurs because of an abnormal acceleration of impulse formation in the AV junction, regardless of the atrial mechanism. It is common to observe that AV JT is initiated by an isolated AV JPC. There are 2 types of AV JT, paroxysmal and nonparoxysmal. The former may be observed in apparently healthy individuals, while the latter always occurs in organic heart diseases and is particularly associated with DI. On the other hand, AV JEBs or JER only appears as a physiologic mechanism to control the ventricles when atrial impulses (either sinus or ectopic) are unable to reach the AV junction. This may occur as a result of various causes, including marked sinus bradycardia, sinus arrest, SA block, and second or third (complete) degree AV block.

The ECG features of each AV junctional beat, regardless of whether it is a response to active or passive impulse formation, are essentially the same, except for the effect on the cardiac rhythm and the time of the onset in the cardiac cycle. In other words, the configurations of the P, QRS, and T complexes of isolated AV junctional beats are identical, regardless of the fundamental mechanism involved.

However, the relationship between atrial and ventricular depolarization will vary depending upon the location of the ectopic pacemaker in the AV junction and the status of the antegrade and retrograde conduction systems. In general, the P waves tend to precede the QRS complexes when the ectopic focus is located in the upper portion of the AV junction and/or when antegrade AV conduction is impaired. Conversely, the QRS complexes tend to precede the P waves when the ectopic focus is located in the lower portion of the AV junction and/or when retrograde VA conduction is impaired. The P wave may not be discernible if it is superimposed on the QRS complex in which the atria and ventricles are activated simultaneously. This may occur when the ectopic focus is located in the middle portion of the AV junction provided that antegrade and retrograde conduction times are identical. P waves may be absent even when the ectopic focus is located in the upper or lower portions of the AV junction if there is a significant impairment of retrograde conduction in the upper portion and of antegrade conduction in the lower portion. In addition, P waves will be absent when there is a complete block of retrograde conduction, regardless of the location of the ectopic focus in the AV junction. Only the P wave may appear, without the QRS complex, in an AV junctional beat when there is a complete block of antegrade conduction. This can occur regardless of the location of the ectopic focus in the AV junction. If there is a block in both antegrade and retrograde conduction, obviously the P and the QRS complexes will be absent. This is a form of exit block.

When P waves are present in AV junctional beats or rhythm (provided that AV dissociation is not present), the P waves are usually inverted in leads II, III, and aVF and upright in lead aVR (Fig. 6–1). This occurs because the atria are activated in a retrograde fashion. The mean electrical axis of the P waves in the frontal plane is usually between −60 and −90° in AV junctional beats or rhythm. The P wave is usually not inverted in lead I (Fig. 6–1). Similarly, the P wave is not inverted in leads $V_5$ or $V_6$.

The P-R or the R-P interval varies depending

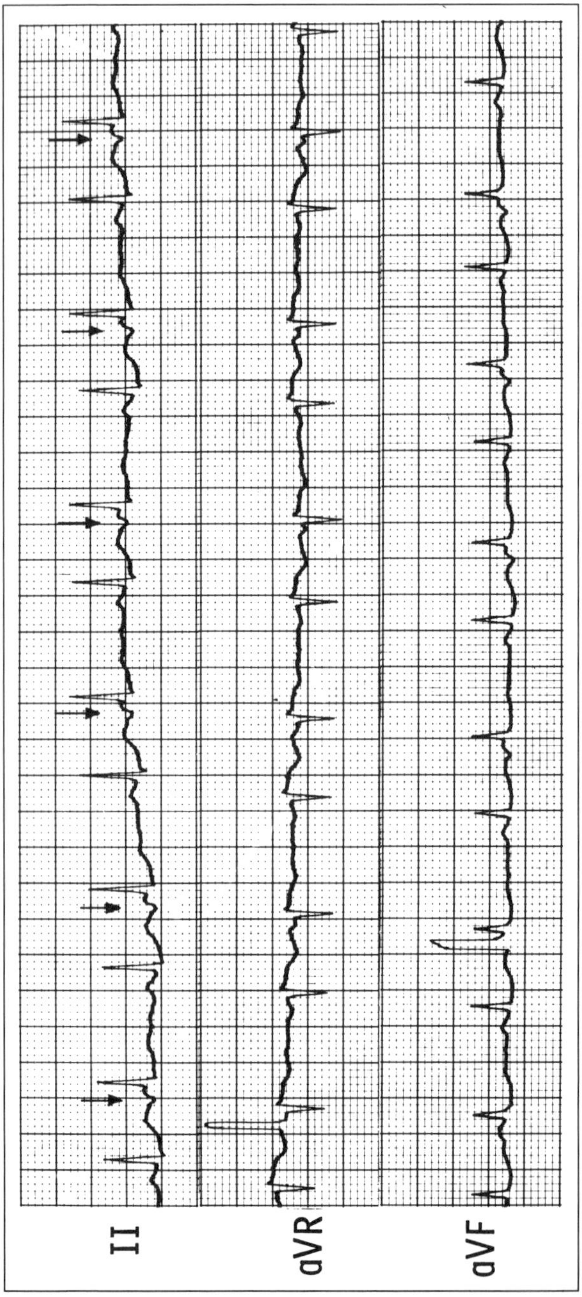


Fig. 6–1. Sinus rhythm with frequent AV JPCs (indicated by arrows) producing AV junctional bigeminy.

upon the location of the ectopic focus in the AV junction and/or the status of antegrade and retrograde conduction. In general, the P-R interval is 0.12 second or less, and the R-P interval is between 0.10 and 0.20 second, provided there is no conduction defect. The reason for the short P-R interval (0.12 second or less) in AV junctional arrhythmias is obvious. Unlike sinus rhythm, the impulse from the ectopic focus in AV junctional arrhythmias does not proceed from the atria to the ventricles. The P-R interval in the AV junctional arrhythmias is a difference of the conduction time between antegrade conduction to the ventricles and retrograde conduction to the atria from the ectopic focus in the AV junction, provided that atrial activation occurs earlier than ventricular. Therefore, the P-R interval in AV junctional arrhythmias is not a true AV conduction time. In general, the P-R interval in AV junctional arrhythmias tends to be shorter when the ectopic pacemaker is located nearer the ventricles and/or when there is some degree of retrograde conduction defect present. The converse holds true for the R-P interval.

Atrioventricular dissociation commonly results when AV junctional beats or rhythm develops. It is discussed in detail later in this chapter.

The QRS complex in AV junctional beats or rhythm is often normal in appearance (Fig. 6–1), but it may be wide and bizarre, either because of aberrant ventricular conduction or preexisting LBBB or RBBB.

Reciprocal beats commonly develop when AV junctional beats or rhythm is present. Reciprocal beats or rhythm will be discussed later in this chapter. Atrioventricular junctional parasystole is a less common AV junctional arrhythmia (Chapter 22).

## ATRIOVENTRICULAR JUNCTIONAL PREMATURE CONTRACTIONS (EXTRASYSTOLES)

Atrioventricular JPCs may arise from any locus in the AV junctional tissue. In most instances, the impulse from the AV junction activates the entire atria, including the sinus node, unless the underlying rhythm is AF or atrial flutter. An ectopic impulse originating from the AV junction is conducted in 2 directions simultaneously. Retrograde conduction activates the atria, whereas antegrade conduction activates the ventricles. Although the onset of retrograde and antegrade conduction is simultaneous, atrial and ventricular activation do not necessarily occur simultaneously. In fact, more often, atrial and ventricular activations are completed at different times.

The sinus node is often prematurely discharged by the ectopic impulse from the AV junction, and the sinus node momentarily loses its inherent automaticity. Propagation of the impulse in the atria from the ectopic focus in the AV junction is always in a retrograde conduction, but conduction below the location of the ectopic focus is identical to that of sinus beats.

### Diagnostic Criteria

An AV JPC is diagnosed when the ectopic P wave, which is conducted in a retrograde fashion and which is preceded by or followed by a normal QRS complex, appears earlier than the cardiac cycles of the basic rhythm (Fig. 6–1).

**Configuration and Mean Axis of Ectopic P Wave:** The configuration of the P wave of the AV JPC is always different from that of the P wave of sinus origin. The P waves in AV JPC are usually inverted in leads II, III, and aVF and almost always upright in leads I and aVR (Fig. 6–1). These P wave changes occur because the atria are activated in a retrograde fashion. The mean axis of the P waves in AV JPCs is between −60 and −90° in the frontal plane. Thus, the P waves in leads I and aVR may be isoelectric or biphasic in AV JPCs.

**Relationship Between Atrial and Ventricular Activation:** The time relationship between atrial and ventricular activation depends upon the location of the ectopic focus in the AV junction and the status of the antegrade and retrograde conduction systems. It is common to observe different degrees of conductivity between antegrade and retrograde conduction. In fact, antegrade conduction may be perfectly normal in the presence of marked impairment of retrograde conduction, or vice versa. Occasionally, antegrade conduction may be completely blocked even when retrograde conduction is normal, or vice versa.

As described previously, the P wave may precede or be followed by the QRS complex or, at times, be superimposed on the QRS complex. The P-R interval is usually 0.12 second or less (Fig. 6–1). However, the P-R interval in AV JPCs or AV JT may be prolonged if an antegrade conduction defect is present. The R-P interval is usually between 0.10 and 0.20 second, unless there is a marked retrograde conduction defect. The R-P interval becomes longer than 0.20 second when retrograde conduction is markedly impaired.

When atrial and ventricular activations are completed simultaneously or when there is a complete block in retrograde conduction, the P wave will be absent. Conversely, only the retrograde P wave of an AV JPC will appear without the QRS complex when there is a complete antegrade block.

**Postectopic Pause:** The postectopic pause varies significantly in AV JPCs because of various factors. When the sinus node is prematurely activated by the ectopic impulse conducted in a retrograde fashion, the postectopic interval in AV JPCs is usually longer than the P-P cycle of the basic rhythm, as seen in APCs. This occurs because the sinus node momentarily loses its inherent automaticity due to suppression by the ectopic impulse. In this circumstance, however, a full compensatory pause does *not* occur (Fig. 6–1).

Not uncommonly, a full compensatory pause is observed when the retrograde impulse from the AV junction fails to discharge the sinus node. This occurs in the following situations:

Sinoatrial interference. In this case, the sinus node produces an impulse as usual just before the ectopic impulse reaches the SA junction. Thus, the 2 impulses, 1 from the sinus node and the other from the AV junction, meet at or near the SA junction. As a result, the AV JPC is manifested by the early appearance of the QRS complex with a retrograde P wave, which occurs slightly earlier than the P-P cycle of the basic rhythm. In other words, the ectopic pacemaker in the AV junction activates both the atria and ventricles without disturbing the sinus node. Thus, the sinus P wave appears following AV JPC in the expected usual cycle.

Atrial interference. In this circumstance, 2 impulses, 1 from the sinus node and the other from the AV junction, meet anywhere in the atria, so that an atrial fusion beat appears. The atrial fusion beat will have a form intermediate between that of an antegrade sinus P wave and a retrograde P wave from the AV junction. The atrial fusion beat may be followed by or preceded by the QRS complex. Rarely, an atrial fusion beat may occur without a QRS complex in an AV JPC when there is a complete antegrade block.

Atrioventricular interference. In this situation, the atria are activated by the sinus node as usual, and only the ventricles are activated by the ectopic focus in the AV junction. Thus, interference occurs in the AV junction. As a result, a sinus P wave appears at its usual position in the cardiac cycle with an independent QRS complex from the AV JPC, leading to momentary AV dissociation.

In general, a full compensatory pause tends to occur when the ectopic focus is located in the lower portion of the AV junction, or when there is impairment or a complete block of retrograde conduction.

Occasionally, AV JPCs may be interpolated. This occurs when the ectopic impulse from the AV junction is unable to activate the atria due to a complete block in retrograde conduction in the presence of a relatively slow basic rhythm and a very short coupling interval. In this case, the sinus P-P cycle is not disturbed and only the QRS complex of the AV JPC is sandwiched between the R-R interval of the basic rhythm. On the other hand, a protection block is considered to be present around the sinus node, as seen in interpolated APC, when an AV JPC is interpolated and its QRS complex is preceded or followed by a retrograde P wave.

**Constant Coupling Intervals:** The coupling interval of AV JPCs is usually constant (Fig. 6–1) because the ectopic impulse discharge in the AV junction is considered to be dependent upon the basic rhythm in some way. This is different from AV junctional parasystole, in which the coupling intervals vary throughout the tracing, because the parasystolic focus produces an independent rhythm (Chapter 22). Although a constant coupling interval is a general rule in AV JPCs, it may vary slightly without having a parasystolic mechanism.

**Configuration of the QRS Complex:** The configuration of the QRS complex in AV JPC is frequently identical with that produced by a normal sinus beat (Fig. 6–1). However, it is not uncommon to observe a wide and bizarre QRS complex due to aberrant ventricular conduction. In general, the degree of aberrant ventricular conduction depends upon the degree of prematurity and the status of the intraventricular conduction system. Thus, aberrant ventricular conduction is prone to develop when the QRS complex of the AV JPC appears early in the cycle (short coupling interval) because the ectopic impulse traverses the ventricles during their relative refractory period.

Besides the degree of prematurity of the AV JPC and the status of the intraventricular conduction system, another factor is often responsible for aberrant ventricular conduction. It tends to occur when the cardiac cyclic length immediately preceding the coupling interval is long. For this reason, aberrant ventricular conduction is frequently observed after AV junctional bigeminy is established. This finding is termed "Ashman's phenomenon" (Chapters 10 and 11).

The QRS complex of the AV JPC may be wide because of a preexisting or rate-dependent BBB.

**Aberrant Atrial Conduction (Chung's Phenomenon):** As seen in APCs, the P wave of the basic rhythm immediately following an AV JPC occasionally has a bizarre configuration, which is different from the P wave of an AV JPC or a P wave of sinus origin. This aberrant atrial conduction is considered to occur because the refractory period of the atria is altered immediately following an AV JPC.

**Frequency of Atrioventricular Junctional Premature Contractions:** An AV JPC may occur as an isolated beat, but it may appear alternately with the basic rhythm (AV junctional bigeminy) as every third beat (AV junctional trigeminy) or every fourth beat (AV junctional quadrigeminy). Atrioventricular JPCs may appear consecutively as 2 or more beats, called "AV junctional group beats." When AV JPCs appear as 3 or more beats consecutively, some investigators call this a short run of AV JT, but, in general, the term AV JT is used when 6 or more AV JPCs occur consecutively.

Atrioventricular JPCs may originate from more than 1 focus and produce ectopic P and/or QRS complexes of different configurations with different coupling intervals. They are termed "multifocal AV JPCs." Frequent AV JPCs may lead to AV JT.

### Mechanism

Atrioventricular JPCs are considered to be produced by the same or a similar mechanism as VPCs, and a detailed description of this mechanism is found in Chapter 7.

### Clinical Significance

Atrioventricular JPCs are a relatively uncommon occurrence in comparison with APCs or VPCs. They may be found in apparently healthy individuals as well as in those with diseased hearts. By and large, the clinical significance of APCs and AV JPCs is considered to be very similar, and they are relatively benign arrhythmias. No active treatment is indicated.

## ATRIOVENTRICULAR JUNCTIONAL ESCAPE BEATS AND RHYTHM

Atrioventricular junctional escape beats and rhythm, like AV JPCs, may originate from any location in the AV junctional tissue. Atrioventricular JEBs may appear singly or consecutively as group beats. Six or more AV JEBs appearing consecutively constitute AV JER. Atrioventricular JEBs and JER appear as a physiologic mechanism and therefore are the most common arrhythmias generated by passive impulse formation.

Under normal circumstances, AV JEBs or JER does not appear because the AV junctional pacemaker is controlled by the sinus node, which produces impulses faster than the AV junction. Thus, the AV junction is continuously depressed by the rapidly discharging sinus impulses. However, AV JEBs or JER appears when the sinus node produces impulses slower than usual (sinus bradycardia) or when the impulse from the sinus node fails to reach the AV junction, as in sinus arrest, SA block, or AV block. One or 2 AV JEBs commonly follow the postectopic pause of either APCs, AV JPCs, or VPCs.

Atrioventricular JEBs or JER may occur in the presence of an ectopic atrial rhythm, including AF, atrial flutter, and AT, when the atrial impulses fail to reach the AV junction due to high degree or complete AV block. Continuous exit block around the ectopic atrial focus also leads to the development of AV JEBs or JER. They may be preceded by or followed by retrograde P waves, depending upon the location of the ectopic pacemaker in the AV junction and the status of the antegrade and retrograde conduction systems. However, more commonly, AV JEBs or JER produces only QRS complexes in the presence of independent atrial activity, thus producing transient or continuous AV dissociation.

The usual rates of AV JER range between 40 and 60 beats/min. When the rate of an AV JER exceeds 60 beats/min, the mechanism involved is considered to be different from escape rhythm, and the former is termed "nonparoxysmal AV JT."

Unlike sinus rhythm, AV JER is usually not influenced by any maneuvers, such as CSS, respiration, exercise, and so on.

## Diagnostic Criteria

**Relationship Between Atrial and Ventricular Activations:** Atrioventricular JEBs or JER may be preceded by or followed by retrograde P waves when the AV junctional pacemaker activates both the atria and ventricles (Fig. 6–2). However, it is common to observe AV JEB or JER manifested by QRS complexes with an independent atrial mechanism (either sinus or ectopic atrial), leading to a transient or continuous AV dissociation (Fig. 6–3).

When the AV junctional escape impulses are able to conduct to both atria and ventricles, the P-R or R-P intervals vary depending upon the location of the ectopic focus in the AV junction and the status of the antegrade and retrograde conduction systems. At times, AV junctional escape impulses activate only a portion of the atria when these impulses meet with the sinus impulses somewhere in the atria. In this circumstance, the P wave will have a form intermediate between that of a sinus P wave and a retrograde AV junctional P wave. This is termed an "atrial fusion (summation) beat." In short, in AV JEBs or JER, the atria may be activated by the AV junctional impulse totally or partially or may not be activated at all. Retrograde conduction to the atria, in AV JEBs or JER, does not occur when the atria are activated by the sinus node just before the AV junctional impulses reach the atria or there is a complete block in retrograde conduction. Needless to say, retrograde activation of the atria by the AV junctional impulses does not occur when the underlying rhythm is AF or atrial flutter (Fig. 6–3).

**Rate:** Since AV JEBs or JER is generated by passive impulse formation, the rate is usually slower than that of normal sinus rhythm. The inherent rates of AV JER range from 40 to 60 beats/min (Figs. 6–2 and 6–3), and rarely it may be as slow as 30 to 35 beats/min. However, it should be noted that an unusually slow AV JER may actually be a misdiagnosis of AV JT with 2:1 or 3:1 exit block. This is particularly prone to develop in the presence of AF, and the underlying cause is often DI.

**Escape Intervals:** It has been shown that AV junctional escape intervals, in most instances, are precisely regular, and they seldom vary more than 0.04 second in duration. However, AV junctional escape intervals may vary occasionally before the AV JER is well established. When the AV junctional escape intervals vary from beat to beat before the AV JER is well established, it is common to observe that its rate

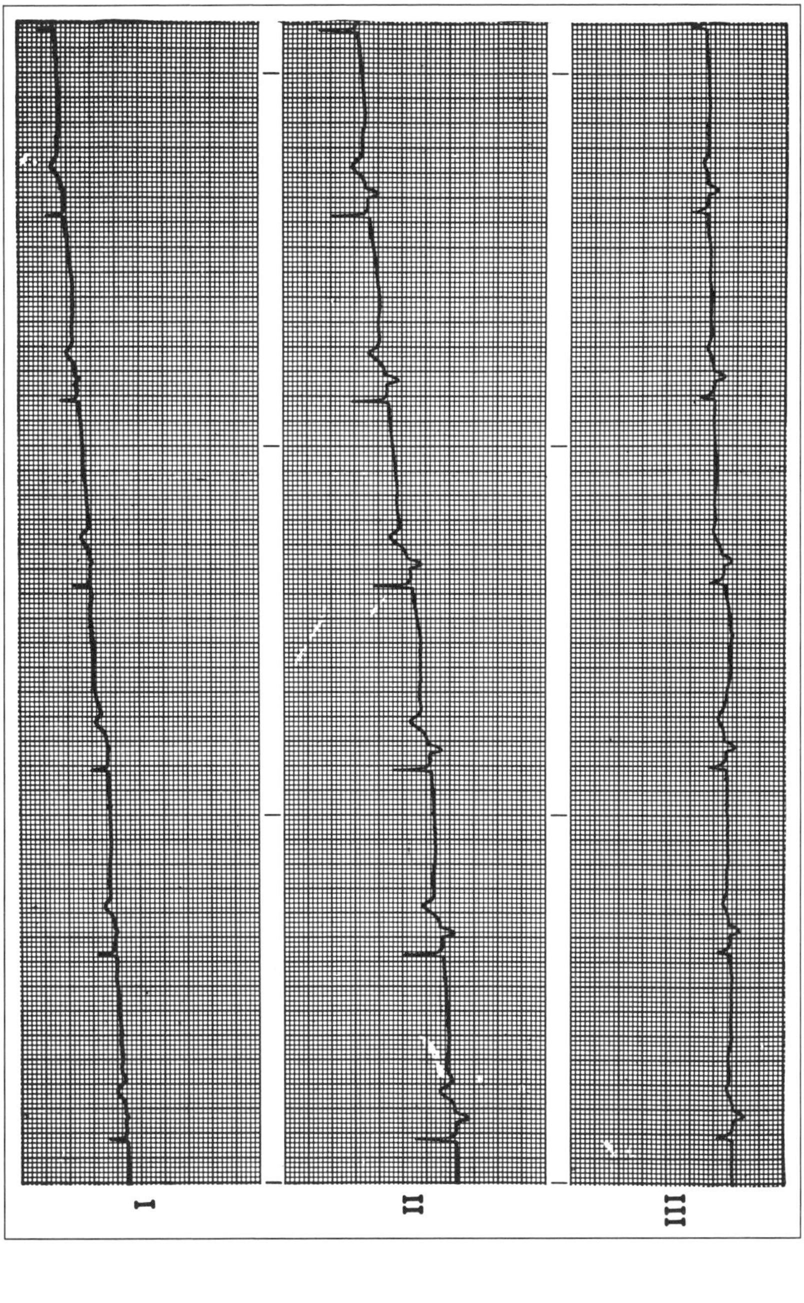


Fig. 6–2. Atrioventricular JER with a rate of 40 beats/min. The underlying process is considered to be advanced SSS.

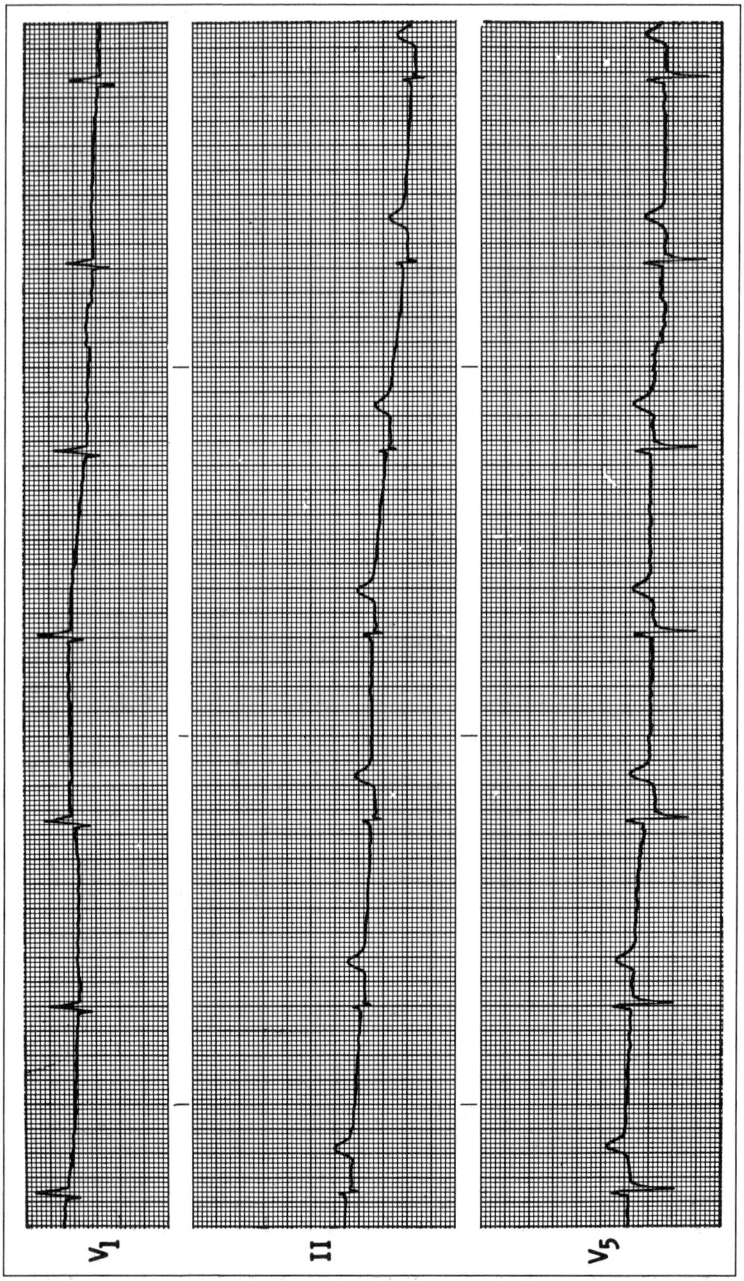


**Fig. 6–3.** Atrial fibrillation with AV JER (rate: 41 beats/min) due to complete AV block as a result of advanced SSS. Incomplete RBBB is diagnosed without any difficulty.

will generally become fixed with faster rate. Occasionally, the reverse occurs. It is not uncommon to observe varying escape intervals when 1 or 2 AV JEBs appear following the postectopic pause of premature beats or second degree AV block or SA block. When 2 or more distinctively different escape intervals appear alternatively or periodically, multifocal AV JERs are considered to be present.

**Configuration of P Waves:** The configuration of the P wave varies depending upon whether the atria are activated by the sinus node or by the AV junction. When the P waves are AV junctional in origin, they are usually inverted in leads II, III, and aVF and upright in lead aVR (Fig. 6–2). The P wave is rarely isoelectric or biphasic in lead aVR. When atrial fusion (summation) beats occur (between sinus and AV junctional impulses), the P wave configuration varies markedly depending upon the degree of the fusion between the 2 impulses. Needless to say, there will be no P wave when the underlying rhythm is AF or atrial flutter (Fig. 6–3).

**Configuration of QRS Complex:** The configuration of the QRS complex in AV JEBs or JER is usually identical to the sinus beat (Figs. 6–2 and 6–3), although it may be broad when there is a preexisting or rate-dependent BBB. Obviously, when the QRS complex is wide and bizarre in AV JER, it closely resembles ventricular escape (idioventricular) rhythm.

## Mechanism

Atrioventricular JEBs or JER always appears whenever atrial impulses (either sinus or ectopic) fail to reach the AV junction. Therefore, the fundamental mechanism for the initiation of AV JEBs or JER is a physiologic mechanism to control the ventricles. Various basic cardiac arrhythmias, including postectopic pause, sinus bradycardia, sinus arrest, SA block, and second and third degree AV block, predispose to the development of the AV JEBs or JER (Figs. 6–2 and 6–3). As a result, AV dissociation is almost always observed (Figs. 2–4 and 6–3), and a pure AV JER (Fig. 6–2), which controls the atria and ventricles, is uncommon.

## Clinical Significance

Atrioventricular JEBs or JER may occur in healthy individuals as well as in those with diseased hearts. When AV JEBs occur occasionally and intermittently following postectopic pauses, sinus bradycardia, sinus arrest, or SA block of short duration, they are insignificant clinically. However, when persisting AV JER is present because of complete AV block, sinus arrest, or SA block of long duration, the patient is often symptomatic. This is particularly true when the underlying heart disease is serious (e.g., acute MI and/or CHF) and/or when drug intoxication (e.g., DI) is present. When the ventricular rate is relatively slow, especially in the presence of underlying AF, the patient often experiences dizziness, mental confusion, and even Adams-Stokes syndrome because of reduced cerebral blood flow. Similarly, a patient with AV JER may develop angina pectoris because of reduced coronary blood flow, and AV JER due to complete AV block frequently produces CHF, which is often refractory to the usual medical management unless an artificial pacemaker is used. A possibility of SSS is very strong when there is persisting AV JER (Fig. 6–2), especially when the rate is very slow (Chapter 14).

The most common cause of AV JEBs or JER in healthy subjects is sinus bradycardia, whereas high degree or complete AV is almost always responsible for the development of AV JER in elderly individuals. When AV JER is found in elderly patients, the underlying atrial mechanism is commonly AF, and frequently DI is responsible for the development of AV block. Atrial fibrillation as an underlying rhythm is, of course, very common in RHD and CAD.

Less commonly, AV JER may be produced by the administration of reserpine (Serpasil), propranolol, or guanethidine (Ismelin), by hyperkalemia, myocarditis of various causes, and systemic diseases, such as rheumatoid and Paget's diseases.

## ATRIOVENTRICULAR JUNCTIONAL TACHYCARDIA

Atrioventricular JT may originate from any location in the AV junctional tissue, as seen in AV JPCs or AV JER. In contrast to AV JER, AV JT appears as an active impulse formation and the rate of AV junctional impulse discharge is accelerated. As a result, the rate is naturally faster than that of AV JER. In other words, AV JT has a rate faster than the inherent rate (40–60 beats/min) of the AV junction.

Atrioventricular JT is divided into 2 major categories (Table 1–1), paroxysmal and nonparoxysmal AV JT. Not only are the nature of the onset and the termination of the 2 forms of AV JT different, but also the usual rates and clinical significance are different. Paroxysmal AV JT produces a rate between 160 and 250 beats/min, which is the same rate range as PAT, and the former may occur in apparently healthy individuals. Conversely, nonparoxysmal AV JT produces a rate between 60 and 150 (commonly between 70 and 130) beats/min, which is the range of normal sinus rhythm and sinus tachycardia, and the former is practically always found in diseased hearts and/or DI.

The ectopic focus in the AV junction may activate both the atria and the ventricles. The P-R and R-P intervals vary in this circumstance depending upon the location of the ectopic focus and the status of the antegrade and retrograde conduction systems. However, in many instances, particularly in nonparoxysmal AV JT, there is an independent atrial mechanism, such as AF, leading to AV dissociation (Fig. 6–4). The QRS complex in the AV JT is often normal, but it may be wide and bizarre because of aberrant ventricular conduction or LBBB or RBBB.

### Diagnostic Criteria

Atrioventricular JT is diagnosed when there is AV junctional rhythm with a rate faster than 60 beats/min.

**Nature of Onset and Termination:** The mode of onset and the termination are different between paroxysmal and nonparoxysmal forms. Paroxysmal AV JT, as the name designates, usually starts abruptly as a paroxysm and may also terminate suddenly (Fig. 6–5). Conversely, nonparoxysmal AV JT persists for long periods of time as long as the underlying causes, such as DI or acute diaphragmatic MI, are present (Figs. 6–4 and 6–6). Both forms of AV JT may

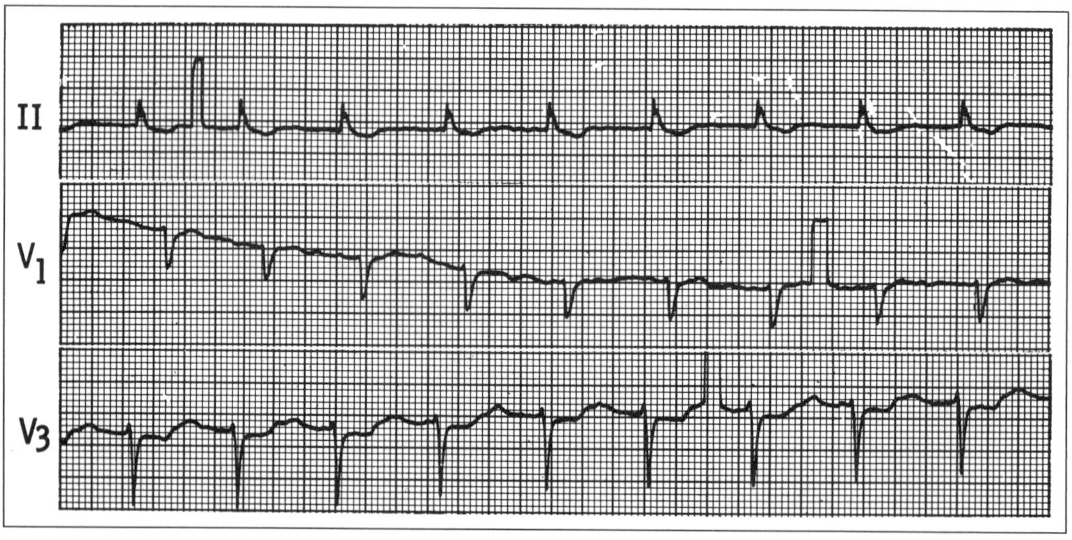


**Fig. 6–4.** Atrial fibrillation with nonparoxysmal AV JT (rate: 86 beats/min) producing complete AV dissociation as a result of DI. Note prominent U waves indicative of hypokalemia.

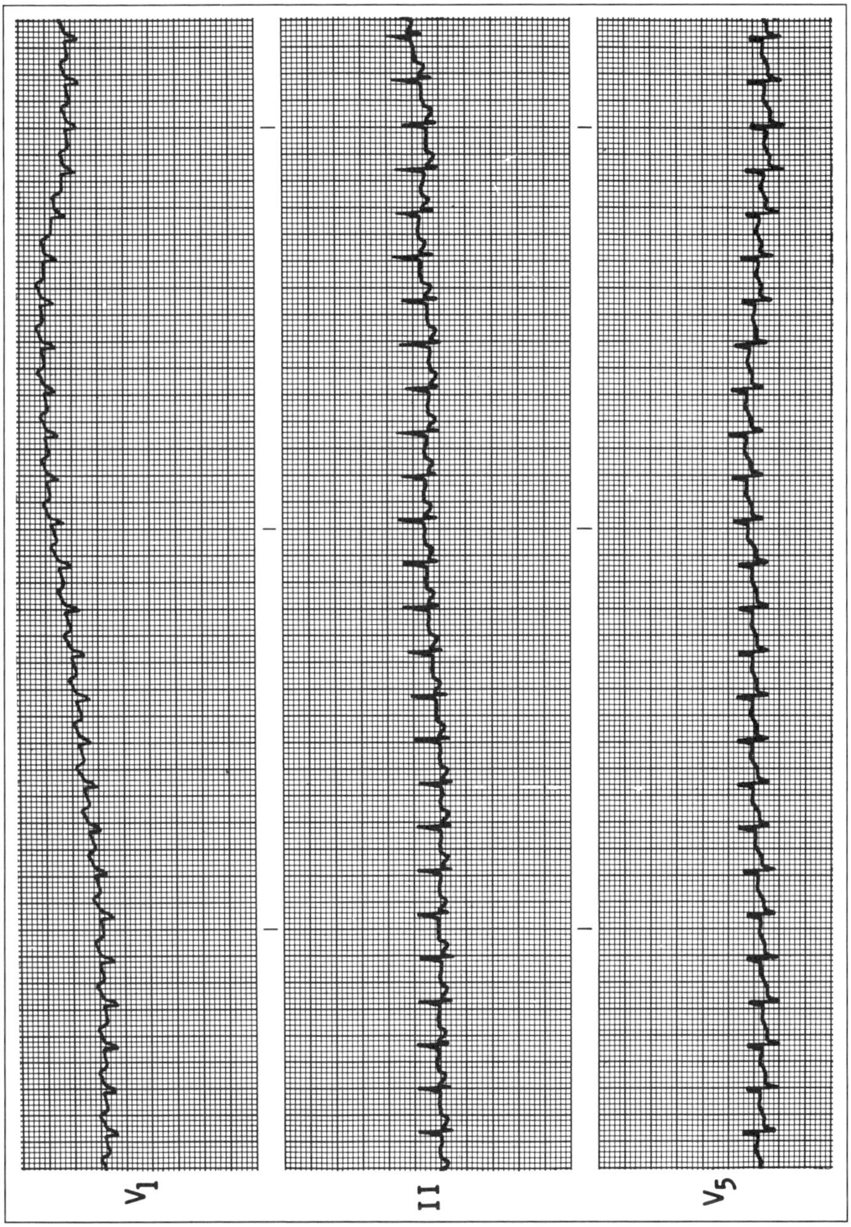


Fig. 6–5. Paroxysmal AV JT with a rate of 188 beats/min.

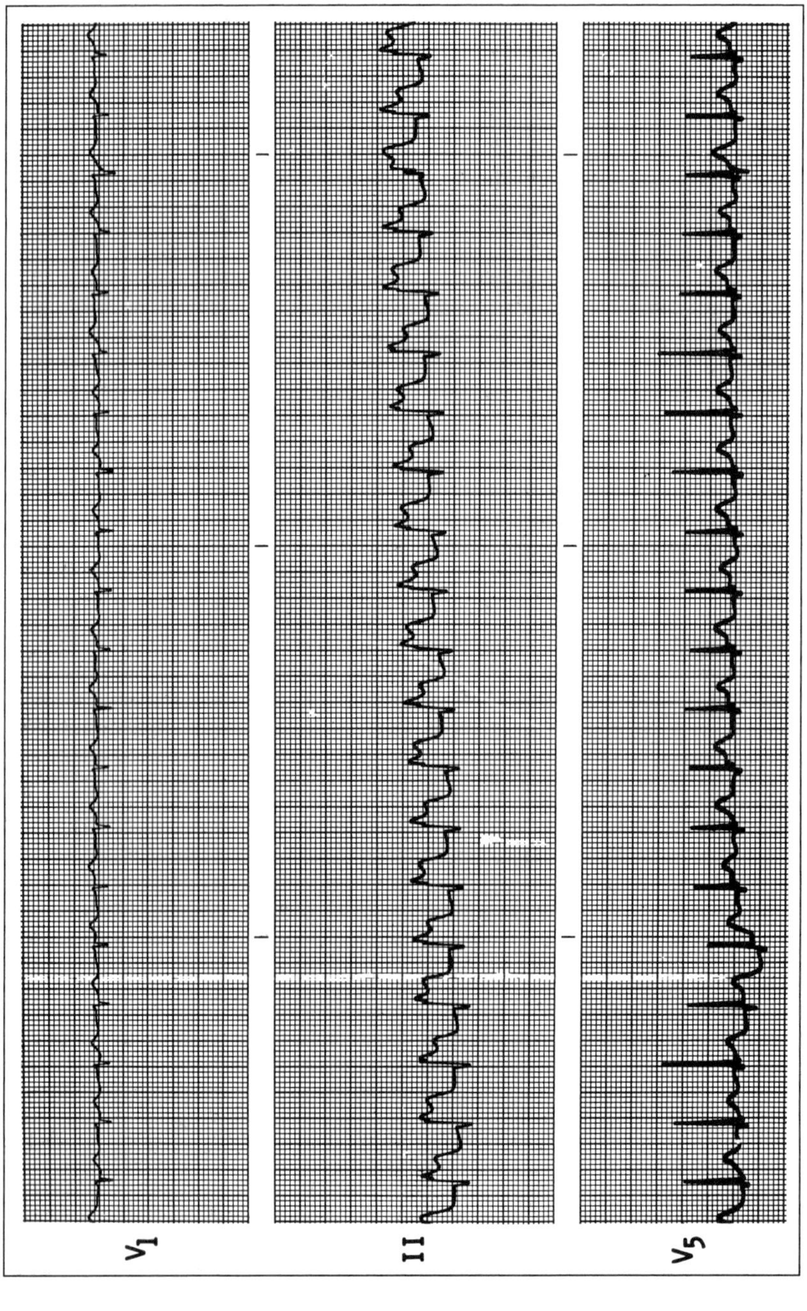


**Fig. 6–6.** Nonparoxysmal AV JT (rate: 126 beats/min) associated with acute diaphragmatic MI.

be initiated by an isolated AV JPC, but this is more common in the paroxysmal form. Not uncommonly, the onset of AV JT, either paroxysmal or nonparoxysmal may be triggered by an impulse from another ectopic focus, either atrial or ventricular. Extremely rarely, AV JT may be initiated by a parasystolic mechanism. In this circumstance, every parasystolic beat may not show in the ECG because of the frequent appearance of exit block. Thus, the long interectopic intervals must be multiples of the shortest interectopic intervals (Chapter 22).

Atrioventricular JT may end spontaneously, by CSS, by digitalization, or by DC shock. Removal of the underlying cause of the tachycardia, especially the nonparoxysmal form, often terminates the rapid heart action.

**Rate:** The ectopic rhythm originating from the AV junction that has a rate faster than 60 beats/min is termed AV JT. The rates found in paroxysmal and nonparoxysmal forms are distinctly different. The rate of the former ranges from 160 to 250 beats/min (Fig. 6–5), and nonparoxysmal AV JT usually produces a rate between 70 and 130 beats/min (Fig. 6–4 and 6–6). Rarely, the rate in nonparoxysmal AV JT may be slower than 70 and faster than 130 beats/min. Therefore, the rates of nonparoxysmal AV JT are essentially within the range of normal sinus rhythm and sinus tachycardia.

It is not uncommon to observe that a direct measurement of the rate in AV JT is not possible. This occurs when there is exit block of varying degrees around the pacemaker in the AV junction. This is especially true if the exit block of Wenckebach phenomenon is present. Furthermore, the rate of the AV JT may only show one half or one third of the actual rate when 2:1 or 3:1 exit block is present.

**Relationship Between Atrial and Ventricular Activation:** In uncomplicated AV JT, the ectopic focus in the AV junction may simultaneously activate the atria and ventricles. This may occur in paroxysmal as well as nonparoxysmal AV JT. In this circumstance, the QRS complex will be preceded or followed by retrograde P waves. The P-R or R-P intervals, as in AV JPCs or AV JER, vary depending upon the location of the ectopic focus in the AV junction and the status of the antegrade and retrograde conduction systems. By and large, uncomplicated AV JT, which controls the atria as well as the ventricles, occurs more commonly in the paroxysmal form.

Atrioventricular JT is manifested by only a QRS complex when the activation of the atria and ventricles coincides or when there is a complete block of retrograde conduction. In most of the latter cases, the atria are controlled by an independent focus in the atria (sinus or ectopic). In this circumstance, AV dissociation naturally results. When there is AF or atrial flutter, AV JT is manifested only by a QRS complex, which again produces AV dissociation (Fig. 6–4). Occasionally, AV JT develops in the presence of independent AT, resulting in double supraventricular tachycardia, which is also a form of AV dissociation. The AV JT associated with AF, atrial flutter, or AT is almost always the nonparoxysmal form and is frequently due to DI (Fig. 6–4).

On extremely rare occasions, the atria and ventricles are activated independently by 2 different pacemakers in the AV junction to produce double AV JT or JER, which also produces AV dissociation. When there is second degree antegrade AV block or retrograde ventriculoatrial (VA) block in AV JT, the P to QRS ratio will vary depending upon the degree of the conduction defect. As seen in sinus rhythm, second degree AV block or VA block may be of Mobitz type I or II. It should be noted that retrograde and antegrade conduction may vary independently.

**Configuration of P Waves:** The configuration of the P waves may vary depending upon whether the atria are activated by the sinus node or an ectopic focus in the atria or the AV junction. When the P waves are of sinus origin, they are usually upright in lead II and inverted in lead aVR, and, of course, the P waves are independent of the QRS complexes. The configuration of the P waves originating from the ectopic focus in the atria is similar to that of sinus P waves. However, the P waves conducted in retrograde fashion from the AV junction will be inverted in leads II, III, and aVF and upright in lead aVR, as seen in isolated AV JPCs or JER. When atrial captured beats occur in the presence of incomplete AV dissociation, retrograde

P waves will appear following the QRS complex of AV JT. When 2 impulses, 1 from the sinus node or ectopic focus in the atria and another from the AV junction, meet in the atria, atrial fusion beats result. The configuration of the atrial fusion beats depends upon the degree to which the atria are activated by the 2 impulses. Needless to say, the P waves will be absent if the underlying atrial mechanism is AF, atrial flutter, or standstill (Fig. 6–4).

**Configuration of QRS Complex:** The configuration of the QRS complex in AV JT is often normal (Figs. 6–4, 6–5, and 6–6). However, the QRS complex may be bizarre and wide when there is aberrant ventricular conduction or BBB. Aberrant ventricular conduction may occur because of a rapid ventricular rate. This is due to the fact that the rapid AV junctional impulses traverse the ventricles during the partially refractory period (usually in paroxysmal form).

**Regularity:** The P-P cycles depend largely upon the origin of the P wave. The P-P cycles are obviously regular when the atria are controlled by regularly discharging sinus or ectopic atrial impulses. In uncomplicated AV JT in which both the atria and ventricles are activated by the AV junctional pacemaker, the P-P and R-R cycles are usually precisely regular. Nevertheless, it is occasionally observed that AV JT may show a slightly irregular cardiac cycle before the AV JT is well established. This is considered to be due to an irregular discharge of impulses from the AV junction during the warming-up period.

The P-P and R-R intervals in AV JT may become irregular when an impairment of retrograde and antegrade conduction or exit block exists. When there is exit block of varying degrees in AV JT, the P-P and R-R intervals show a marked irregularity. When there is 2:1 or 3:1 exit block, long P-P or R-R intervals are usually multiples of short P-P or R-R cycles.

## Mechanisms

There are numerous clinical and experimental investigative evidences to support the close relationship between AV JT and isolated AV JPCs. Paroxysmal tachycardia, regardless of whether it is atrial, AV junctional, or ventricular, is considered to be generated by the same or a similar mechanism, with different origins of the ectopic impulses (a detailed description is found in Chapter 7). In rare cases, AV JT may be due to a parasystolic mechanism (Chapter 22). By and large, the reentry phenomenon is considered to be responsible for the production of various ectopic tachycardias.

## Clinical Significance

Paroxysmal AV JT may occur in healthy individuals as well as in those with diseased hearts, but it is much more common in the former. In contrast, nonparoxysmal AV JT practically always occurs in diseased hearts and/or DI. In addition, the underlying rhythm is often chronic AF. The underlying heart disease is commonly CAD, RHD, or cardiomyopathy. The most common cause of nonparoxysmal AV JT, especially in the presence of AF, is DI (Fig. 6–4), which accounts for approximately 60% of the total incidence of nonparoxysmal AV JT. The next most common cause is acute diaphragmatic MI (Fig. 6–6), which accounts for about 20%. Less commonly, nonparoxysmal AV JT may be associated with myocarditis, myocardiopathy, hypertensive heart disease, and congenital heart disease, such as Ebstein's disease.

Mostly healthy subjects can tolerate paroxysmal AV JT for long periods of time, unless the ventricular rate is extremely rapid. Paroxysmal AV JT often terminates spontaneously or otherwise by CSS, digitalization, or DC shock.

On the other hand, nonparoxysmal AV JT, even with a relatively slow ventricular rate, may produce or aggravate CHF or angina pectoris due to a reduction of the cardiac output and subsequent impairment of the coronary blood flow. Practically all patients with nonparoxysmal AV JT in the presence of AF (Fig. 6–4) suffer from advanced CHF and/or severe DI.

Various symptoms may be produced by AV JT, including palpitations, a tight feeling in the chest, or actual chest pain, weakness, dizziness, anxiety, apprehension, or at times, a feeling of impending death. True fainting episodes are rare. In nonparoxysmal AV JT, many patients show various signs and symptoms of CHF and/or DI.

## ATRIOVENTRICULAR DISSOCIATION

### Definition

By definition, AV dissociation indicates that the atria and ventricles beat independently, so that the P waves or AF or atrial flutter waves and the QRS complexes do not have any relationship. The various etiologies responsible for the development of AV dissociation are listed in Table 6–1. It should be emphasized that AV dissociation is by no means a complete description of the cardiac arrhythmia because it is always a consequence of some other cardiac mechanism.

### Diagnostic Criteria and Mechanisms

Atrioventricular dissociation is diagnosed when the atria and ventricles beat independently. There are 3 basic major rhythm disturbances that produce AV dissociation: (1) slowing or impairment of sinus impulse formation or impairment of the conduction at the SA junction, (2) acceleration of impulse formation in the AV junction or ventricles, and (3) AV conduction disturbance, including artificial pacemaker-induced ventricular rhythm. In AV dissociation, the atrial mechanism may be AF, atrial flutter, or AT. In rare instances of AV dissociation, both the atria and ventricles are activated independently by 2 or more different pacemakers in the AV junction to produce double or triple AV JTs or JERs. When there are 1 or more atrial or ventricular fusion or captured beats in AV dissociation, the term "incomplete AV dissociation" is used. If no captured beats exist, "complete AV dissociation" is the end result.

**Disturbances of Sinus Impulse Formation and Conduction:** The inherent rate of the primary pacemaker (sinus node) in normal adults is between 60 and 100 beats/min; that of the AV node is 40–60 beats, and that of the ventricles 30–40 beats. Whenever the primary pacemaker produces an impulse more slowly than usual (sinus bradycardia) or fails to conduct impulses to the AV junction due to block at the SA junctional tissue (SA block) or fails to produce an impulse (sinus arrest or pause), the AV junction or ventricles may take over, producing AV JER or ventricular escape (idioventricular) rhythm (VER), respectively (Fig. 6–7). Almost always, in this situation, AV JER appears because of the faster inherent rate in the AV junction as compared with the ventricles. At times, AV JEBs may occur alternately with the ventricular captured beats (normally conducted sinus beats) in marked sinus bradycardia. This ECG finding has been termed "A-V junctional escape-bigeminy."

The atria and ventricles would beat independently, but at a similar rate, if the rate of the primary pacemaker slowed to the level of AV JER. This type of AV dissociation may be observed in healthy young adults without any evidence of heart disease (Fig. 6–7). On the other hand, it may be observed during the administration of various drugs, including digitalis, propranolol, reserpine, and guanethidine. It has little clinical significance. However, if the mechanism is sinus arrest or SA block, it is almost always due to serious cardiac disease and/or DI. Atrioventricular dissociation almost always appears, but as a temporary phenomenon, when intermittent and brief sinus arrest or SA block occurs. For a similar reason, AV dissociation may temporarily develop following the pause after any premature ectopic impulse when AV JEBs arise to control the ventricles. However, 1 of the lower pacemakers (AV node or ventricles) may take over the entire cardiac activity if SA block or sinus arrest persists for a long period of time.

**Acceleration of Impulse Formation in Atrioventricular Junction or Ventricles:** In this instance, the AV junction or ventricles initiate impulses at a faster rate, regardless of the atrial activity (either sinus or ectopic atrial), thus re-

**TABLE 6–1. Causes of AV dissociation**

| DISTURBANCES OF SINUS IMPULSE FORMATION & CONDUCTION | | | ACCELERATION OF IMPULSE INFORMATION IN THE AV JUNCTION OR VENTRICLES | | AV CONDUCTION DISTURBANCES | |
|---|---|---|---|---|---|---|
| Sinus Bradycardia | Sinus Arrest | SA Block | AV Junctional Tachycardia | Ventricular Tachycardia | Complete (or Advanced) AV Block | Artificial Pacemaker-induced Ventricular Rhythm |
| 1. Sinus bradycardia with AV junctional escape rhythm | 1. Sinus arrest with AV junctional escape rhythm | 1. SA block with AV junctional escape rhythm | 1. Sinus rhythm with AV junctional tachycardia | 1. Sinus rhythm with ventricular tachycardia | 1. Sinus rhythm with AV junctional or ventricular escape rhythm | 1. Sinus rhythm with artificial pacemaker-induced ventricular rhythm |
| 2. Sinus bradycardia with ventricular escape rhythm | 2. Sinus arrest with ventricular escape rhythm | 2. SA block with ventricular escape rhythm | 2. Atrial fibrillation with AV junctional tachycardia | 2. Atrial fibrillation with ventricular tachycardia | 2. Atrial fibrillation with AV junctional or ventricular escape rhythm | 2. Atrial fibrillation with artificial pacemaker-induced ventricular rhythm |
| | | | 3. Atrial flutter with AV junctional tachycardia | 3. Atrial flutter with ventricular tachycardia | 3. Atrial flutter with AV junctional or ventricular escape rhythm | 3. Atrial flutter with artificial pacemaker-induced ventricular rhythm |
| | | | 4. Atrial tachycardia with AV junctional tachycardia | 4. Atrial tachycardia with ventricular tachycardia | 4. Atrial tachycardia with AV junctional or ventricular escape rhythm | 4. Atrial tachycardia with artificial pacemaker-induced ventricular rhythm |
| | | | 5. Multiple AV junctional tachycardia | 5. AV junctional tachycardia with ventricular tachycardia | 5. AV junctional tachycardia with AV junctional or ventricular escape rhythm | 5. AV nodal tachycardia with artificial pacemaker-induced ventricular rhythm |

→ AV dissociation

Reproduced with permission from Chung: Principles of Cardiac Arrhythmias, 3rd ed., Baltimore, Williams & Wilkins, 1983.

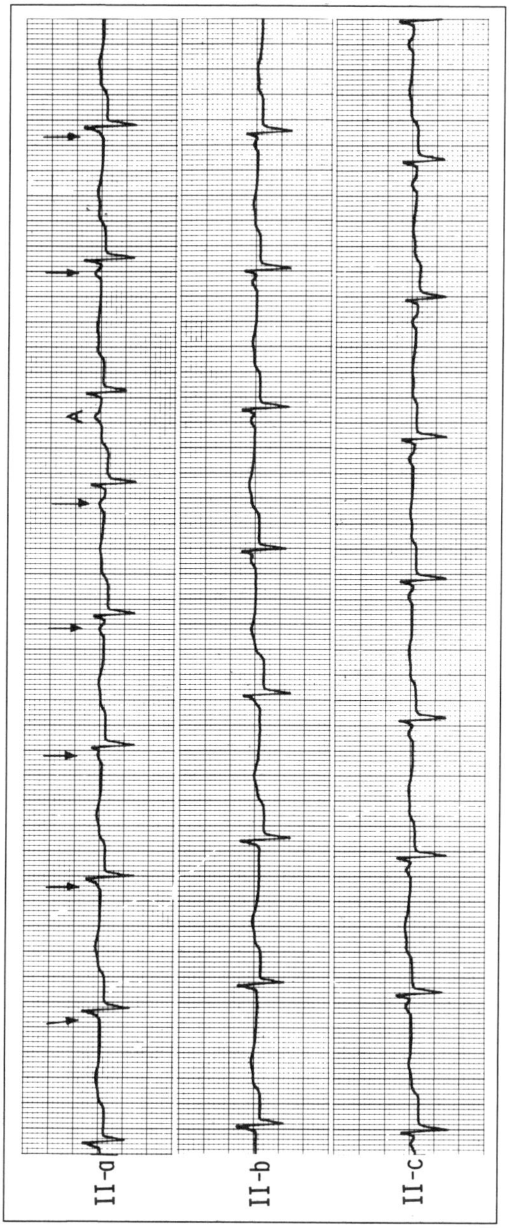


Fig. 6–7. Sinus bradycardia (indicated by arrows) with an APC (A) and intermittent AV JER producing incomplete AV dissociation. Note that the atrial and ventricular rates are almost the same (rate: 54 beats/min) but independent in most areas. Leads II-a, II-b, and II-c are continuous.

sulting in AV dissociation (Fig. 6–4). Rapid ectopic pacemaker action may appear as a paroxysmal or nonparoxysmal tachycardia.

Ventricular tachycardia and, rarely, ventricular flutter may be associated with AV dissociation, but it is quite difficult and often impossible to detect the atrial activity (either sinus or ectopic) because, during the paroxysms, the atrial waves are usually superimposed on the bizarre and wide QRS complexes.

**Atrioventricular Conduction Disturbances:** Whenever the atrial impulse (either sinus or ectopic) is not conducted to the AV junction and ventricles due to a block in the AV junctional tissue, in the common bundle, or in the bilateral bundles, AV JER or VER develops to control the ventricles as a physiologic mechanism. In this instance, the atrial rate is faster than, and is also independent of, the ventricular rate (Figs. 2–4 and 6–3). Often AV block and SA block develop in the same patient. This is particularly common in acute diaphragmatic MI and DI.

When the ventricles are controlled by an artificial pacemaker independent of the atrial mechanism, AV dissociation will, of course, result.

**Captured Beats:** If the mechanism of AV dissociation is not complete AV block, whenever any chamber is *not* in the refractory state, 1 of the 2 pacemakers may activate the entire heart. In other words, the sinus or ectopic atrial pacemaker may control the ventricles when they are not in a refractory phase. This is termed "ventricular captured beats" (Fig. 6–7). Ventricular captured beats in the presence of AV dissociation merely indicate normally conducted sinus or atrial (i.e., fibrillation) beats. Likewise, an ectopic pacemaker in the AV junction or ventricles or an artificial pacemaker that controls the ventricles may activate the atria in a retrograde fashion when the atria are not in a refractory phase. This phenomenon is termed "atrial captured beats." It should be noted that the atrial captured beat originating from the AV junction (rarely ventricles) may be followed by a reciprocal beat due to a reentry phenomenon. Reciprocal beats are discussed later in this chapter. If the captured impulse in the atria or ventricles simultaneously meets with an impulse from another pacemaker, partial atrial or ventricular captured beats develop, and are called "atrial" or "ventricular fusion beats," respectively. Recognition of captured beats is not difficult because they occur prematurely with a constant P-R or R-P relationship when the atrial mechanism is not fibrillation or flutter. When the underlying atrial mechanism is AF or atrial flutter, in the presence of AV dissociation, ventricular captured beats are, actually, normally conducted ordinary AF or atrial flutter beats. Often, ventricular captured beats exhibit aberrant ventricular conduction because of a short coupling interval Once a captured beat occurs, 1 pacemaker may control the entire heart either temporarily or continuously. Ventricular captured beats are very common in the presence of underlying AF because AV JT or AV JER often occurs intermittently or periodically. Needless to say, it is impossible for atrial captured beats to occur when the underlying rhythm is AF or atrial flutter, since the atria are constantly activated by 1 or more rapidly discharging atrial ectopic foci.

Atrial or ventricular captured beats may occur in double or triple AV JTs or JERs when antegrade or retrograde conduction is not completely blocked. For a similar reason, atrial or ventricular fusion beats may be observed in double or triple AV JTs or JERs and in artificial pacemaker-induced ventricular rhythm, unless there is a complete block in antegrade or retrograde conduction.

In any event, whenever a captured beat (either complete or partial) is present, this should be termed "incomplete AV dissociation" because the atria and ventricles have some relationship to each other even though only momentarily. In the presence of intermittent complete AV block, captured beats may intermittently occur, and this situation has been called "high degree" or "advanced AV block." This is also a form of incomplete AV dissociation.

If there are no captured beats and the atria and ventricles beat independently throughout, this should be called "complete AV dissociation."

**Ectopic Atrial Mechanism:** In AV dissociation, the atria are not necessarily controlled by the sinus node, and likewise the ventricles may be controlled by either the AV junction or the ventricles. Therefore, the atrial mechanism may be AF, atrial flutter or AT. Under these circumstances, either complete or incomplete AV dissociation may develop. For example, AF or atrial flutter with AV JER or VER due to complete or high degree AV block may be present (Fig. 6–3). Atrial fibrillation, atrial flutter or AT with AV JT or VT may also be present (Fig. 6–4).

**Multiple Atrioventricular Junctional Rhythm or Tachycardia:** In a rare form of AV dissociation, the atria and ventricles are controlled by 2 different pacemakers in the AV junctional tissue. In this instance, the atria are activated in retrograde fashion. Occasionally, the atria may be intermittently activated by the sinus node in the presence of double AV JTs or JERs, resulting in triple rhythm. In this case, atrial fusion beats may be observed, placed between antegrade sinus and retrograde AV junctional impulses. Each pacemaker at the AV junction may produce an AV JT or JER.

## Clinical Significance

The clinical significance of AV dissociation depends largely upon the basic rhythm disturbance. When the basic rhythm disorder is sinus bradycardia or sinus arrhythmia, there is no clinical significance. In contrast to this, when the basic disorder is nonparoxysmal AV JT or high degree or complete AV block, serious underlying heart disease is usually found. Especially when nonparoxysmal AV JT or JER develops in the presence of an underlying AF or atrial flutter, DI is almost always responsible, and often there is intractable CHF. When VT is associated with AV dissociation, advanced heart disease is nearly always present, and immediate treatment is needed.

In short, AV dissociation per se does not indicate or exclude organic heart disease, and AV dissociation per se does not require treatment. The treatment of AV dissociation is primarily directed toward the basic rhythm disorder and the fundamental underlying heart disease and/or drug (e.g., digitalis) toxicity.

# RECIPROCAL BEATS AND RHYTHM

Reciprocal beats and rhythm (echo beats and rhythm) are considered to be generated by a specific form of reentry phenomenon. This arrhythmia nearly always arises from AV JT or JER (Fig. 6–8). Occasionally, reciprocal beats may be initiated by AV JPCs or VPCs, and, rarely, APCs or even sinus beats may be followed by reciprocal beats.

A reciprocal beat is diagnosed when a retrograde P wave is noted to be sandwiched between 2 closely spaced QRS complexes, the first of which originates from an ectopic focus (commonly, the AV node). As a result, the QRS complex following the retrograde P wave appears earlier than the usual R-R cycle of the basic rhythm. Since reciprocal beats and rhythm are almost always initiated by AV JT or JER, the underlying cause is frequently DI.

## Diagnostic Criteria

**Configuration of P Wave:** In uncomplicated reciprocal beat, the P wave that is sandwiched between 2 closely spaced QRS complexes usually has the appearance of a retrograde P wave (Fig. 6–8). At times, the sandwiched P wave may have different degrees of atrial fusion. This occurs when the atria are simultaneously activated by 1 impulse conducted in a retrograde fashion (reciprocal impulse) from the AV junction and another impulse from the sinus node, in the presence of AV dissociation. Of course, there will be no P wave seen in a reciprocal beat when the underlying atrial mechanism is AF or atrial flutter. Similarly, the sandwiched P wave will be absent from a reciprocal beat when there is a block in retrograde conduction.

**R-P and P-R Intervals:** Since reciprocal beats commonly occur in AV JT or JER with delayed retrograde conduction, the R-P intervals are always longer than 0.20 second. When progressive lengthening of the R-P intervals occurs because of a delayed retrograde conduction with Wenckebach phenomenon, reciprocal beats are prone to follow the longest R-P interval of each sequence. The P-R interval of a reciprocal beat

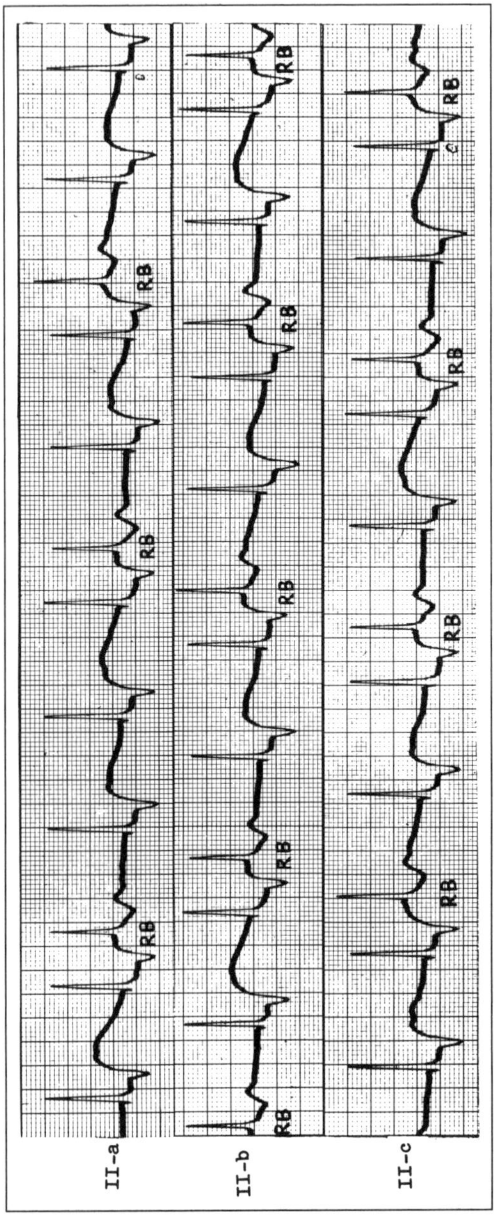


**Fig. 6–8.** Atrioventricular JER (ventricular rate: 57 beats/min) with Wenckebach VA block and frequent reciprocal beats (RB). Note that the R-P intervals progressively lengthen until a reciprocal beat occurs. Leads II-a, II-b, and II-c are continuous.

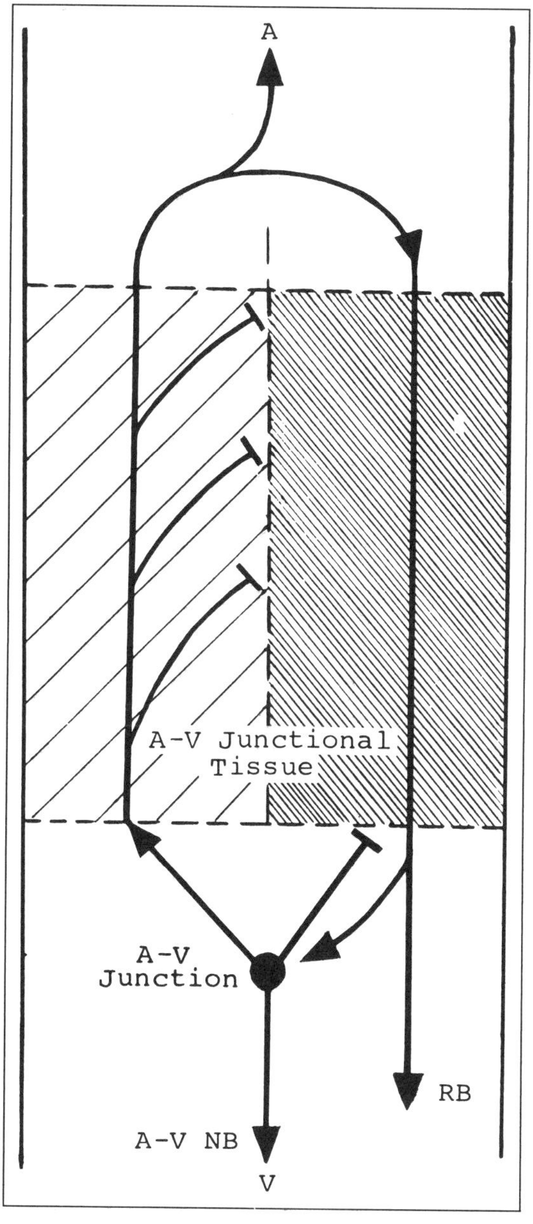


Fig. 6–9. This diagram illustrates the mechanism of reciprocal beats. The genesis of a reciprocal beat is considered to be a specific form of reentry phenomenon occurring in the AV junctional tissues. One assumes that there is a longitudinal dissociation present in the AV junctional fibers, which have different degrees of depressed conductivity. Thus, some longitudinal fibers (closely hatched area) are more depressed than others (widely hatched area). Consequently, unidirectional block of retrograde conduction occurs in the more depressed fibers, in addition to a generalized delay in retrograde conduction in the whole of the AV junctional fibers. The impulse originating from the AV junction is conducted in both directions, toward the ventricles (V; antegrade) and toward the atria (A; retrograde). The retrograde impulse will soon reach the depressed AV junctional fibers. The retrograde impulse is completely blocked at the more depressed fibers (closely hatched area), while it is conducted at a slower speed than usual in a retrograde fashion in the remaining, less depressed fibers (widely hatched area). In the meantime, the more depressed longitudinal fibers (closely hatched area), which were previously refractory to the retrograde impulse, recover their conductivity. As a result, the retrograde impulse splits before reaching the atria (A). One impulse continues in a retrograde direction to the atria, and another retraces its steps in an antegrade direction toward the AV junction. When the time required (the R-R interval that includes the sandwiched P wave) for the retrograde conduction of the AV junctional impulse (R-P interval) and the subsequent antegrade conduction of the reentry impulse (P-R interval) is sufficient for the ventricles to recover from their initial response to the AV junctional impulse, a second ventricular complex, namely, the reciprocal beat (RB), will result.

may be prolonged, and it may exceed the R-P interval. However, as a rule, the R-P interval is longer than the P-R interval in reciprocal beats.

**R-R Interval:** The R-R interval that includes the sandwiched P wave is usually 0.50 second or less. However, it may be slightly longer than 0.50 second when there is a marked conduction delay in retrograde and/or antegrade conduction.

**Frequency:** Reciprocal beat may appear as an isolated beat, but it may occur at every other, third, or fourth beat, leading to regular irregularity. It has been reported that reciprocal beats may occur consecutively to produce reciprocal rhythm or tachycardia, but differentiation of these from AV JT or JER is often difficult or impossible.

**Aberrant Ventricular Conduction:** The QRS complex following the sandwiched P wave in reciprocal beat may be normal in configuration. However, the QRS complex may have a wide and bizarre contour because of aberrant ventricular conduction. This occurs because the impulse following the sandwiched P wave reaches the ventricles during their relative refractory period due to the short R-R interval containing the sandwiched P wave.

**Reciprocal Beats or Rhythm in Atrial Fibrillation or Atrial Flutter:** The characteristic sandwiched retrograde P wave will, of course, be absent when the underlying rhythm is AF or atrial flutter. Nevertheless, other features of reciprocal beats may be observed, although the rhythm is often difficult to diagnose with certainty. Reciprocal beats associated with AV JT in the presence of AF often produce regular irregularity of the ventricular rhythm.

### Mechanism

The fundamental mechanism (Fig. 6–9) responsible for the genesis of reciprocal beats is considered to be a specific form of a reentry phenomenon occurring in the AV junctional tissue. One assumes that there is a longitudinal dissociation present in the AV junctional fibers, which have different degrees of depressed conductivity. Thus, some of the longitudinal fibers are more markedly depressed than others. Consequently, unidirectional block of retrograde conduction occurs in the more depressed fibers, in addition to a generalized delay in retrograde conduction in the entire AV junctional fibers. The impulse originating from the AV node is conducted in both directions, toward the ventricles (antegrade) and toward the atria (retrograde). The retrograde impulse will soon reach the depressed AV junctional fibers. The retrograde impulse is completely blocked in the more depressed fibers, while it is conducted at a slower speed than usual in a retrograde fashion in the remaining, less depressed fibers. The R-P interval in a reciprocal beat is consequently prolonged (longer than 0.20 second) because of the delayed retrograde conduction. In the meantime, the more depressed longitudinal fibers, which were previously refractory to the retrograde impulse, recover their conductivity. As a result, the retrograde impulse splits before reaching the atria; 1 impulse continues in a retrograde direction to the atria, and another retraces its steps in an antegrade direction toward the AV node. In other words, the antegrade impulse traverses down the longitudinal fibers, which are now responsive but were previously refractory. When the time required (the R-R interval that includes the sandwiched P wave) for the retrograde conduction of the AV nodal impulse (R-P interval) and the subsequent antegrade conduction of the reentry impulse (P-R interval) is sufficient for the ventricles to recover from their initial response to the AV nodal impulse, a second ventricular complex, namely, the reciprocal beat, will result.

### Clinical Significance

Since reciprocal beats frequently occur in the presence of AV JT or JER, their clinical significance is often similar to that of the latter. In general, the fundamental cause for the development of reciprocal beats and rhythm is commonly DI. This is particularly true when the underlying rhythm is AF.

## ATRIOVENTRICULAR JUNCTIONAL PARASYSTOLE

Atrioventricular junctional parasystole is an uncommon AV junctional arrhythmia, which is discussed in Chapter 22.

# Chapter 7

# Ventricular Arrhythmias

Ventricular arrhythmias may be generated by either active or passive impulse formation. A relatively uncommon ventricular arrhythmia is produced by a parasystolic mechanism (Chapter 22). Active impulse formation from a ventricular focus may produce a VPC, VT, ventricular flutter, and VF. These ventricular arrhythmias occur regardless of the underlying cardiac rhythm. In contrast to this, passive impulse formation of the ventricles occurs when the AV junction fails to produce an impulse passively in spite of the fact that atrial impulses are unable to reach the ventricles (commonly due to high degree or complete AV block) in the expected time or when the AV block is distal to the AV node. The rhythm generated by passive impulse formation by the ventricles is termed "ventricular escape rhythm (VER)" or "idioventricular rhythm." Ventricular arrhythmias, regardless of the fundamental mechanism, may originate from any location in the ventricles. The configuration of the QRS complex in ventricular arrhythmias is greatly influenced by the location of the ectopic focus. The configuration may be almost normal and resemble a sinus beat or may be so bizarre that the duration of the QRS complex may exceed 0.16 second.

The most common ventricular arrhythmia and, in fact, the most common ectopic beats encountered in human hearts are, without doubt, VPCs. Since VPCs may be observed in almost every individual some time during his or her life, even without demonstrable heart disease, the occasional occurrence of this arrhythmia is insignificant clinically.

Ventricular tachyarrhythmias, including VT, ventricular flutter, and VF, are almost always found in serious heart disease, and often they are fatal unless immediately treated. These arrhythmias are frequently initiated by an isolated VPC, particularly multifocal in origin. It is commonly observed that VT may transform to ventricular flutter and VF, or vice versa, in the same patient.

## VENTRICULAR PREMATURE CONTRACTIONS (EXTRASYSTOLES)

Ventricular premature contractions are the most common cardiac arrhythmias and may be observed in practically every individual some time during his life. This arrhythmia is uncommon in children, but its incidence increases with age, even without demonstrable heart disease. Although VPCs are commonly found in healthy adults, especially following excessive ingestion of coffee or tea, heavy smoking, or emotional excitement the frequent occurrence of this arrhythmia, particularly when it is multifocal in origin, nearly always indicates organic heart disease and/or digitalis intoxication (DI).

Ventricular premature contractions may originate from a single focus or from multiple foci anywhere in the ventricles. They may occur rarely, occasionally, or frequently and regularly or irregularly. There may be 2 or more consecutive VPCs, which may lead to VT, ventricular flutter, or VF. When VPCs occur consecutively, the finding is called "ventricular group beats." Any underlying cardiac rhythm may be present concomitantly with VPCs. This arrhythmia is almost always followed by a full compensatory pause, and interpolated VPCs are only occasionally observed, especially when the basic cardiac rhythm is slow.

### Diagnostic Criteria

Ventricular premature contractions are diagnosed when a wide and bizarre QRS complex

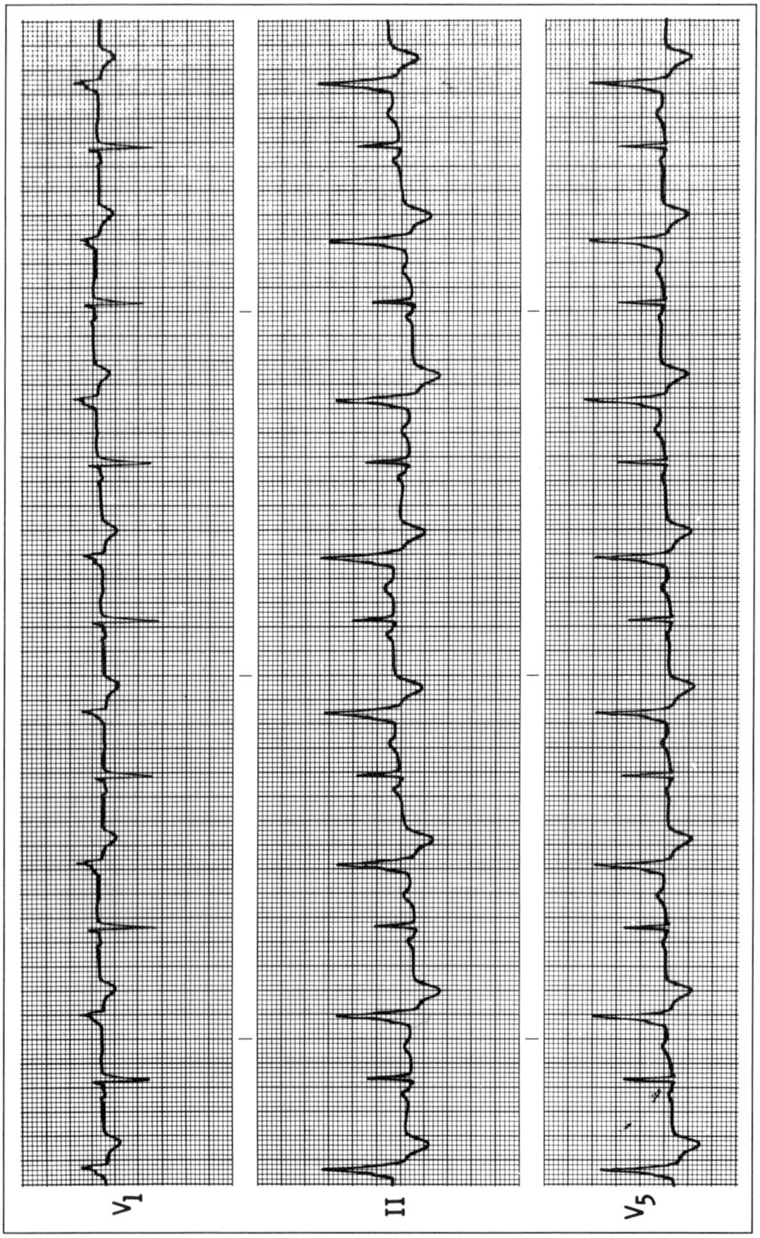


Fig. 7–1. Sinus rhythm with frequent VPCs producing ventricular bigeminy.

appears prematurely without a preceding ectopic P wave. A full compensatory pause almost always follows this arrhythmia.

**Configuration of QRS Complex and ST, T Waves:** The duration of the QRS complex is nearly always 0.12 second or more in a VPC because of the abnormal propagation of the ectopic impulse in the ventricles as a result of the asynchronous onset of the excitation in the 2 ventricles (Fig. 7–1). Thus, the configuration of the QRS complex often resembles either an LBBB or an RBBB. By and large, a VPC originating from the left ventricle resembles the QRS complex of RBBB. Conversely, an LBBB pattern will be observed when the ventricular ectopic focus is in the right ventricle. However, a VPC arising from the neighborhood of the bifurcation of the AV (common) bundle has a QRS complex that resembles a sinus beat. Although various investigative studies have been carried out in regard to the determination of the origin of a VPC, its practical value is very limited. In addition to the location of the ectopic focus, any underlying myocardial disease and/or preexisting intraventricular conduction defect can influence the degree of bizarre configuration. It has been shown that when the QRS complex exceeds 0.16 second, significant underlying organic heart disease is strongly suggested. Furthermore, a VPC with a short coupling interval tends to be more bizarre. This is observed because the impulse from the VPC traverses the ventricles during the partial refractory period. In general, the QRS configuration is apt to be more bizarre when the ectopic focus is located distally from the bifurcation of the AV (common) bundle, when the coupling interval is short, and when the underlying myocardial disease and/or intraventricular conduction disturbance exists.

The configuration of the QRS complex of a unifocal VPC is usually identical in each given lead (Fig. 7–1). When the impulses arise from 2 or more ventricular foci, the term "multifocal" VPCs is used. In this case, 2 or more different QRS complexes with different coupling intervals are observed in the same lead (Fig. 7–2).

When a VPC occurs late in the cycle of the basic rhythm, a ventricular fusion beat may be observed. This occurs because the sinus impulse meets with the ventricular ectopic impulse somewhere in the ventricles because of the long coupling interval. The configuration of the ventricular fusion beat will be intermediate between that of the sinus and ectopic beats, and its configuration will vary depending upon the portion of the ventricles activated by the 2 impulses. Ventricular fusion beats tend to occur when the rate of the basic rhythm is relatively rapid. Needless to say, ventricular fusion beats are much more common in ventricular parasystole because of its independency from the basic rhythm (Chapter 22).

Characteristically, secondary ST, T wave changes are observed in VPCs. Notably, the direction of the ST segment and T wave deviation is always opposite to that of the QRS complex (Fig. 7–1).

**Constant Coupling Interval:** The coupling interval of unifocal VPCs is usually constant (Fig. 7–1) because the impulse formation in the ventricle is dependent upon the preceding beat of the basic rhythm. However, the coupling intervals will vary when VPCs arise from 2 or more foci (Fig. 7–2). In contrast to fixed coupling intervals in VPCs, ventricular parasystole characteristically produces varying coupling intervals (Chapter 22).

**Frequency:** Ventricular premature contractions may appear rarely, occasionally, or frequently and regularly or irregularly. When VPCs occur at the rate of 30 or more beats/hour, the occurrence is said to be frequent. When VPCs occur regularly, they may alternate with the basic beats (ventricular bigeminy; Fig. 7–1), with every third beat (ventricular trigeminy), or with every fourth beat (ventricular quadrigeminy). The term "ventricular group beats" is used when 2 or more consecutive VPCs appear (Fig. 7–3). Ventricular tachycardia is said to be present if 6 or more consecutive VPCs appear.

**Postectopic Pause:** One of the characteristic features of VPCs is the full compensatory pause that follows (Figs. 7–1 and 7–2). A full compensatory pause is said to exist when the R-R interval containing the VPC is 2 times the R-R interval of the basic rhythm (Fig. 7–1). This phenomenon is observed as long as the sinus node is not prematurely discharged by the ven-

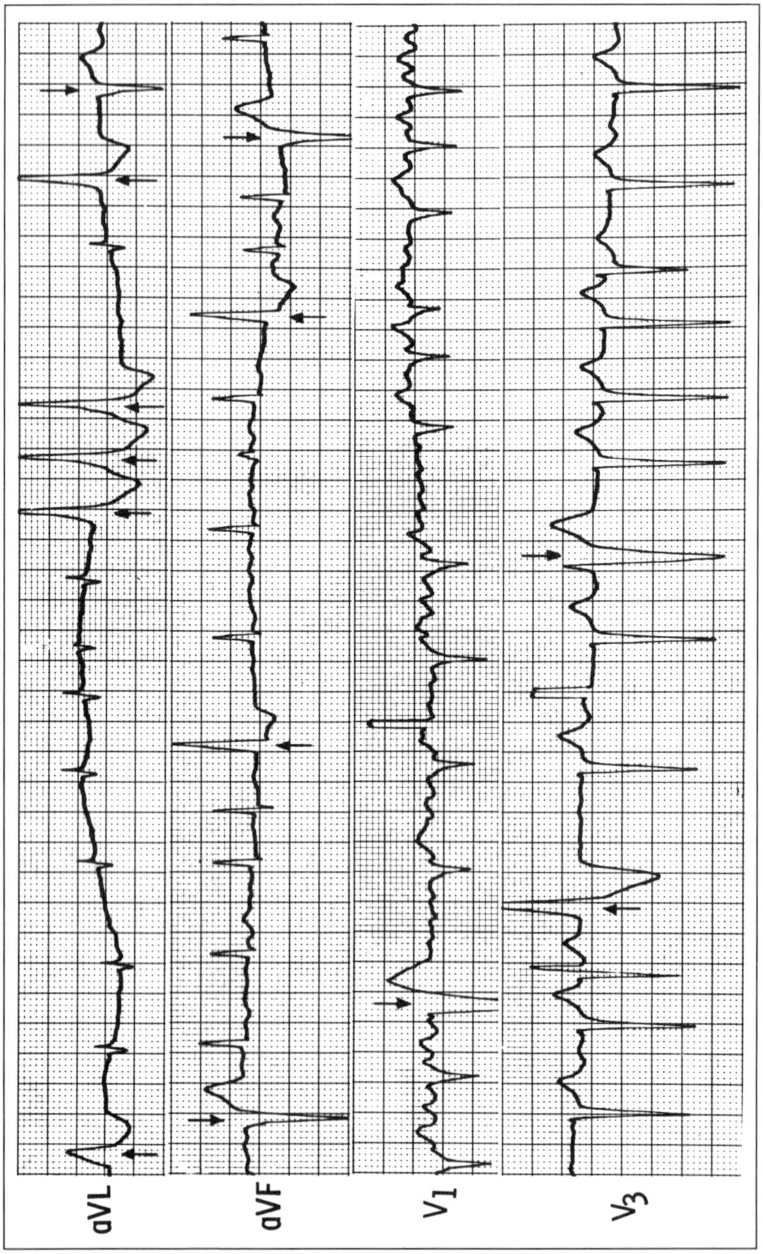


**Fig. 7–2.** Atrial flutter-fibrillation with frequent multifocal VPCs and ventricular group beats (indicated by arrows).

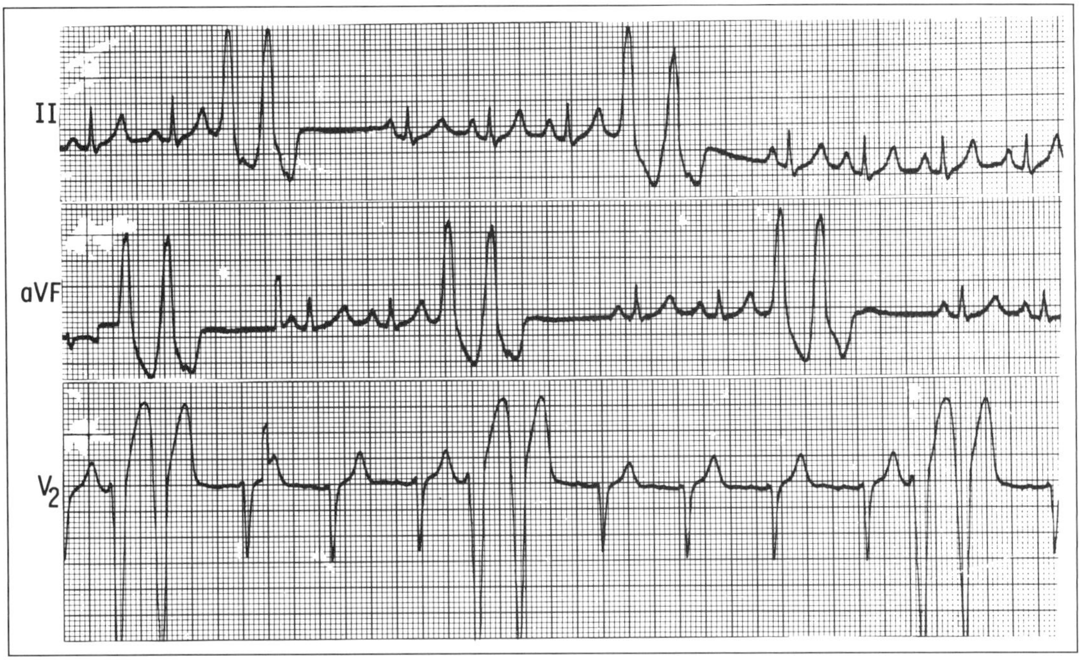


**Fig. 7–3.** Sinus rhythm with frequent VPCs and ventricular group beats (2 in a row).

tricular ectopic impulse. In other words, a full compensatory pause is observed when the ventricular ectopic impulse meets with the sinus impulse at the SA junction (SA interference), in the atria (atrial interference), at the AV junction (AV interference), and in the ventricles (ventricular interference). A detailed explanation of these findings is diagrammatically shown in Figure 7–4. When atrial or ventricular interference occurs, an atrial or ventricular fusion beat will result, respectively. Interference commonly occurs in the AV junction so that the sinus node controls the atria while the ventricles are independently activated by a ventricular ectopic focus. In this case, the sinus P wave is not usually discernible because the P wave is superimposed on a portion of the bizarre QRS complex or the ST segment and T wave of the VPC. By and large, the site of the interference is determined by the degree of the prematurity of the ventricular ectopic beat and/or the rate of the basic rhythm. A full compensatory pause cannot be measured precisely when the basic rhythm is irregular, as in sinus arrhythmia. When the underlying rhythm is AF or atrial flutter, a long pause follows the VPC (Fig. 7–5) and is analogous to a full compensatory pause during sinus rhythm.

Not uncommonly, the impulse from the VPC may activate the atria in a retrograde fashion. In this case, inverted P waves in leads II, III, and aVF and an upright P wave in lead aVR are observed following the QRS complex of the VPCs. Under this circumstance, the sinus node may be passively and prematurely activated by the ventricular ectopic impulse. When a retrograde P wave follows the QRS complex of a VPC, the retrograde P wave usually occurs earlier than a sinus P wave would be anticipated, and the P-P interval from the ectopic to the subsequent sinus P wave is usually longer than the P-P cycle of the basic rhythm (Fig. 7–4). The R-P interval in this case is around 0.20 second, and it is generally constant. When the R-P interval is markedly prolonged because of an impaired retrograde conduction, a reciprocal beat may follow a VPC. A full compensatory pause is usually observed when the interference occurs

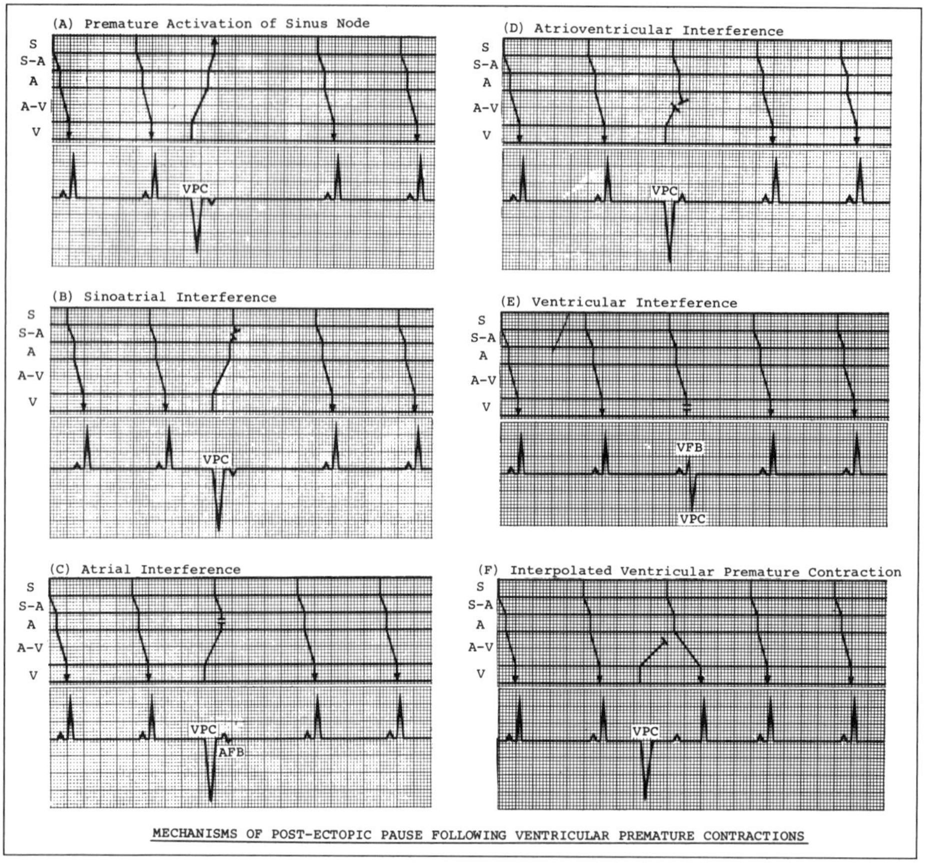


**Fig. 7–4.** Mechanism of postectopic pauses following VPCs. **A.** Premature activation of sinus node by a retrograde impulse from ventricular ectopic focus. **B.** Sinoatrial interference. **C.** Atrial interference (atrial fusion beat). **D.** Atrioventricular interference. **E.** Ventricular interference (ventricular fusion beat). **F.** Interpolated VPC. AFB = atrial fusion beat; VFB = ventricular fusion beat. A detailed description is found in the text.

at the SA junction (Fig. 7–4). However, a period longer than a full compensatory pause may be observed when the sinus node is prematurely activated by the ventricular impulse because the sinus node will be momentarily suppressed (Fig. 7–4). It should be noted that the sinus P wave immediately following a VPC may resemble a retrograde P wave when the P wave is superimposed on a portion of the ST segment or T wave.

On rare occasions, a VPC may be interpolated, especially when the basic rhythm is relatively slow (Figs. 7–4 and 7–6). An interpolated VPC is a true extra beat because the VPC is sandwiched between 2 QRS complexes of the basic rhythm. A full compensatory pause is, of course, not observed in this instance, but the R-R interval containing the VPC is often slightly longer than the remaining R-R intervals. This is observed because the longer P-R interval of the sinus beat immediately following VPC is due to concealed VA (retrograde) conduction (Figs. 7–4 and 7–6). An interpolated VPC is not uncommon in fixed-rate artificial pacemaker-induced ventricular rhythm.

**Postectopic T Wave Changes:** Occasionally, the T wave of the sinus beat immediately following a VPC may show alteration of its contour, amplitude, and/or direction (Fig. 7–7). This phenomenon is termed "postectopic T wave change." On rare occasions, 2 or more successive sinus beats following a VPC may

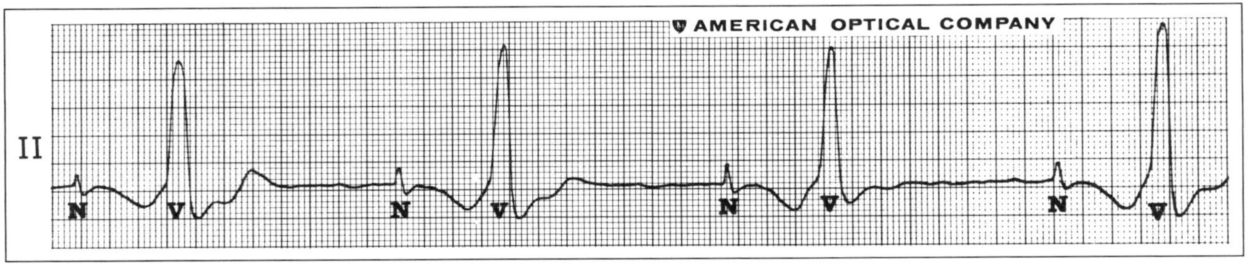


**Fig. 7–5.** Atrial fibrillation with AV JER (N) due to complete AV block and frequent VPCs (V) causing ventricular bigeminy. These rhythm disturbances are digitalis induced.

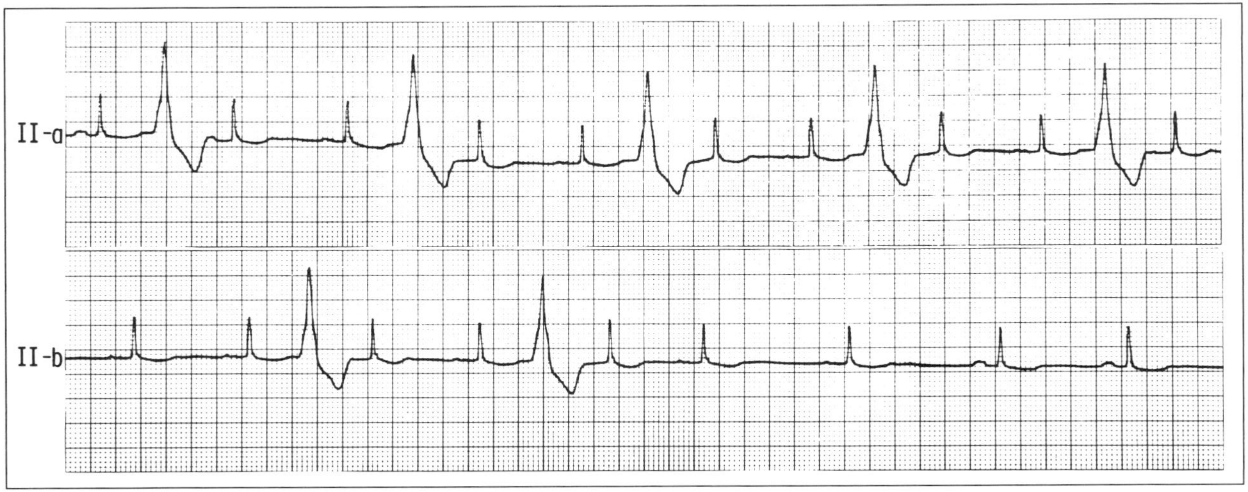


**Fig. 7–6.** Sinus arrhythmia with wandering atrial pacemaker and frequent interpolated VPCs. Leads II-a and II-b are continuous.

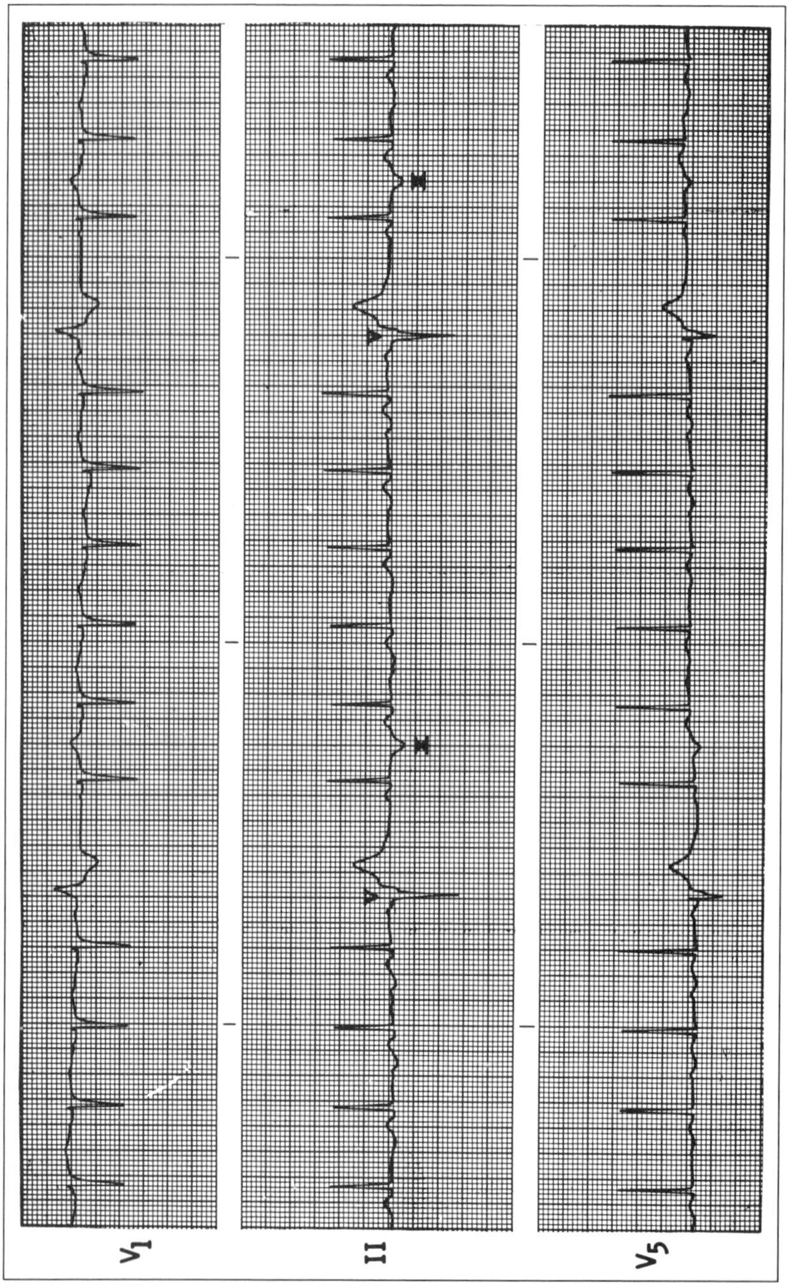


**Fig. 7–7.** Sinus rhythm with frequent VPCs (V) followed by postectopic T wave change (X).

show postectopic T wave changes. The mechanism of the postectopic T wave change is not clearly understood, but it is considered to be due to alteration of the ventricular repolarization process related to a preceding postectopic pause. Thus, postectopic T wave changes are much more common following an interpolated VPC than a full compensatory pause. The recognition of postectopic T wave changes is important clinically because this phenomenon is almost always indicative of organic heart disease.

**Postectopic Aberrant Ventricular and Atrial Conduction:** The QRS complex of the sinus beat following a VPC occasionally shows a slightly or markedly deformed configuration. This is considered to be due to the fact that ventricular activation by the sinus impulse immediately following the VPC is carried out during a partial refractory period. This is a form of aberrant ventricular conduction. This aberrant ventricular conduction is commonly associated with postectopic T wave changes and commonly found following an interpolated VPC.

Extremely rarely, the P wave of the sinus beat following a VPC may have a deformed configuration. This is termed "aberrant atrial conduction" (Chung's phenomenon). This phenomenon may be observed in 2 or more consecutive sinus beats following a VPC.

## Mechanisms

Since the fundamental mechanisms involved in the production of premature beat, either atrial, AV junctional, or ventricular, are considered to be very similar or even identical, a detailed description will be given at this time. The ectopic pacemaker, regardless of its location, is unable to produce its inherent escape impulse under normal circumstance because the ectopic pacemaker is constantly suppressed by the primary pacemaker (sinus node), which has a faster inherent rate. The ectopic pacemaker may produce an escape impulse (passive impulse formation) whenever the impulse from the primary pacemaker does not reach the AV junction at the expected time for any reason (e.g., marked sinus bradycardia, SA block, AV block, and so on). However, active impulse formation occurs when the excitability of the heart is altered. This will be manifested by a premature beat (extrasystole) or by tachyarrhythmias of various origins.

Generally, a premature contraction, regardless of the location of the ectopic focus, has a constant coupling interval because it is in some way dependent upon the preceding beat of the basic rhythm.

Among the various postulated mechanisms for premature contractions, 2 theories are acceptable to most investigators. Both of these theories assume a focal origin of the ectopic impulse resulting from stimulation by the preceding beat of the basic rhythm. The 2 theories include the reentry phenomenon and enhancement of a subthreshold level of activity.

**Reentry Theory:** This theory assumes that there is a focal depression of conductivity involving the vicinity of the ectopic focus resulting in localized refractoriness. Because of this localized refractoriness, the impulse of the basic cardiac rhythm is able to traverse to an area that is nonrefractory, producing a normal beat. Meanwhile, the localized area that was refractory recovers its responsiveness and becomes excitable again. At this point, an impulse of the basic rhythm reaches the previously refractory segment and is able to penetrate it. By the time the previously depressed area has undergone depolarization and the initially excited area has emerged from its absolute refractory state, the excitation impulse once again traverses the myocardium. As a result, the beat appears prematurely and has a constant coupling interval (Fig. 7–8). The reentry phenomenon may explain some cases of premature contractions with slightly varying coupling intervals when an unequal velocity of the ectopic impulse via the reentry pathway is postulated. However, it should be emphasized that varying coupling intervals are commonly caused by a parasystolic mechanism that produces an independent ectopic rhythm in contrast to the dependent rhythm in ordinary premature beats (Chapter 22).

**Theory of Enhancement of Subthreshold Activity:** This theory assumes that the premature

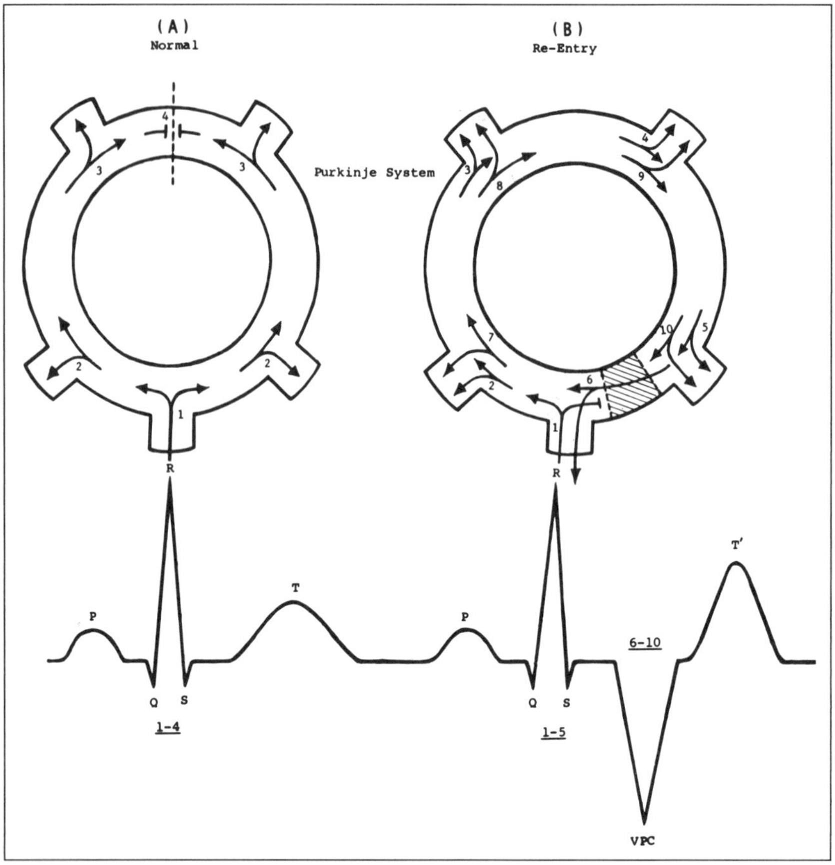


**Fig. 7–8.** Diagram showing reentry phenomenon responsible for the production of premature contractions (extrasystoles). **A.** The normal excitation of the Purkinje system. The impulse is assumed to enter at point 1, where it splits, one impulse being conducted in a clockwise direction and the other counterclockwise. Subsequently, these impulses spread in opposite directions (points 2 and 3) via the Purkinje system and finally meet and obliterate each other at point 4. It is during the spread of excitation via the Purkinje system ring (points 1, 2, 3, 4) that the QRS complex is produced. **B.** The reentry mechanism. In this diagram, the clockwise spread of the impulse is essentially the same as occurs in normal fibers (points 1, 2, 3, 4, 5). A counterclockwise spread of the impulse is prevented by the refractory segment of Purkinje fibers (hatched area). The normal QRS complex is produced by a clockwise spread of the impulse (points 1, 2, 3, 4, 5). When a depressed segment (hatched area) recovers its responsiveness and becomes excitable again, the excitation impulse reenters the circular ring of the Purkinje system and spreads once again (points 6, 7, 8, 9, 10). As a result, a VPC is produced.

beat is produced as a result of some enhancement of a focus of subthreshold activity by the preceding impulse of the basic rhythm. Presumably, a localized metabolic disturbance occurs that would produce some increase in focal excitability. If there is superimposed further increment of focal excitability induced by the trigger impulse of the basic rhythm on this subthreshold background, the level of excitability in the ectopic focus becomes transiently suprathreshold. At this instant, an ectopic focus becomes transiently suprathreshold, and an ectopic impulse is discharged. It should be noted that the exact mechanism by which the trigger impulse of the basic rhythm increases excitability within an ectopic focus is not completely understood. One possibility is that a chemical change occurs within the ectopic focus due to a transient circulatory effect initiated by the trigger impulse of the basic rhythm. On the other hand, this increment of subthreshold excitability could conceivably be related to the phenomenon of Wedensky facilitation. This phenomenon, which was demonstrated in nerve preparations in 1903, simply states that the excitability within an area distal to a partially or completely blocked impulse due to scar tissue or depressed muscle blocks can become momentarily increased. Whether this abrupt enhancement of excitability is sufficient to create suprathreshold excitability and the resulting discharge of the ectopic focus seems to be largely dependent upon other fluctuations within the subthreshold environment.

The Wedensky phenomenon is a form of the supernormal phase of conduction and excitability. Scherf and Schott were the first to introduce the concept of the supernormal phase into clinical electrocardiography, particularly as it applies to the genesis of premature contractions. The supernormal phase of excitability of cardiac tissue can be accepted for the genesis of premature contractions occurring near the end of the T wave of the preceding beats. However, premature beats occurring late in the cardiac cycle are difficult to explain on the basis of a supernormal phase of excitability because the duration of the supernormal excitability is only a few hundredths of a second near the end of the T wave.

## Clinical Significance

Ventricular premature contractions may be observed in any healthy subject at some time during his or her life. Common predisposing factors for the production of VPCs in healthy individuals include excessive use of coffee or tea, heavy smoking, and emotional disturbances. This arrhythmia is rather uncommon during childhood, and its incidence increases with age. The presence of VPCs by no means indicates any organic heart disease.

On the other hand, various organic heart diseases and drug (e.g., digitalis) intoxications are frequently associated with VPCs. In general, frequently appearing (30 beats or more per hour) or multifocal VPCs or ventricular group beats are often indicative of organic heart disease. The following features of VPCs are frequently observed in various clinical entities:

1. When the frequency of the VPCs increases with exercise, organic heart disease (usually CAD) is said to be present. Conversely, VPCs become less frequent or even disappear during exercise in healthy subjects in most cases.
2. When VPCs are multifocal or this arrhythmia coexists with other ectopic arrhythmias, organic heart disease and/or DI is often responsible (Figs. 7–2 and 7–5).
3. Ventricular bigeminy during digitalization is almost always pathognomonic of DI. This is particularly true when ventricular bigeminy occurs in the presence of AF with AV JER or JT (Fig. 7–5).
4. Ventricular premature contractions, which occur early in the cardiac cycle so that they are superimposed on the top of the T wave of the preceding beat (R-on-T phenomenon), may initiate VT, ventricular flutter, or VF (Fig. 7–9). In addition, ventricular group beats often lead to ventricular tachyarrhythmias. These phenomena are extremely common during the first 48–72 hours after acute MI.
5. Postectopic T wave changes are usually indicative of organic heart disease (Fig. 7–7).

The most common causes of frequent and multifocal VPCs are CAD, especially acute MI, and DI. Cardiomyopathy and MVP syndrome also frequently produce VPCs. Occasionally appearing VPCs usually do not produce any clinical symptoms, although sensitive individuals may experience an unpleasant feeling in the chest, skipped heartbeats, and palpitations. In general, the clinical signs and symptoms are greatly influenced by the underlying cause, the nature and severity of the heart disease, and/or the degree of DI if present.

Treatment of this arrhythmia also differs depending upon the cause. Treatment is usually not needed when the VPCs occur occasionally in healthy subjects. However, the causative factor (e.g., excessive coffee) should be omitted if possible when this arrhythmia occurs fre-

A.

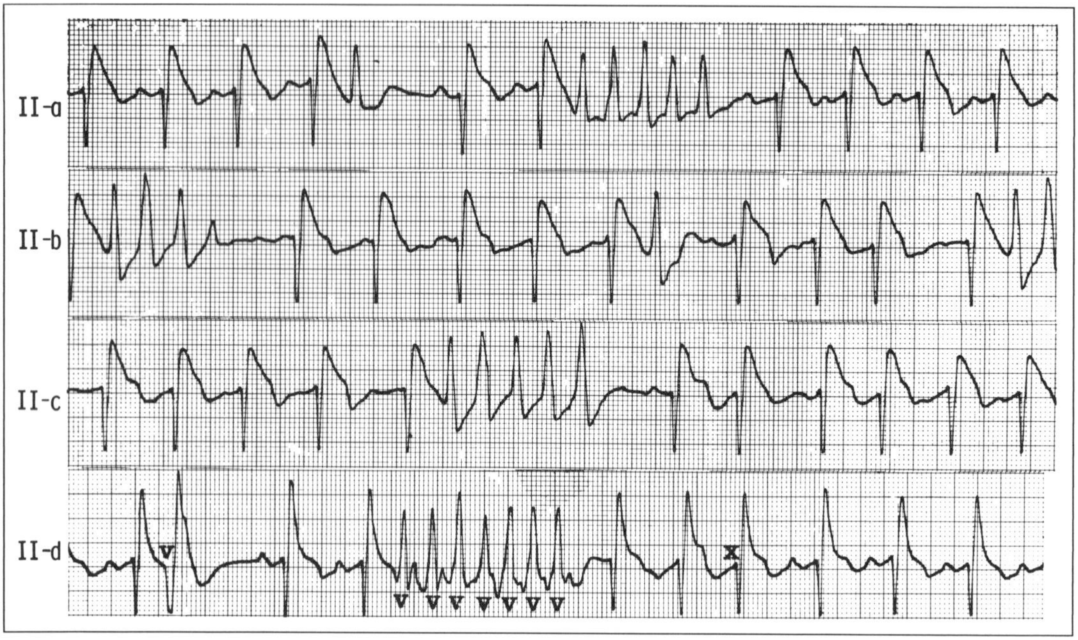


B.

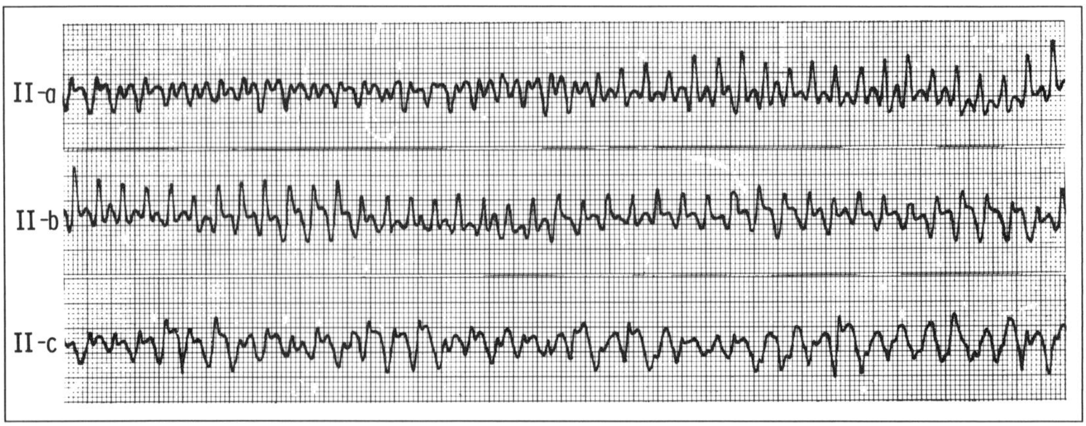


**Fig. 7–9. A** and **B** were obtained from the same patient with acute diaphragmatic MI. **A.** The rhythm is sinus with first degree AV block, APCs (X), and frequent VPCs (V) with group beats and a short run of VT. Leads II-a, II-b, II-c, and II-d are continuous. **B.** Soon after the tracing **A** was taken, the patient developed VF as a result of frequent VPCs with the R-on-T phenomenon. Leads II-a, II-b, and II-c are continuous.

quently. Otherwise, various antiarrhythmic agents (e.g., quinidine, procainamide, propranolol) may be tried when VPCs persist. When VPCs are associated with acute MI, the intravenous injection of lidocaine (Xylocaine) followed by continuous slow intravenous infusion is the treatment of choice. Needless to say, digitalis should be discontinued immediately when the arrhythmia is considered to be digitalis induced. In addition, phenytoin (Dilantin) and potassium are equally effective in abolishing digitalis-induced VPCs.

## VENTRICULAR TACHYCARDIA

The term "ventricular tachycardia (VT)" is used when 6 or more consecutive VPCs occur. Ventricular tachycardia, like isolated VPCs, may originate from any ventricular location. Since cardiac impulses originating from a ventricular focus are transmitted in an abnormal fashion, the QRS complex in VT is usually bizarre and wide (0.12 second or more). Ventricular tachycardia may occur transiently as a short paroxysm, or it may persist for a long time as long as the underlying cause is not corrected. Between bouts of VT, 1 or more sinus beats or isolated VPCs may occur intermittently. The atrial mechanism is often sinus, but it may be any ectopic rhythm, such as AF, atrial flutter, or AT, although identification of the atrial mechanism is often difficult.

By and large, there are 3 forms of VT. The most common form is paroxysmal VT, which has often a paroxysmal nature (Fig. 7–10) and usually has rapid rates (180–250 beats/min), similar to those in PAT or paroxysmal AV JT. A less common form is nonparoxysmal VT (idioventricular or accelerated ventricular rhythm), which is analogous to nonparoxysmal AV JT. Nonparoxysmal VT (Fig. 7–11) is almost always found in acute MI (usually in the first 24–72 hours), and it has relatively slow rates (70–130 beats/min). This form of VT is considered to be produced by an acceleration of the impulse formation of idioventricular pacemaker. A rare form of VT is considered to be generated by a parasystolic mechanism (Fig. 7–12), and the usual rates are similar to those of nonparoxysmal VT. The R-R intervals may be precisely regular, but it is not uncommon to observe a slight irregularity. Ventricular tachycardia is commonly unifocal, but it may originate from 2 or more independent ventricular foci. It is nearly always found in patients with advanced organic heart disease. Ventricular flutter or VF may follow VT, and the outcome is frequently fatal.

### Diagnostic Criteria

Ventricular tachycardia is diagnosed when the ventricles beat rapidly, usually unrelated to the atrial mechanism, and the QRS complex is wide (0.12 second or more) and bizarre.

**Nature of Onset and Termination:** Paroxysmal VT is usually paroxysmal in nature, and thus, the onset and the termination of the arrhythmia are generally abrupt. The duration of the paroxysm may be so short that several normally conducted sinus beats, or isolated or grouped VPCs, may occur between paroxysms. The initiation of paroxysmal VT is frequently triggered by an isolated ventricular premature beat (Fig. 7–10). Conversely, an isolated VPC commonly occurs following the termination of VT (Fig. 7–10). Following the termination of VT, a posttachycardia pause often follows because the sinus or other ectopic pacemaker requires a warming-up period after continuous suppression of pacemaking function by the ventricular impulses. Ventricular tachycardia may occur transiently, but it may persist for a long period of time until the underlying cause is treated. It may terminate spontaneously, but it is often terminated by antiarrhythmic drug therapy or by DC shock. Nonparoxysmal or parasystolic VT is usually not paroxysmal (Figs. 7–11 and 7–12).

**Rates:** The paroxysmal form of VT usually produces ventricular rates between 180 and 250 beats/min (Fig. 7–10), which are similar to those found in paroxysmal AT or AV JT. However, a ventricular rate faster than 200 beats/min is uncommon in VT. Occasionally, the ventricular rate may be slower than 160 beats/min

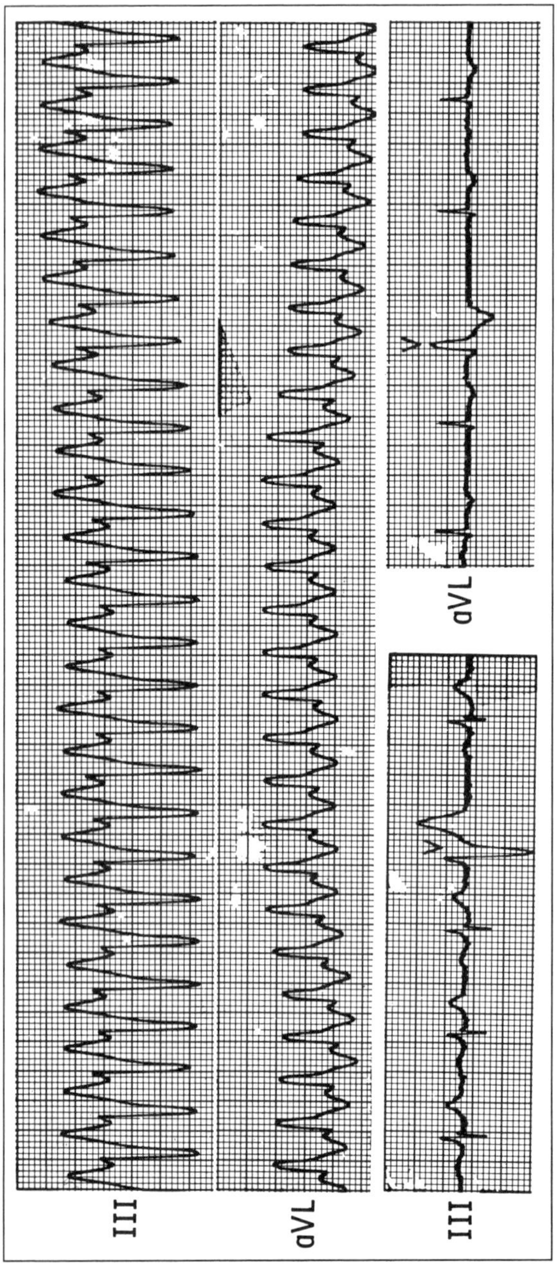


**Fig. 7–10.** Paroxysmal VT with a rate of 214 beats/min. Note that the configuration of VPCs (V) and VT complex is identical.

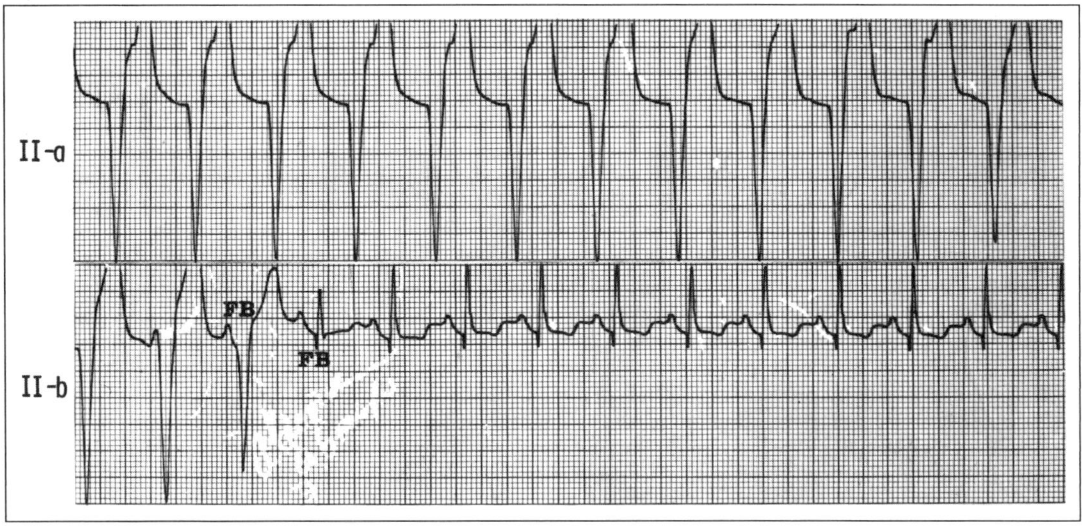


**Fig. 7–11.** Sinus rhythm with intermittent nonparoxysmal VT (rate: 96 beats/min). Note ventricular fusion beats (FB). Leads II-a and II-b are continuous.

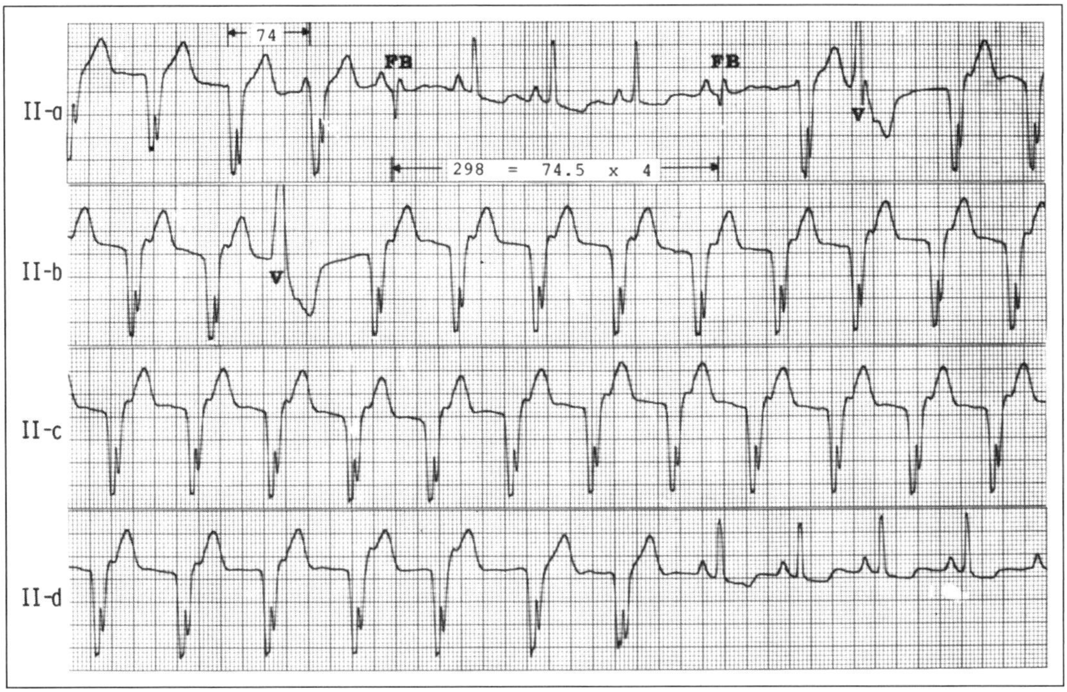


**Fig. 7–12.** Sinus rhythm with intermittent parasystolic VT (rate: 78 beats/min) and VPCs (V). Note that a long interectopic interval is a multiple of the shortest interectopic interval. There are occasional ventricular fusion beats (FB). Leads II-a, II-b, II-c, and II-d are continuous.

or even as slow as 70–130 beats/min, especially in nonparoxysmal or parasystolic VT (Figs. 7–11 and 7–12).

**Relationship Between Atrial and Ventricular Activations:** In most instances of VT, the atrial and ventricular activities are independent throughout to produce complete AV dissociation. The atrial mechanism is commonly sinus and the atrial rate is often rapid (sinus tachycardia), although it is slower than the ventricular rate. Rarely, the atrial mechanism may be an unusually slow sinus bradycardia, especially when the underlying cause is acute diaphragmatic MI. When the atrial mechanism is sinus, the sinus impulses occasionally may be conducted to the ventricles. In this case, the sinus impulse may capture the ventricles partially when the sinus impulse meets with the impulse from the ventricular ectopic focus, resulting in a ventricular fusion beat (partial ventricular captured beat). Extremely rarely, impulses from the ventricular focus may activate the atria in a retrograde fashion (atrial captured beats). A partial atrial captured beat (atrial fusion beat) may also occur when 2 impulses, 1 from the sinus node and another from the ventricles, meet simultaneously in the atria. As described previously, the term "incomplete AV dissociation" is used when 1 or more captured beats (ventricular or atrial; complete or partial) are present (Chapter 6).

At times, the atrial mechanism in VT may be an ectopic rhythm, including AF, atrial flutter, or AT. Under these circumstances, of course, complete or incomplete AV dissociation will result, as seen with the sinus mechanism in the atria.

**Configuration of QRS Complex:** Unifocal VT usually produces a constant configuration of the QRS complex (Fig. 7–10). However, it is not uncommon to observe that the contour of the QRS complex may be altered slightly from beat to beat in unifocal VT. This occurs because of different degrees of superimposition of the atrial and ventricular activities. A marked variation of the contour may be due to various degrees of ventricular fusion beat. When ventricular complexes exhibit a markedly different contour from beat to beat, the term "multiform VT" is used. Multiform VT is said to occur more frequently in advanced organic heart disease and is often a precursor of ventricular flutter or VF.

On rare occasions, the direction of the QRS complex in VT may change alternately or periodically (Fig. 7–13). This is called "bidirectional VT," which is almost a pathognomonic feature of advanced DI. In bidirectional VT, the impulse is said to occur from a single focus when the R-R intervals are constant, regardless of the direction of the QRS complex. Conversely, 2 ventricular foci are said to be present when 2 different R-R cycles are observed, associated with different QRS complexes. It is of interest that the configuration of the QRS complexes in isolated VPCs and in VT is often identical. This indicates that the same ventricular focus produces the single VPC as well as VT (Fig. 7–10). Secondary ST, T wave changes are always observed in VT, as in isolated VPCs.

When the VT is originating from the ventricular septum, the QRS complex is often relatively narrow. The term "fascicular VT" is commonly used under this circumstance when the QRS complex is relatively narrow with incomplete RBBB pattern (Fig. 7–14).

In ordinary VT, it is always possible to distinguish between the S-T, T waves and the QRS complex (Fig. 7–10) because VT is nothing but consecutively appearing VPCs. However, the boundary between the end of the QRS complex and the ST, T waves may become ill defined when VT begins to transform to ventricular flutter or VF. This type of VT has been termed "prefibrillatory" or "preflutter" VT (Fig. 7–9). In this circumstance, ventricular flutter or VF will soon be the result in most instances (Fig. 7–9).

**Regularity of R-R Cycles:** The R-R intervals in VT may be precisely regular, but they may be slightly irregular. Grossly irregular ventricular cycles are extremely unusual unless multifocal VT is present. Markedly irregular R-R intervals indicate AF with LBBB or RBBB or aberrant ventricular conduction rather than VT (Chapter 11). Atrial fibrillation with WPW syndrome often produces wide and bizarre QRS complexes that closely resemble VT (Chapter 13). Two or more distinctly different R-R cycles occurring with different QRS complexes indicate that 2 or more ectopic foci are present in the ventricles.

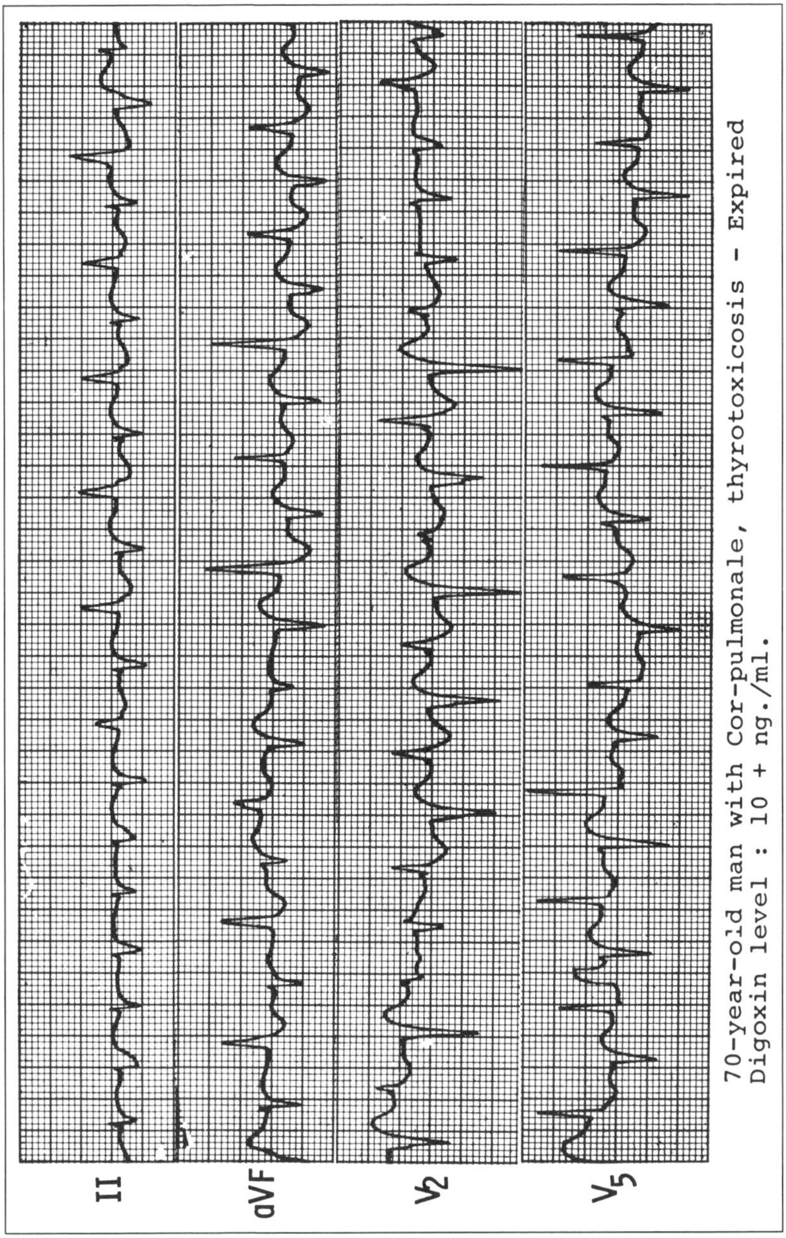


Fig. 7–13. Atrial fibrillation with bidirectional VT (rate: 173 beats/min) producing complete AV dissociation as a result of far advanced digitalis toxicity.

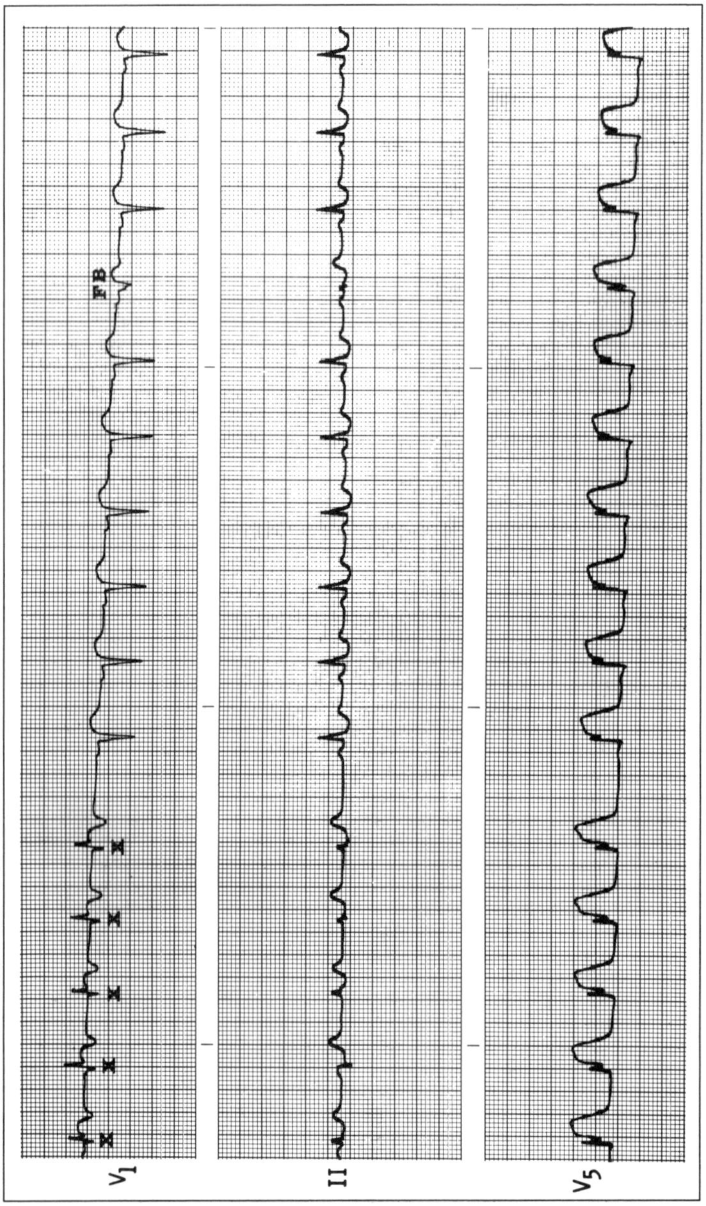


**Fig. 7–14.** Sinus rhythm with intermittent fascicular tachycardia (X) (rate: 92 beats/min) in a patient with acute anterior MI. Note a ventricular fusion beat (FB).

## Mechanisms

The fundamental mechanism of paroxysmal VT is considered to be closely related to that of VPCs. As described earlier in this chapter, the 2 most popular theories regarding the genesis of premature beats as well as most tachycardias are the reentry phenomenon (Fig. 7–8) and the enhancement of subthreshold activity. Rarely, VT may be due to a parasystolic mechanism (Fig. 7–12), in which the ventricular rate is usually much slower than that of ordinary VT. Nonparoxysmal VT is considered to be produced by an acceleration of the impulse formation of an idioventricular pacemaker. Ventricular tachycardia is commonly unifocal, but it may originate from 2 or more foci. By and large, frequent VPCs often lead to VT, ventricular flutter, or VF, especially in patients with acute MI (Fig. 7–9).

## Clinical Significance

Although VT is said to occur occasionally in healthy individuals without demonstrable heart disease, it is nearly always found in people with advanced organic heart disease. The most common cause of VT is CAD, particularly acute MI. The second most common cause is probably DI. Multiform or multifocal VT is said to occur more in serious heart disease than uniform and unifocal VT. In addition, VT may occur in various other heart diseases, including RHD and hypertensive heart disease, and cardiomyopathy.

Intractable CHF is frequently present in VT. In this circumstance, the severe CHF is often an ideal ground to induce VT, and the latter, in turn, frequently produces or aggravates the CHF.

Symptoms and signs in VT vary depending upon the nature and severity of the underlying heart disease, such as acute MI and CHF. Accordingly, various symptoms and signs of CHF, acute MI, and DI are frequently present. Not uncommonly, the patient may experience a feeling of impending death.

Various drugs have been used for the treatment of VT in addition to the ready availability of DC shock. The drugs commonly used include lidocaine (Xylocaine), procainamide (Pronestyl), phenytoin (Dilantin), quinidine, and beta-adrenergic blocking agents and calcium blockers. Direct current shock is extremely effective in the treatment of VT from any cause except DI. The treatment of choice for VT is different depending upon the etiologic factor. For instance, the drug of choice for the treatment of VT associated with acute MI is lidocaine (Xylocaine), given by direct intravenous injection and followed by a continuous intravenous infusion. On the other hand, VT induced by digitalis is treated either by intravenous injection of phenytoin (Dilantin) or intravenous infusion of potassium. Frequently, procainamide may be used in place of lidocaine or phenytoin. Quinidine or beta-adrenergic blocking agents are also often used when the above agents prove to be ineffective. On rare occasions, the use of an artificial pacemaker is a lifesaving measure in the treatment of drug-resistant VT. In certain cases with refractory VT, a special form of surgical approach is carried out with varying degree of success. It should be emphasized that elimination of the direct cause (e.g., DI) is an extremely important aspect of treatment. On the other hand, nonparoxysmal or parasystolic VT requires no treatment in most cases because the rate is relatively slow and the tachycardia is usually self-limited.

# TORSADE DE POINTES

Torsade de pointes is an atypical VT that occurs most frequently during quinidine therapy (Fig. 7–15) but may be induced by other etiologic factors. It is important to recognize this atypical VT because the clinical significance as well as the therapeutic approach are considerably different from those of ordinary VT, and there is a rather unique QRS morphology during the tachycardia. The term "torsade de pointes" was popularized by Dessertenne when the arrhythmia was described for the first time in 1966. Characteristically, torsade de pointes is manifested by a long Q-T interval, polymor-

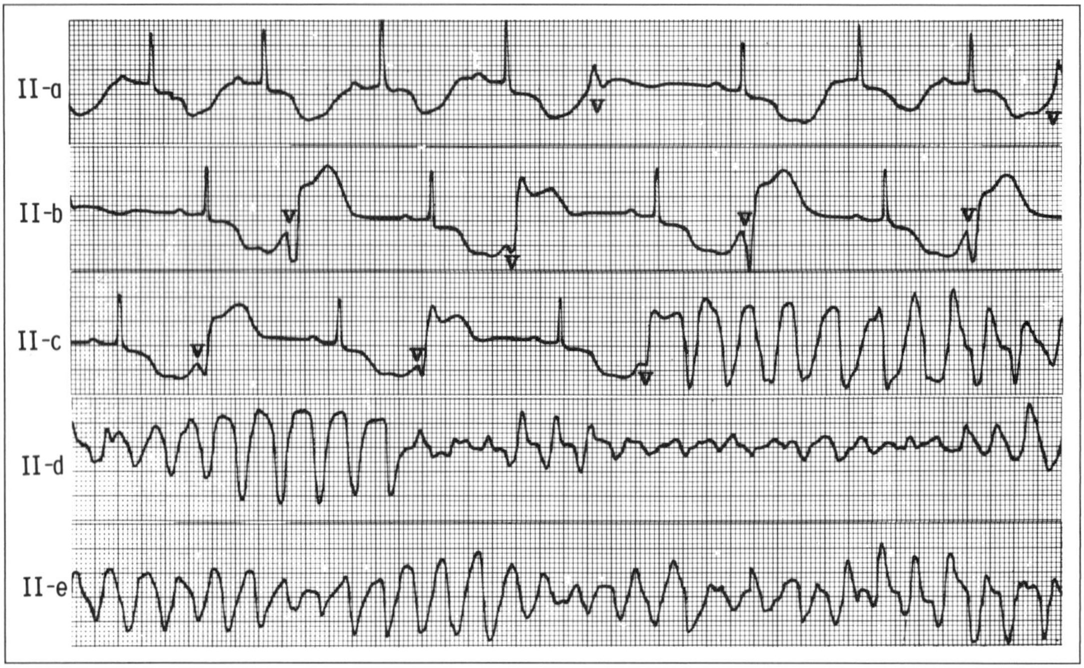


**Fig. 7–15.** Sinus rhythm with first degree AV block and frequent VPCs (V) with R-on-T phenomenon leading to multiform VT (torsade de pointes) and VF. The ECG abnormalities are fundamentally caused by quinidine-induced prolonged Q-T interval with broad T wave. Leads II-a, II-b, II-c, II-d, and II-e are continuous.

phous QRS complexes with varying R-R intervals, and fluctuating QRS axes (Fig. 7–15). As a rule, VT is initiated by a VPC occurring relatively late during ventricular repolarization, but the arrhythmia may be terminated spontaneously.

It has been shown repeatedly that the conventional mode of therapy for this VT may not only be ineffective but may also be hazardous in most cases. Isoproterenol infusion is the usually recommended initial therapy for torsade de pointes, primarily because the drug shortens the ventricular repolarization time. When isoproterenol is ineffective or contraindicated, however, ventricular pacing is considered to be a safe and reliable method for the treatment of the arrhythmia.

Torsade de pointes frequently causes recurrent episodes of syncope or near-syncope, and this consequence is considered to be the most serious complication of quinidine therapy. In addition, torsade de pointes has been reported during other antiarrhythmic drug therapy (e.g., procainamide and disopyramide). The arrhythmia may also occur in cases of electrolyte disturbances, congenital Q-T prolongation syndrome, and CAD, even in the absence of any antiarrhythmic drug effect.

## Nomenclature

Beside the most popular term, torsade de pointes, the arrhythmia has been given various names, including ventricular fibrillo-flutter, ectopic VT, paroxysmal VF, transient recurrent VF, atypical VT, repetitive paroxysmal tachycardia, delayed repolarization arrhythmia, cardiac ballet, and polymorphous VT. The French term, "torsade de pointes," seems to be appropriate because of Dessertenne's original contribution.

## Etiology

Although the precise underlying mechanism of this arrhythmia (Table 7–1) is not clearly understood, it is known to be most frequently observed during quinidine and quinidine-like antiarrhythmic drug therapy. In addition, the arrhythmia has been encountered during therapy with other drugs (e.g., prenylamine, phenothiazines, amitryptiline) and various clinical circumstances, including hypokalemia, hypomagnesemia, and congenital prolonged Q-T syndrome.

Torsade de pointes is almost always associated with prolongation of the Q-T interval, and a VPC usually initiates the tachycardia. Since the U wave is considered to be a portion of the repolarization process in the ventricular Purkinje system, the prolongation of the Q-U interval may have the same significance as the Q-T interval prolongation and may also reflect increased asynchrony of ventricular repolarization. In a practical sense, it is often difficult or even impossible to distinguish between the Q-T interval and the Q-U interval in many cases, especially when only a short ECG rhythm strip is available for interpretation.

**TABLE 7–1. Possible causes of torsade de pointes**

A. *Drug induced*
  1. Antiarrhythmic drugs
     Quinidine, procainamide, disopyramide, ajmaline, amiodarone, and lidocaine
  2. Other drugs
     Prenylamine, phenothiazines, tricyclic antidepressant drugs

B. *Nondrug induced*
  1. Congenital Q-T prolongation syndrome
     a. Jervell-Lange-Nielson syndrome
     b. Romano-Ward syndrome
  2. Electrolyte disturbances
     a. Hypokalemia
     b. Hypomagnesemia
  3. Intrinsic cardiac diseases
     a. Myocardial ischemia and infarction
     b. Myocarditis
     c. Bradyarrhythmias
        (1) Marked sinus bradycardia (e.g., sick sinus syndrome)
        (2) Advanced or complete AV block
     d. Mitral valve prolapse syndrome (MVPS)
  4. Liquid protein diets
  5. Central nervous system disorders (e.g., subarachnoid hemorrhage)
  6. Hypothermia

Reproduced with permission from Chung: Principles of Cardiac Arrhythmias, 3rd ed. Baltimore, Williams & Wilkins, 1983.

It can be said that the vulnerable period of the ventricles will be prolonged proportionally to the duration of the T wave. Since the prolonged Q-T interval responsible for the production of torsade de pointes is invariably associated with a markedly broad T wave, any cardiac impulse (commonly VPCs) may easily provoke VT and VF (the R-on-T phenomenon) even if a ventricular ectopic beat occurs during the late portion of the cardiac cycle. As a matter of fact, torsade de pointes often transforms to VF in many cases. Hence, in reality, the arrhythmia is prefibrillatory multiform VT.

## Electrocardiographic Manifestations and Diagnosis

The characteristic ECG features of torsade de pointes are as follows (Fig. 7–15):

1. During sinus rhythm (at times, ectopic rhythms, such as AF), the Q-T interval is markedly prolonged (often more than 0.60 sec) with very broad T waves.
2. The arrhythmia is often initiated by a VPC with a long coupling interval and the R-on-T phenomenon.
3. The arrhythmia consists of large and bizarre multiform QRS complexes with a frequency of 100–180 beats/min (at times, as rapid as 200–300 beats/min).
4. The amplitude and the direction of the QRS complexes frequently vary from beat to beat, leading to a picture of a torsion around an isoelectric line. Consequently, the French name "torsade de pointes" (torsion of pointes) was given to describe the arrhythmia
5. The arrhythmia may terminate spontaneously and may repeat itself after several seconds or minutes. On the other hand, the arrhythmia often transforms to VF, and sudden death may occur.

Most patients experience near-syncopal or syncopal episodes that are due to the sudden onset of this ventricular arrhythmia. It is extremely important to emphasize that the arrhythmia is not responsive to conventional antiarrhythmic drug therapy in most cases. In fact, commonly used antiarrhythmic agents often aggravate this clinical situation.

### Treatment

The conventional antiarrhythmic drugs, such as procainamide, quinidine, and disopyramide, should be avoided in the treatment of torsade de pointes, since these agents often aggravate the arrhythmia, leading to deterioration of the clinical circumstance.

The general guidelines for the therapeutic approach to torsade de pointes are:

1. To correct the underlying cause if recognized
2. To use pharmacologic agents that shorten the refractory period of the ventricular myocardium
3. To institute an artificial cardiac pacing

It is extremely important to correct or to eliminate the underlying cause if possible as soon as the diagnosis of torsade de pointes is made. The causative drugs (e.g., quinidine) should be discontinued immediately, and any electrolyte imbalance should be corrected. The most suitable drugs in the treatment of this ventricular arrhythmia should be the agents that do not prolong the Q-T interval, including propranolol, lidocaine, and phenytoin. The aim of pharmacologic therapy for this arrhythmia is to shorten the repolarization period of the ventricles, thereby preventing the possibility of the reentry circuit. Thus, the recommended drug of choice in this clinical situation is isoproterenol.

When the above-mentioned drug therapy is shown to be ineffective, artificial cardiac pacing is the next step. In most cases, a temporary pacemaker with slight overdrive pacing rate (rate: 80–120 beats/min) is used. Fortunately, the artificial pacing is effective in suppressing torsade de pointes in most cases. If the pacing is unsuccessful, however, cardioversion may be indicated.

When advanced or complete AV block coexists with this ventricular arrhythmia (a form of bradytachyarrhythmia syndrome), the use of artificial pacing is even more beneficial. In the majority of cases, a pacing rate ranging from 80 to 120 beats/min is effective, but the most suitable pacing rate should be determined for a given patient. It has been suggested that the ventricular pacing should be considered as the treatment of choice for torsade de pointes before trying various antiarrhythmic drugs, even in patients without coexisting AV block.

## VENTRICULAR FLUTTER AND FIBRILLATION

Ventricular flutter and VF are, needless to say, the worst cardiac arrhythmias encountered in the human heart. They are the commonest causes of sudden death and are particularly associated with acute MI, advanced cardiomyopathy, and/or DI. When ventricular flutter or VF occurs in acute MI, sudden death frequently results even before symptoms or anatomic alteration of the myocardium develops. Ventricular flutter and VF often coexist or transform from one to the other, and a pure form of ventricular flutter is relatively uncommon. Because of the frequent association of ventricular flutter and VF, the mixed form is called "ventricular flutter-fibrillation," which is analogous to atrial flutter-fibrillation.

### Diagnostic Criteria

In both ventricular flutter and VF, the distinction between the QRS complex and the S-T, T waves is absent. Instead, a regular and consecutive undulation occurs in ventricular flutter (Fig. 7–16), whereas a grossly irregular undulation of varying amplitude is present in VF (Fig. 7–17).

**Configuration of QRS Complex, ST, T Complexes:** The characteristic feature of pure ventricular flutter is regularly occurring un-

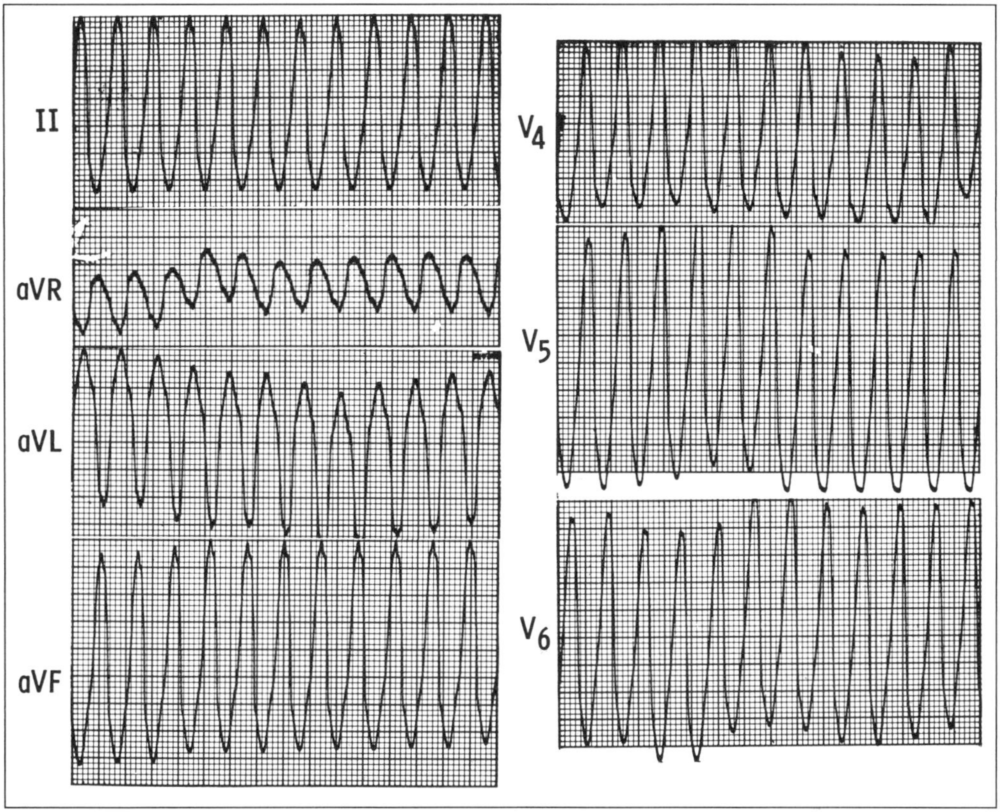


Fig. 7–16. Ventricular flutter with a rate of 214 beats/min.

dulations of equal amplitude throughout (Fig. 7–16). Thus, a separation of QRS complex from ST segment and T wave is not possible. Each flutter wave consists of a round upper and lower end that corresponds to the ordinary R and S (or QS) waves. Consequently, the ECG tracing of ventricular flutter is almost the same regardless of whether or not it is read upside down. The amplitude of the undulation may be large or small depending upon the status of the ventricular myocardium. In general, when ventricular flutter occurs in an apparently healthy individual (e.g., following electrocution), the amplitude of the flutter is large. In contrast to this, the amplitude is very small in a severely damaged heart, especially in an acute MI. When the amplitude of the ventricular flutter wave becomes progressively lower, VF often follows. The term "ventricular flutter-fibrillation" is used when a mixed form of ventricular flutter and VF is observed.

In VF, an irregularly irregular ventricular rhythm of varying configuration occurs (Fig. 7–17). The VF wave replaces the ordinary QRS, ST, and T complexes. In contrast to ventricular flutter, the configuration of the VF wave may show a sharp or round upper and lower end, although the contour and amplitude vary throughout. As in ventricular flutter, when cardiac function progressively deteriorates, the amplitude of the fibrillation wave becomes progressively smaller, particularly immediately before death.

**Rate:** The ventricular rate in ventricular flutter is usually between 180 and 250 beats/min (Fig. 7–16), which is in the same range as ordinary VT. However, the rate of ventricular flutter may become faster than 250 and slower

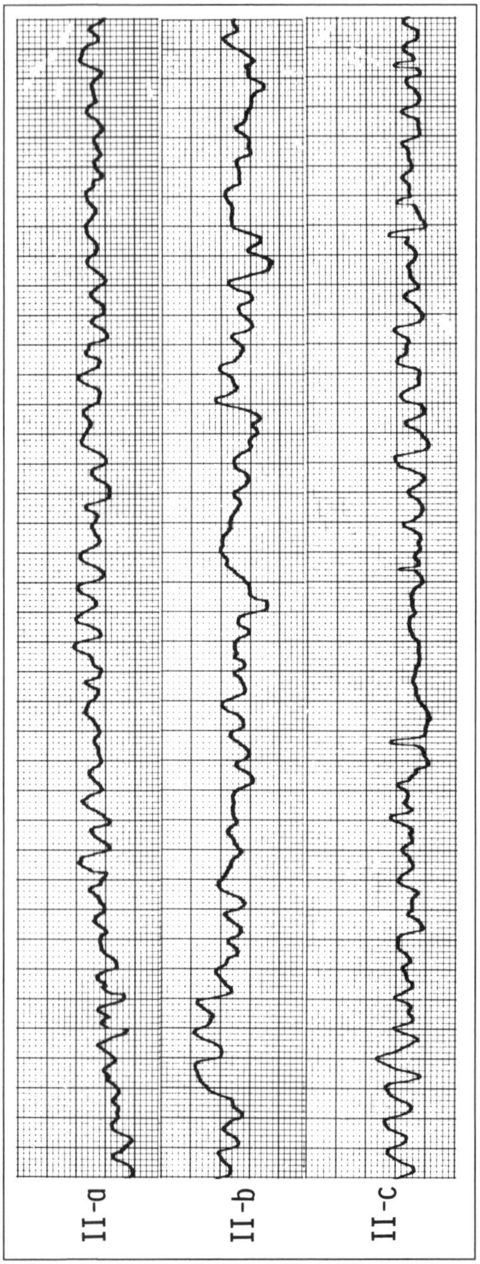


**Fig. 7–17.** Ventricular fibrillation. Leads II-a, II-b, and II-c are continuous.

than 180 beats/min just before the arrhythmia transforms to VF.

In VF, the ventricular rate has an extremely wide range (Fig. 7–17) in that it may be as slow as 150 beats/min or as fast as 500 beats/min. The ventricular rate may be extremely slow just before death.

**Relationship Between Atrial and Ventricular Activities:** In general, it is impossible to determine the atrial mechanism in either ventricular flutter or VF because of the wide and bizarre ventricular waves. However, it is quite possible that any atrial mechanism may be present independent of the ventricular mechanism.

### Mechanisms

The fundamental mechanisms responsible for the development of ventricular flutter and VF are considered to be essentially the same as those for atrial flutter and AF, except that the ectopic focus (or foci) is (are) located in the ventricles in the former. Many theories have been proposed to explain the genesis of flutter and fibrillation, and, among them, 4 theories are still considered to be strong possibilities. These theories are: (1) the theory of circus movement, (2) the theory of multiple reentry phenomenon, (3) the theory of unifocal impulse formation, and (4) the theory of multifocal impulse formation. A detailed description of the mechanisms of flutter and fibrillation is given in Chapter 5.

### Clinical Significance

Although ventricular flutter or VF has been occasionally reported in individuals without apparent cause, these arrhythmias nearly always occur in serious organic heart diseases. The most common underlying heart disease is CAD, especially acute MI. The next most common cause is DI. In addition, ventricular flutter or VF may be found in various other heart diseases, including RHD, cardiomyopathy, cardiac trauma (penetrating or blunt), thyrotoxicosis, during cardiac surgery, cardiac catheterization, quinidine or Pronestyl toxicity, marked hyperkalemia, hypercalcemia, hypokalemia, and following electrocution. These arrhythmias are often fatal in spite of all available medical measures. Ventricular flutter or VF frequently develops during the terminal stages of various noncardiac diseases. Intractable CHF may precede ventricular flutter or VF.

The treatment of choice for ventricular flutter or VF is, without doubt, DC shock. When these arrhythmias are terminated, the same medical treatment outlined for VT should be carried out. An artificial pacemaker is occasionally used for the treatment of drug-resistant or DC shock-resistant ventricular flutter or VF. It is extremely important to eliminate the direct cause (i.e., drug toxicity or electrolyte imbalance), if possible. An investigational device, an implantable automatic minidefibrillator, has been utilized in selected patients with recurrent ventricular flutter or VF, with a favorable result.

## CHAOTIC RHYTHM

The term "chaotic rhythm" has been used to designate multifocal ventricular rhythms with extremely unstable mechanisms. Thus, chaotic rhythm often consists of a period of VT, VF, or ventricular flutter, multifocal VPCs, high degree or complete AV block, ventricular escape (idioventricular) rhythm, and ventricular standstill. By precise definition, each portion of the ECG tracing usually shows a specific cardiac arrhythmia (e.g., VT or idioventricular rhythm). However, at times, some parts of the chaotic rhythm cannot be described specifically, particularly immediately before death. In the dying heart, the ventricles may be controlled by 2 or more ventricular foci. For example, a portion of the ventricles may have VF or ventricular flutter, whereas the remaining portion of the ventricles may have ventricular escape rhythm (VER). In this circumstance, the term "ventricular dissociation" may be used. In a practical sense, whenever the term "chaotic rhythm" is used, the predominant cardiac rhythm consists of ventricular flutter, VF and VER.

## VENTRICULAR ESCAPE (IDIOVENTRICULAR) BEATS AND RHYTHM

Ventricular escape (idioventricular) beats and rhythm, like VPCs or VT, may originate from any location in the ventricles. Ventricular escape beats (VEBs) may appear singly or consecutively as group beats. When 6 or more consecutive VEBs appear, the term "ventricular escape rhythm" (VER) is used. These are generated by passive impulse formation in the ventricles when the AV junction is unable to produce escape impulses despite the fact that the sinus or atrial impulses do not reach the AV junction in the expected time or when the site of complete AV block is distal to the His bundle.

Under normal circumstances, like AV JER, VER does not appear, because these subsidiary pacemakers are controlled by the sinus node, which has a faster inherent rate. Thus, the AV junctional as well as the ventricular pacemakers are continuously depressed by the rapidly discharging sinus impulses. The most common cause of VER is complete infranodal AV block often resulting from BBBB (Fig. 2–4). Less commonly, VEBs or VER may occur following sinus arrest (pause) or SA block when the AV junction is unable to produce escape impulses. They may occur in the presence of an ectopic atrial rhythm, including AF, atrial flutter and AT, when the atrial impulses fail to reach the ventricles due to high degree or complete infra-nodal AV block frequently resulting from BBBB. Not uncommonly, VER may occur without the presence of definite atrial activity in the terminal stages of advanced heart disease. Extremely rarely, VEBs or VER may be followed by a retrograde P wave when the impulses from the ventricular ectopic focus activate the atria in a retrograde fashion. The usual rates of VER range from 30 to 40 beats/min but may be as slow as 15–20 beats/min. This arrhythmia is nearly always found in advanced heart disease, especially in elderly individuals, and is often a terminal cardiac arrhythmia.

### Diagnostic Criteria

**Configuration of QRS Complex:** The configuration of the QRS complex in VEBs or VER is essentially the same as that of VPCs or VT. Thus, the configuration varies depending upon the location of the ectopic focus in the ventricles. However, in general, the contour of the QRS complex in VEBs or VER is often more bizarre, particularly in the terminal stages of advanced heart disease. The duration of the QRS complex nearly always exceeds 0.16 second. Two or more different configurations of the QRS complexes may be observed when the VER originates from 2 or more different ventricular foci.

**Rate:** The usual rate in VER is between 30 and 40 beats/min (Fig. 2–4), but it may be slightly faster than 40 beats/min. At times, it may be as slow as 15–20 beats/min. In the terminal stage, the rate of VER becomes extremely unstable, and it usually progressively slows, especially immediately prior to death.

**Relationship between Atrial and Ventricular Activations:** The atrial and ventricular activations are nearly always independent in VER, leading to complete AV dissociation (Fig. 2–4). However, atrial activity is usually not discernible in VER when this arrhythmia occurs in a dying heart. In this case, atrial standstill is most likely present, although fine AF cannot be excluded. On the other hand, a slow undulation may coexist with VER in the dying heart. In this circumstance, it is uncertain whether the undulation represents atrial activity or independent ventricular activity. On rare occasions, a retrograde P wave may follow VEBs or VER when the atria are activated by the ventricular escape focus in a retrograde fashion. This is called an "atrial captured beat."

**Escape Intervals:** The ventricular escape intervals may be regular (Fig. 2–4), but more commonly they are irregular. The irregular ventricular escape intervals may be due to multifocal ventricular foci or to a unifocal ventricular focus with a varying rate of impulse discharge. The escape intervals usually become progressively longer in the dying heart.

### Mechanisms

Ventricular escape beats or rhythm commonly results from high degree or complete infranodal AV block usually secondary to BBBB. As described previously, VER is generated by passive impulse formation in the ventricles when the sinus or atrial impulses fail to reach the ventricles at the expected time. On the other hand, VER is frequently observed in the dying heart without discernible atrial activity. The mechanisms of complete AV block and BBBB are discussed in Chapters 8 and 9.

### Clinical Significance

Since VER is usually found in advanced heart disease, this is one of the worst cardiac arrhythmias. Adams-Stokes syndrome and/or severe CHF is frequently observed because of the slow ventricular rate and the frequently coexisting VT, ventricular flutter and VF, in addition to markedly advanced heart disease. In fact, VER, particularly without discernible atrial activity, is usually a terminal arrhythmia in the dying heart. The clinical significance of complete AV block, including BBBB, is described in Chapters 8 and 9.

The treatment of VER varies depending upon the nature and severity of the underlying heart disease. In general, a permanent artificial pacemaker is often a life-saving measure.

## VENTRICULAR STANDSTILL (ARREST)

Ventricular standstill (arrest), like atrial standstill (arrest), is usually the consequence of some other cardiac arrhythmia. The term "ventricular standstill" is used when no QRS complex is observed for a few seconds or longer. Ventricular standstill may occur in the presence of any atrial activity (sinus or ectopic), but both atrial and ventricular activities may be absent altogether. Ventricular standstill results when a subsidiary pacemaker fails to produce an escape impulse during sinus arrest or SA block. Sinus arrest often follows after spontaneous termination of an ectopic tachycardia or even after a single ectopic beat because of the depression of the pacemaking function in the sinus node. In this circumstance, ventricular standstill frequently results because the subsidiary pacemaker also may not produce an escape impulse at the expected time. Ventricular standstill may be produced by CSS during supraventricular tachyarrhythmias. In addition, posttachyarrhythmia ventricular pause is extremely common following the termination of atrial, AV junctional, or ventricular tachyarrhythmias either by drugs or DC shock. Not uncommonly, ventricular standstill may result in high degree or complete AV block when concealed AV conduction occurs, leading to suppression of a subsidiary pacemaker. On rare occasions, ventricular standstill may occur suddenly during sinus rhythm. In the dying heart, ventricular standstill eventually results following VT, ventricular flutter, VF, or slow VER.

The clinical significance of ventricular standstill varies markedly depending upon the duration of the pause, and the nature and severity of the underlying heart disease. In general, ventricular standstill of short duration following a bout of ectopic tachycardia is usually insignificant clinically. In contrast to this, ventricular standstill of long duration is often fatal unless a faster cardiac rhythm is restored immediately. Ventricular standstill may be observed in any type of heart disease, but the most common heart disease is CAD, especially in acute MI. The second most common cause is probably advanced DI. However, it should be noted that ventricular standstill eventually results in the dying patient regardless of the underlying cause. Adams-Stokes syndrome is observed in practically every patient when ventricular standstill occurs for a long duration. In addition, CHF is also very common because of the insufficient cardiac output and the advanced heart disease in most cases. Cardiopulmonary resuscitation and the use of an artificial pacemaker are often life-saving procedures when ventricular standstill occurs in long duration regardless of the etiology.

## VENTRICULAR PARASYSTOLE

Ventricular parasystole is a rather uncommon ventricular arrhythmia. The configuration of the QRS complex in ventricular parasystole is essentially the same as that of an ordinary VPC, but the former produces an independent ventricular rhythm in the presence of any underlying rhythm. A detailed description of ventricular parasystole is found in Chapter 22.

# Chapter 8

# Atrioventricular Conduction Disturbances

Conduction disturbances may occur anywhere in the heart and are ordinarily expressed as a heart block. In general, impairment of conduction is divided into 4 major categories according to the location of the block. They are:

1. Sinoatrial (SA) block (conduction disturbance at the SA junctional tissue)
2. Intraatrial block (conduction disturbance within the atria)
3. Atrioventricular (AV) block (conduction disturbance at the AV junctional tissue, His bundle, or both bundle branches)
4. Intraventricular block (conduction disturbance within the ventricles or bundle branch system)

Among these conduction disturbances, AV block and intraventricular block are commonly observed and may be associated with a block anywhere else in the heart. Although a precise definition of AV block is a conduction disturbance occurring at the AV junction, the term "heart block" has been used loosely to designate AV block.

Atrioventricular block is characterized by an abnormally prolonged AV conduction time (P-R interval) or failure of conduction of one or more atrial impulses (either sinus or ectopic) due to a prolonged refractory period in the AV junctional tissue. Thus, true AV block must be distinguished from functional AV block, which occurs as a physiologic mechanism. For example, when a sinus P wave that falls outside the Q-T interval of the preceding ventricular beat fails to conduct to the ventricles or conducts slowly (P-R interval of 0.21 second or longer), a true AV block is said to be present. On the other hand, atrial flutter with 2:1 AV conduction (Fig. 5–11) commonly occurs due to a functional rather than a true AV block. This occurs because the AV junctional tissue is unable to respond to the rapid atrial rate due to its longer refractory period. For a similar reason, the P wave of an APC often fails to conduct to the ventricles when the P wave appears soon after the QRS complex of the preceding beat. These alterations of the AV conduction in an APC are functional (physiologic) and, therefore, are not a manifestation of a true AV block.

It has been shown that the normal absolute refractory period of the AV junctional tissue corresponds approximately to the initial half of the Q-T interval, whereas the relative refractory period corresponds to the second half of the Q-T interval. In general, the duration of the refractory period of the AV junction is directly related to the length of the preceding cardiac cycle. Thus, it can be said that the longer the preceding cycle length, the longer the duration of the refractory period of the beat following that cycle, whereas the shorter the preceding cycle, the shorter the duration of the refractory period. This electrophysiologic finding is termed "Ashman's phenomenon" (Chapter 11).

Atrioventricular block is divided into 2 major categories, incomplete (partial) and complete AV block. Incomplete AV block includes first, second, and high degree AV block. Atrioventricular block may occur transiently, intermittently, or permanently, and 1 type may change to another from time to time even in the same individual. In general, the following classification of AV block is used according to the degree of the AV conduction disturbance:

*First degree AV block.* First degree AV block is characterized by a prolonged P-R interval (0.21 second or more in adults and 0.18 second or more in children) in which every atrial impulse reaches the ventricles.

*Second degree AV block.* Second degree AV

block is diagnosed when some of the atrial impulses fail to reach the ventricles so that QRS complexes are unexpectedly dropped. Atrioventricular conduction ratios are used to compare the number of impulses conducted to the atria to those conducted to the ventricles. For instance, 4:3 AV block indicates that for every 4 atrial impulses, 3 are conducted to the ventricles. There are 2 types of second degree AV block. The common type is Wenckebach (Mobitz type I) second degree AV block. In this type, the P-R interval of each successively conducted beat lengthens progressively until a P wave is not followed by a QRS complex (blocked P wave). The uncommon type is characterized by the occurrence of a blocked P wave and otherwise constant P-R intervals in all conducted beats (Mobitz type II AV block). Atrioventricular conduction ratios may be 3:2, 4:3, 5:4, 6:5, and so on in either Mobitz type I or II AV block. The AV ratio may be fixed or may vary throughout the tracing. Two to one A-V block is diagnosed when every other atrial impulse is blocked. It should be noted that Mobitz type I (Wenckebach) AV block represents AV nodal block, whereas Mobitz type II AV block is infranodal block (usually a manifestation of incomplete TFB).

*Advanced (or high degree) AV block.* Advanced AV block is diagnosed when a blocked P wave occurs in more than a 2:1 AV ratio. Thus, 3:1, 4:1, 5:1, 6:1, and so on AV block belongs to this category. Atrioventricular conduction ratios of the even numbers, such as 4:1 or 6:1 AV block, are much more common than that of the odd numbers, such as 3:1 or 5:1 AV block. In advanced AV block, AV JEBs (less commonly VEBs) frequently appear as a physiologic mechanism, leading to incomplete AV dissociation.

*Complete (third degree) AV block.* Complete AV block indicates that none of the atrial impulses are conducted to the ventricles. Consequently, in almost every case, AV JEB or rarely, VER appears to control the ventricles. In complete AV block, atrial and ventricular activities are independent, leading to complete AV dissociation (Chapter 6). Complete AV block may be due to a block in the AV node (AV nodal block), in the His bundle (intra-His block), or in the bilateral bundle branches (infra-His block).

It has been pointed out that Mobitz type II AV block is due to partial BBBB in most cases and frequently is a precursor of complete AV (infranodal) block. An AV conduction disturbance is frequently bidirectional, but it may be unidirectional. For example, antegrade AV conduction may be impaired in the presence of normal retrograde VA conduction, or vice versa.

## FIRST DEGREE ATRIOVENTRICULAR BLOCK

First degree AV block is the most common conduction disturbance. This may occur in apparently healthy subjects as well as in those with diseased hearts. First degree AV block is extremely common in elderly individuals without clinical evidence of heart disease. On the other hand, first degree AV block may be observed in acute myocarditis, acute diaphragmatic MI, and mild DI. First degree AV block is considered to be the most common and the earliest finding in acute rheumatic fever in children.

### Diagnostic Criteria

The diagnostic feature of first degree AV block is a prolongation of the P-R interval. Thus, first degree AV block is diagnosed when the P-R interval is 0.21 second or longer in adults or 0.18 second or longer in children. In first degree AV block, each atrial impulse must be conducted to the ventricles. In general, the P-R intervals are constant throughout, but they may be altered in length when there is a significant change in heart rate. The P-R interval during longer cardiac cycle is often shorter, and the P-R interval during shorter cardiac cycle is often longer.

The P-R interval may be prolonged as much as 0.80 second, and, extremely rarely, it may exceed the P-P cycle.

### Mechanism

First degree AV block, in the majority of cases, is considered to be due to a prolongation of the relative refractory period in the AV junction, which extends to the end of the cycle. The prolonged refractory period is more marked in the earlier portion of the cardiac cycle. Less commonly, a prolongation of the P-R interval may be produced when there is an impairment of conduction in the common (AV) bundle (His bundle). In addition, theoretically impaired conduction in the left and right bundle branches of equal degree also produces a prolonged P-R interval. When the impairment of conductivity in the right and left bundle branches is unequal in degree, a prolonged P-R interval of varying degree, associated with a QRS complex of varying configuration, may result. On the other hand, a wide P wave due either to a marked left atrial enlargement or to an intraatrial conduction defect also produces a prolonged P-R interval.

### Clinical Significance

First degree AV block may be observed in apparently healthy individuals, but it is more commonly found in diseased hearts. Elderly individuals without demonstrable heart disease often have first degree AV block that is considered to be due to chronic degenerative changes in the AV conduction system. Therefore, first degree AV block in elderly subjects (above age 60) is clinically insignificant. However, first degree AV block with acute onset is often due to DI, acute diaphragmatic MI, and acute myocarditis. Less commonly, first degree AV block may be found in healthy young adults and children as a result of increased vagal tone. Under this circumstance, intermittent Wenckebach AV block may also occur.

Treatment of first degree AV block per se is usually not indicated, but the underlying cause (e.g., DI) must be corrected, if possible. Any patient with first degree AV block of recent onset should be observed closely for possible development of higher degree AV block.

## SECOND DEGREE ATRIOVENTRICULAR BLOCK

The term "incomplete AV block" has been loosely used to designate second degree AV block without specifying its degree or type. Thus, the term "incomplete AV block" often implies that it is second degree AV block. However, the type and AV conduction ratio should be specified in second degree AV block, since the fundamental mechanisms and their clinical significance are often different.

Second degree AV block was initially described independently in 1899 by Wenckebach and in 1906 by Hay. Subsequently, second degree AV block was divided into 2 major categories, in 1924, by Mobitz, who called the 2 categories Mobitz types I and II. Mobitz type I AV block is called also Wenckebach AV block. Remember that Wenckebach AV block represents AV nodal block, whereas Mobitz type II AV block is infranodal block, which commonly results from a partial TFB.

Second degree AV block is diagnosed when a P wave (either sinus or ectopic) is blocked. In other words, a P wave is not followed by QRS-T complexes because of an abnormally prolonged refractory period in the AV junction. Mobitz type I AV block (Wenckebach AV block) is characterized by a progressive lengthening of the P-R intervals until a blocked P wave occurs. The occurrence of a blocked P wave, preceded by a progressive lengthening of the P-R intervals, is termed "Wenckebach phenomenon" or "period." It should be noted that Wenckebach phenomenon may occur anywhere in the heart. On the other hand, Mobitz type II AV block is characterized by the occurrence of a blocked P wave without the preceding Wenckebach period.

The blocked P wave may occur occasionally or frequently, periodically, and regularly or irregularly. The ratio of the AV conduction is expressed according to the numbers of the P waves versus the numbers of the conducted QRS complexes. For example, when 1 of 4 atrial impulses is blocked, the AV ratio is expressed as 4:3 AV block.

Second degree AV block occurs when the refractory periods of the AV junctional tissue, both absolute and relative, are abnormally prolonged but do not occupy the entire cardiac cycle. In Mobitz type I (Wenckebach) AV block, the absolute and relative refractory periods of the AV junction are said to be prolonged to an equal or unequal degree. On the other hand, Mobitz type II AV block actually represents incomplete BBBB (partial TFB) (see Chapter 9).

Two to one AV block is another form of second degree AV block, which may be a variant of either Mobitz type I or II AV block. When 2:1 AV block is associated with LBBB, RBBB, or BFB, the block represents a variant of Mobitz type II AV block. On the other hand, 2:1 AV block with normal QRS complexes represents a variant of Wenckebach AV block in most cases.

Two or more consecutively appearing blocked P waves, such as 3:1 or 4:1 AV block, are termed "high degree or advanced" AV block. At times, 2:1 AV block becomes 3:1 AV block when the atrial rate is increased by exercise or certain drugs. For example, the ventricular rate may be 65 beats/min when the atrial rate is 130 beats/min with 2:1 AV block. As the atrial rate is increased to 150 beats/min, the ventricular rate may actually be reduced to 50 beats/min because of 3:1 AV block. This occurs when more atrial impulses arrive in the AV junction, which has a prolonged absolute refractory period, so that the AV junction is able to accept only every third atrial impulse. Advanced AV block is discussed later in this chapter.

## Diagnostic Criteria

**Mobitz Type I Atrioventricular Block (Wenckebach Atrioventricular Block):** Mobitz type I AV block (Wenckebach AV block) is a rather common form of second degree AV block. This type of AV block is diagnosed when the P-R intervals become progressively prolonged until a P wave is not followed by a QRS complex.

*P-R Intervals:* Wenckebach AV block is characterized by a progressive lengthening of the P-R intervals until a blocked P wave occurs (Fig. 8–1). Following the blocked P wave, the same cycle is again repeated (Fig. 8–1). The P-R interval following the pause (blocked P wave) is the shortest of all and may be within normal limits or longer than 0.20 second. Conversely, the P-R interval immediately preceding the blocked P wave is the longest that occurs during the Wenckebach period. The maximal increment in the P-R interval occurs between the first and the second conducted beats following the pause, and the increment in the length of the P-R intervals becomes less and less thereafter until the blocked P wave occurs (Fig. 8–1). The fundamental mechanism responsible for the alteration of the P-R intervals in Wenckebach AV block (Fig. 8–2) is discussed later in this chapter, under Mechanism. Occasionally, a characteristic feature of the Wenckebach period may be altered, particularly in the last beat preceding the blocked P wave or the first beat following the blocked P wave. That is, the last P-R interval before the pause may be much longer than expected or the first P-R interval following the blocked P wave may fail to shorten. This type of unexpected AV conduction occurs during the critical transitional phase between the absolute and relative refractory phase of the AV junction. This critical phase is the most unstable portion in the entire refractory period of the AV junction. Under this circumstance, ordinarily, the P wave is blocked, but, less commonly, the P-R interval may be unexpectedly prolonged or the atrial impulse may penetrate the AV junction but be unable to be conducted to the ventricles (concealed AV conduction). In addition, an exceptionally unexpected alteration of the P-R interval may be due to supernormal AV conduction in the depressed AV junctional tissue.

*Ratio of the Atrioventricular Conduction:* Atrioventricular conduction ratio in the Wenckebach AV block may be fixed or may change from time to time. Common AV conduction ratios are either 3:2 or 4:3 AV block, indicating that every 2 of 3, or 3 of 4 atrial impulses are conducted to the ventricles, respectively. Less commonly, the AV conduction ratio may be 5:4, 6:5, 7:6, 8:7, and so on. When the AV conduction ratio is fixed, the ventricular rhythm shows a regular irregularity. On the other hand, the ventricular rhythm is markedly irregular when the AV conduction ratios vary in Wenckebach AV block. The AV conduction ratio may be unexpectedly altered when concealed AV conduction and/or supernormal AV conduction occurs.

*R-R Intervals:* A characteristic R-R cycle is observed during the Wenckebach period. The

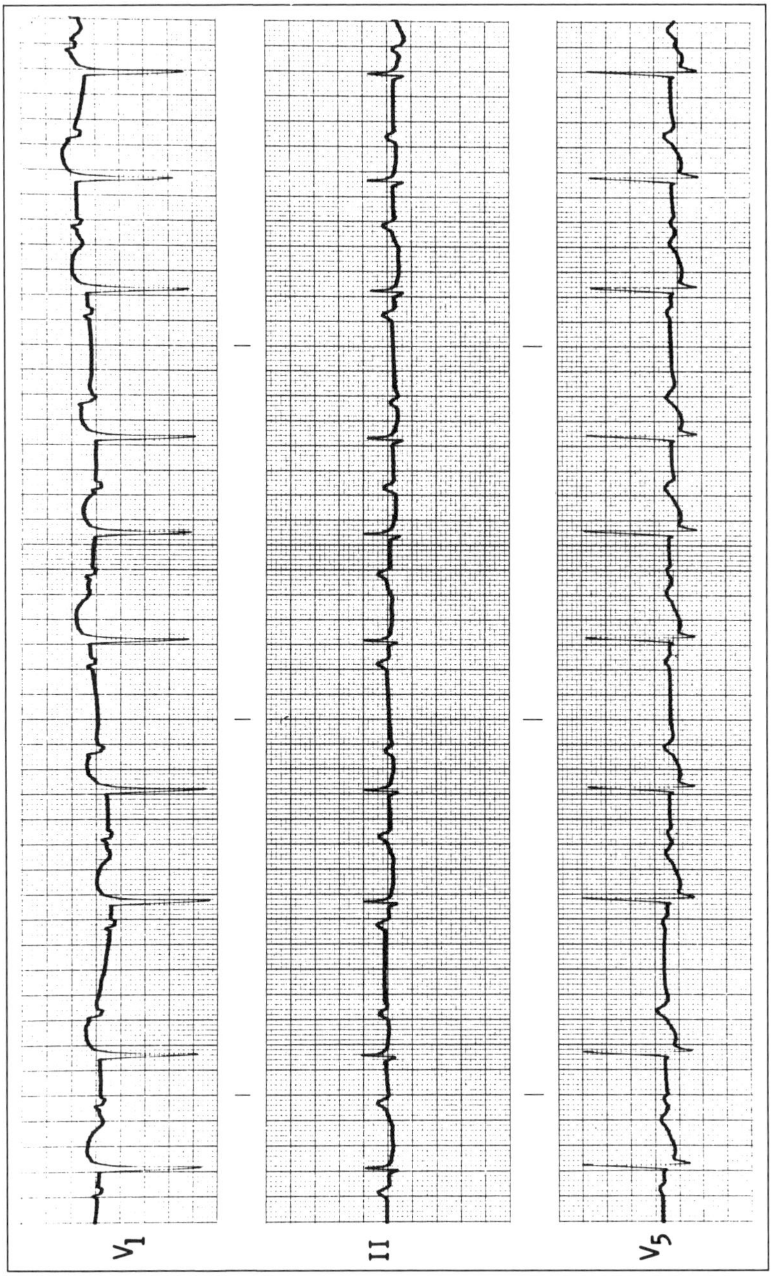


Fig. 8–1. Sinus rhythm with Wenckebach AV block (AV conduction ratios vary from 3:2 to 4:3). Left ventricular hypertrophy and left atrial hypertrophy are diagnosed.

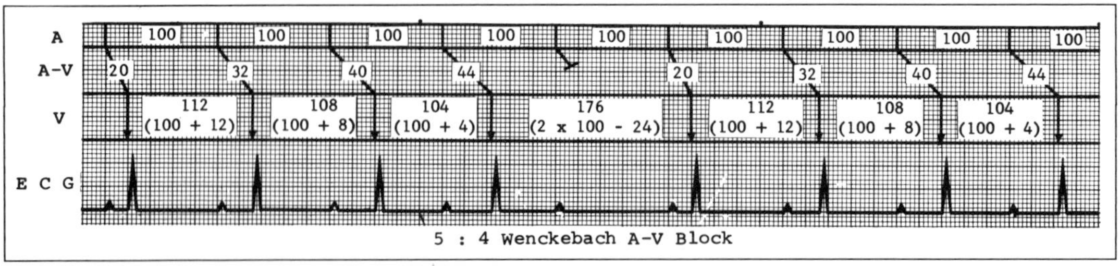


**Fig. 8–2.** This diagram illustrates Mobitz type I (Wenckebach) AV block. The numbers represent hundredths of a second. The numbers in the upper row represent the atrial cycle (P-P interval ) with a rate of 60/min. The numbers within the oblique lines at AV level indicate the AV conduction time (P-R interval). The progressive lengthening of the P-R intervals is apparent until a blocked atrial impulse (dropped P wave) occurs. Following this blocked atrial impulse, the P-R interval shortens to its original value (0.20 second), and the sequence is repeated. The numbers in the lower row represent the duration of successive ventricular cycles. The progressive shortening of the ventricular cycle length (R-R interval) is due to the progressive increment of AV conduction before the blocked atrial impulse and the decrement immediately following the blocked P wave. The numbers in the parentheses in the lower row indicate the degree of increment or decrement in the ventricular cycle length.

R-R interval that includes the blocked P wave is the longest found during the Wenckebach period, but it is shorter than 2 cycles of the P-P interval (Fig. 8–2). This occurs because the R-R interval including the blocked P wave is actually 2 P-P intervals minus the decrement in the P-R interval between the conducted sinus beats preceding and following the pause (Fig. 8–2). The R-R interval immediately following the pause is the second longest during the Wenckebach period because of a maximal increment in the P-R interval. The R-R intervals thereafter become shorter and shorter in successively conducted beats because the degree of the increment in the P-R intervals becomes less and less until a blocked P wave occurs (Fig. 8–2). When the AV conduction ratio is fixed, the ventricular rhythm characteristically shows a regular irregularity (Fig. 8–1). Ventricular pseudobigeminy will result when the AV conduction ratio is fixed (e.g., 4:3 or 3:2).

*Atrial Mechanism:* The atrial mechanism is commonly sinus (Fig. 8–1), but it may be AT or atrial flutter (Fig. 5–8). In the latter case, the Wenckebach phenomenon may be functional (physiologic) due to the extremely rapid atrial rate because of the longer refractory period in the AV junction. Rarely, AV JT with Wenckebach AV block may be observed.

*P-P Intervals:* The P-P intervals are regular in Wenckebach AV block, but they may be irregular when ordinary sinus arrhythmia is present. In addition, the P-P intervals may become periodically irregular when ventriculophasic sinus arrhythmia exists. Diagnostic criteria of Wenckebach (Mobitz type I) AV block are summarized as follows:

1. Progressive lengthening of P-R intervals followed by a blocked P wave
2. Progressive shortening of R-R intervals followed by a blocked P wave
3. The longest R-R interval is shorter than 2 cycles of the P-P interval
4. Regular irregularity of the R-R cycles when the AV ratio is fixed

**Mobitz Type II Atrioventricular Block:** Mobitz type II AV block is a much less common form of second degree AV block than is Wenckebach (Mobitz type I) AV block. Mobitz type II AV block is diagnosed when blocked P waves occur periodically without a preceding Wenckebach phenomenon (Fig. 8–3). When 2:1 AV block persists, a differentiation of Mobitz types I and II is not possible unless a transitional change from or to a lesser degree (3:2) AV block or higher degree AV block (3:1, 4:1, and so on) with occasional ventricular captured beats is observed in the same ECG tracing. However, in a practical sense, 2:1 AV block is a variant of Mobitz type II AV block when the QRS complexes demonstrate LBBB, RBBB, or BFB (Fig. 8–4). On the other hand, 2:1 AV block with normal QRS complexes represents a

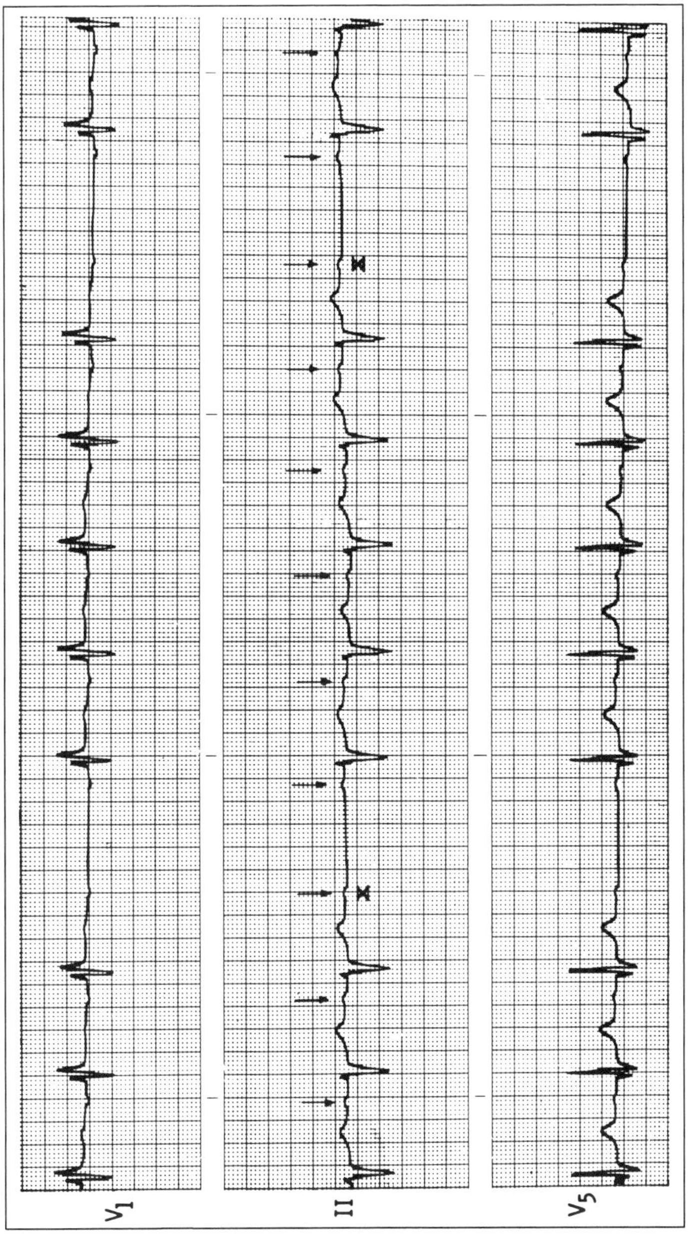


Fig. 8–3. Arrows indicate sinus P waves. The rhythm is sinus with Mobitz type II AV block. X indicates a blocked P wave. RBBB with left anterior hemiblock is indicative of BFB. In addition, old posterolateral MI is suggested.

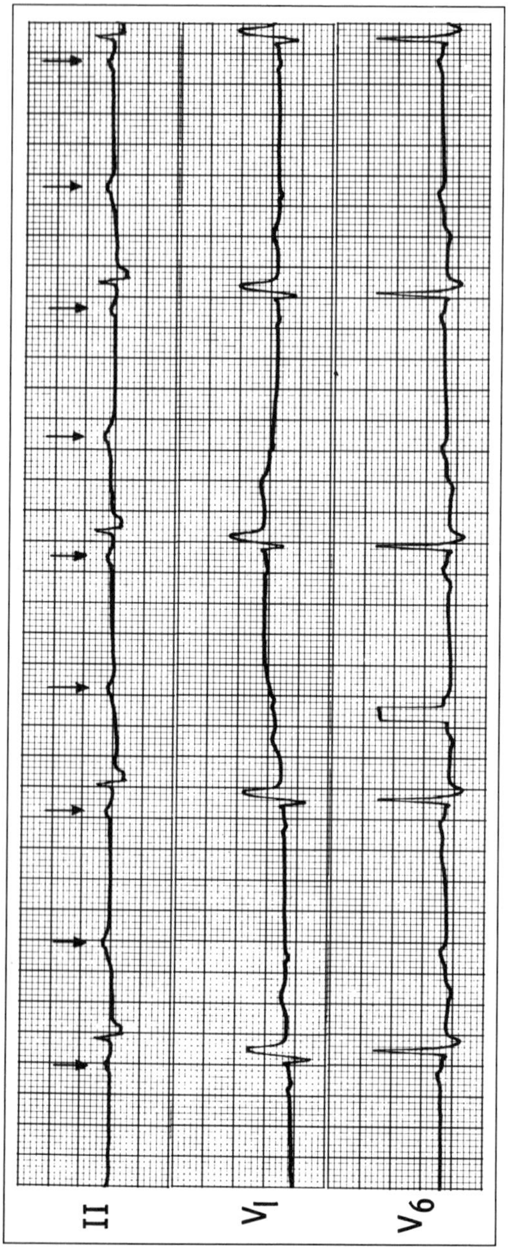


Fig. 8–4. Arrows indicate sinus P waves. The rhythm is sinus with 2:1 AV block associated with RBBB. In this case, 2:1 AV block is considered to be a variant of Mobitz type II AV block (infranodal AV block).

variant of Wenckebach AV block (Fig. 8–5) in most cases.

*P-R Intervals:* The P-R intervals of all the conducted beats in Mobitz type II AV block are always constant (Fig. 8–3).

*Ratio of Atrioventricular Conduction:* The AV conduction ratio, like Wenckebach AV block, may be fixed or may vary. The AV ratio is commonly 3:2 or 4:3, and less commonly 5:4, 6:5, 7:6, or 8:7 AV conduction may be observed. Mobitz type II AV block (e.g., 3:2 or 4:3 AV block) may change to or from 2:1 AV block on the same ECG tracing.

*R-R Intervals:* The R-R intervals including the blocked P wave are usually 2 times the P-P (or R-R) interval of the conducted beats (Fig. 8–3). The R-R intervals of all conducted beats, other than the R-R interval including the blocked P wave, are constant (Fig. 8–3) unless sinus arrhythmia is present.

*P-P Intervals:* The P-P intervals in Mobitz type II AV block are constant unless sinus arrhythmia exists. On the other hand, short and long P-P intervals may occur alternatively in 2:1 AV block because of ventriculophasic sinus arrhythmia. In this case, the P-P interval including the QRS complex is shorter than that without the QRS complex. On rare occasions, the reverse phenomenon may occur.

*Atrial Mechanism:* The atrial mechanism is usually sinus, but it may be AT.

Diagnostic criteria of Mobitz type II AV block are summarized as follows:

1. Periodic occurrence of a blocked P wave without Wenckebach phenomenon
2. Constant P-R intervals in all conducted beats
3. The R-R interval including the blocked P wave is multiples of the P-P interval
4. Regular irregularity of the R-R cycles when the AV ratio is fixed
5. Common association with LBBB, RBBB, or BFB

## Mechanism

**Mobitz Type I Atrioventricular Block (Wenckebach Atrioventricular Block):** Mobitz type I AV block is considered to be due to a prolongation of the absolute and relative refractory periods in the AV junction to an equal or unequal degree. The characteristic feature of the Wenckebach phenomenon (progressive lengthening of P-R intervals until a blocked P wave occurs) is explained as follows (Fig. 8–2):

The maximal increment of the P-R interval occurs in the second conducted beat following the pause. This is observed because the refractory period of the AV junction is directly related to the length of the preceding R-R interval. The longest R-R interval (pause) induces a marked increase in the length of the refractory period in the AV junction, leading to a maximal increment of the P-R interval in the second conducted beat.

Following the maximal increment of the P-R interval in the second conducted beat, the P-R intervals in the subsequent beats progressively lengthen until a blocked P wave occurs, but the degree of the increment in the P-R intervals becomes less and less. Consequently, the R-R intervals following the pause progressively shorten until a blocked P wave occurs. The progressive shortening of the R-R intervals is considered to be due to 2 opposing effects on the refractoriness in the AV junction. They are a shortening effect due to the shorter cycle lengths per se and a lengthening effect consequent to the increasing fatigue (refractoriness) of the AV junctional tissue.

During the Wenckebach period, the R-R interval of each consecutively conducted beat is equal in length to the P-P interval plus the increment of the P-R interval between the 2 successively conducted beats. Conversely, the R-R interval that includes the blocked P wave (pause) is equal in length to 2 P-P intervals minus the decrement in the P-R interval between the conducted sinus beats preceding and following the pause. As a result, the longest R-R interval (pause), which contains the blocked P wave, is usually shorter than 2 short R-R intervals or 2 P-P intervals. For a similar reason, the R-R interval of the first beat following the pause is longer than the R-R interval of the last beat preceding the pause.

When the P-P cycles vary because of sinus arrhythmia, the above-mentioned characteristic features of the Wenckebach period may be somewhat altered. In addition, ventriculophasic

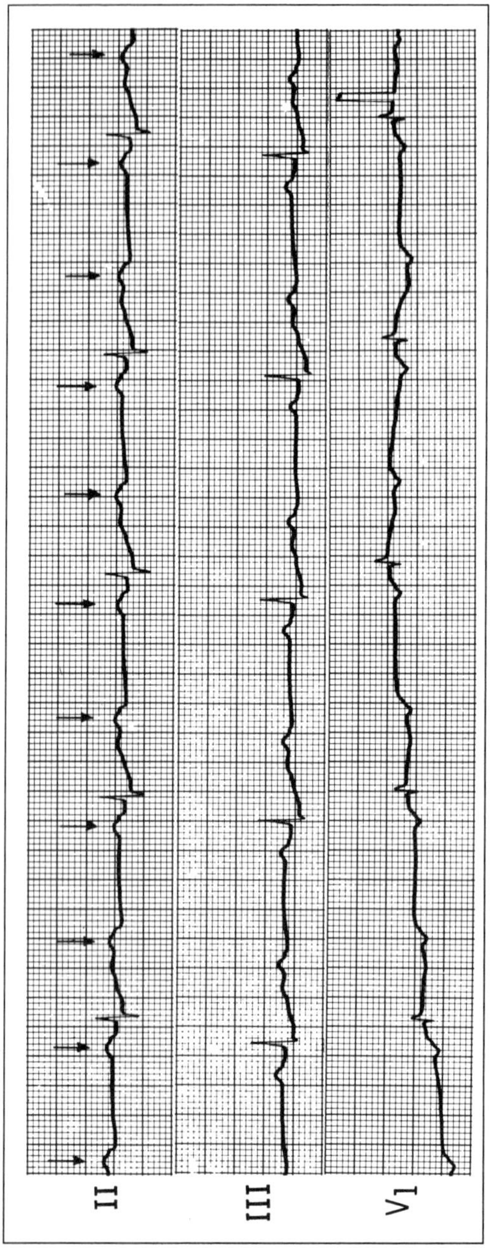


**Fig. 8–5.** Arrows indicate sinus P waves. The rhythm is sinus with 2:1 AV block. In this case, 2:1 AV block is considered to be a variant of Wenckebach (Mobitz type I) AV block (AV nodal block). Broad P waves indicate left atrial enlargement.

sinus arrhythmia also may produce an alteration of the Wenckebach period. Occasionally, an unexpectedly long or short P-R interval or unexpectedly conducted or blocked P wave may occur in Wenckebach AV block because of concealed AV conduction and/or supernormal AV conduction. In these circumstances, the characteristic Wenckebach period will be again altered. It should be pointed out again that Wenckebach AV block represents AV nodal block.

**Mobitz Type II AV Block:** Mobitz type II AV block is considered to be due to a block distal to the AV node. Therefore, Mobitz type II AV block represents infranodal block, which is nearly always due to incomplete BBBB (partial TFB). Rarely, Mobitz type II AV block is due to a block within the His bundle (intra-His block). Mobitz type II AV block is nearly always associated with hemiblocks, LBBB, RBBB, or BFB (Fig. 8–3). Mobitz type II AV block is often a precursor of complete AV (infranodal) block as a result of complete BBBB (complete TFB).

## Clinical Significance

The clinical significances of Mobitz types I and II AV block are quite different. In general, Mobitz type I AV block (Wenckebach AV block) produces no or very little symptoms. In contrast to this, Mobitz type II AV block is often associated with a high incidence of CHF and/or Adams-Stokes syndrome. Some sensitive patients may experience palpitation or skipped heartbeats that may resemble or be identical to the feeling induced by premature contractions (e.g., VPCs). When blocked P waves occur frequently and the ventricular rate becomes slow, particularly in Mobitz type II AV block, patients may experience dizziness, fainting, or even complete unconsciousness. Because of the nature of Mobitz type II AV block, high degree or complete AV block often follows.

Mobitz type I AV block (Wenckebach AV block) is often transient in nature, and this type of AV block may be induced by mild DI or acute infection (e.g., acute rheumatic fever, diphtheria, scarlet fever, and many other forms of bacterial, viral, and fungal infection). Acute diaphragmatic MI is often associated with Mobitz type I AV block because of a transient ischemic change occurring in the AV junction. In addition, Wenckebach AV block may be observed occasionally in healthy children and young adults as a result of increased vagal tone. Since the commonest cause of acute diaphragmatic MI is occlusion of the right coronary artery, which also supplies the AV junction, Mobitz type I AV block often occurs under this circumstance. On the other hand, acute anteroseptal MI is commonly associated with Mobitz type II AV block or even complete AV block (infranodal block) because of irreversible changes (necrosis) in the bifurcation or the bundle branches or both. Cardiac surgery of various types may induce a transient or permanent AV block of varying degrees.

Mobitz type I AV block (Wenckebach AV block) per se usually does not require treatment. Conversely, a permanent artificial pacemaker is highly recommended for the treatment of Mobitz type II AV block because of irreversible damage in the conduction system and a higher incidence of the Adams-Stokes syndrome. Removal or treatment of the direct cause of the AV block (e.g., DI, infections) is extremely important to prevent the development of a higher degree AV block. When there is CHF, it should be treated accordingly.

The prognosis in Mobitz type I AV block is generally good, whereas Mobitz type II AV block has a serious outcome. However, the nature and severity of underlying heart disease directly influence the prognosis.

# HIGH DEGREE (ADVANCED) ATRIOVENTRICULAR BLOCK

High degree (advanced) AV block is diagnosed when the AV conduction ratio is 3:1 or more. Thus, high degree AV block is between second degree AV block and complete AV block and is the most advanced incomplete AV block. It is not uncommon to observe that complete AV block is initiated by high degree AV block. Common AV conduction ratios are even numbers, such as 4:1, 6:1, 8:1 conduction, and the AV conduction ratios of odd numbers, such as 3:1, 5:1, 7:1, are relatively uncommon. Because of a slow ventricular rhythm in high degree AV block, AV JEBs or, less commonly, VEBs appear to control the ventricles as a physiologic mechanism. It is the rule rather than the exception to observe 1 or more AV JEBs when AV conduction ratios are 4:1 or higher. When AV conduction ratios further increase in high degree AV block, the numbers of the AV JEBs exceed those of the conducted beats. In this circumstance, conducted beats (ventricular captured beats) may occur very rarely, and otherwise the ECG tracing shows complete AV block (Fig. 8–6). Some investigators designate this extremely advanced AV block as "almost complete AV block." High degree AV block may be due to a block in the AV node (AV nodal block), within the His bundle (intra-His block), or distal to the His bundle (infra-His block).

In high degree AV block, incomplete AV dissociation usually results because the AV JEBs (less commonly VEBs) and the sinus P waves are independent except for the conducted beats (ventricular captured beats). The atrial mechanism in high degree AV block may be an ectopic rhythm, such as AF, atrial flutter, or AT (Fig. 5–19). A detailed description of the relationship between high degree AV block and incomplete AV dissociation is found in Chapter 6.

## Diagnostic Criteria

By definition, high degree (advanced) AV block indicates that the AV conduction ratio is 3:1 or more.

**Atrioventricular Conduction Ratio:** Common AV conduction ratios in high degree AV block are 4:1, 6:1, 8:1, 10:1, and so on. Less commonly, the AV conduction ratios are odd numbers, such as 3:1, 5:1, and 7:1. When con-

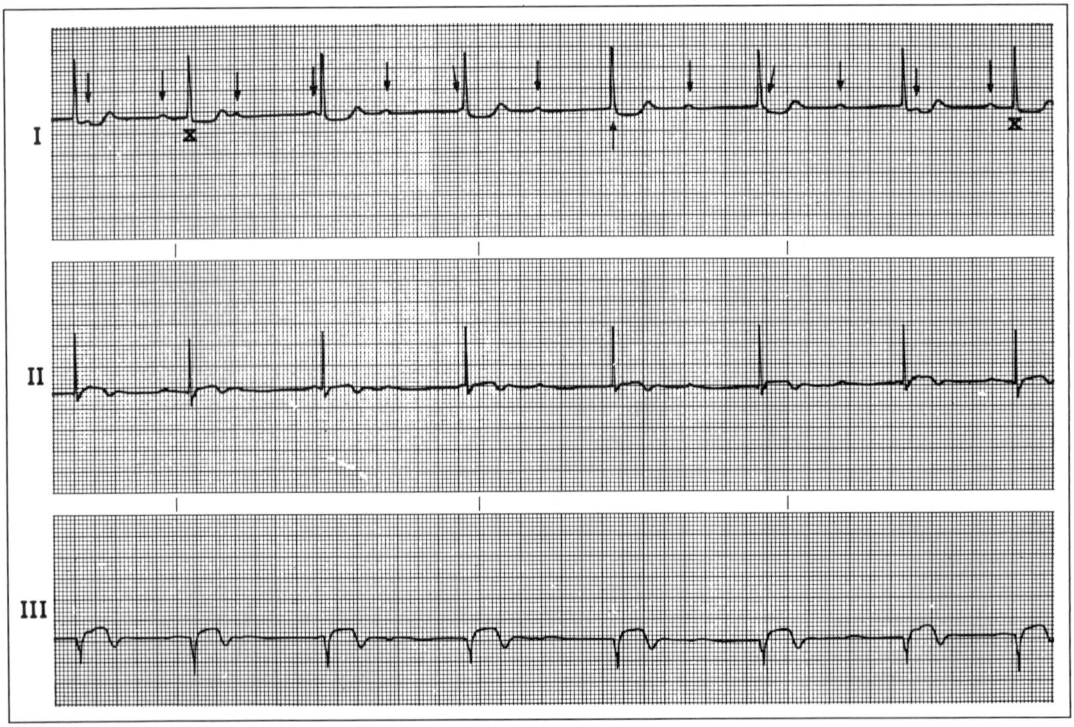


**Fig. 8–6.** Arrows indicate sinus P waves. This ECG tracing reveals sinus rhythm (atrial rate: 78 beats/min) with advanced AV block producing predominantly AV JER (ventricular rate: 42 beats/min) in a patient with acute diaphragmatic MI. Note that there are 2 ventricular captured beats (normally conducted sinus beats, marked X). Under this circumstance, the AV block represents AV nodal block, which is usually transient in acute diaphragmatic MI.

ducted beats appear only occasionally, an exact AV conduction ratio is difficult or, at times, impossible to determine, especially when dealing with a limited length of the ECG tracing. It is not uncommon to observe only 1 or 2 conducted beats (ventricular captured beats) in a whole tracing (Fig. 8–6). Needless to say, in this case, AV JER or VER is present to control the ventricles and is independent of the P waves, resulting in incomplete AV dissociation (Fig. 8–6). Thus, the AV block in this situation is nearly complete. High degree or complete AV block is 1 of the 3 major underlying rhythm disorders responsible for the production of AV dissociation (Chapter 6).

**P-R Intervals:** As seen in second degree AV block, the P-R intervals of the conducted beats in high degree AV block may be normal, but they may be markedly prolonged. In general, the P-R intervals of the conducted beats are constant, unless Wenckebach phenomenon, concealed AV conduction, or supernormal AV conduction occurs.

**Atrial Mechanism:** The atria may be controlled by the sinus node, but it is not uncommon for the atrial mechanism to be an ectopic rhythm, such as AF, atrial flutter, or AT.

**Atrioventricular Dissociation:** One or more AV JEBs commonly occur to control the ventricles in high degree AV block. This results in incomplete AV dissociation (Fig. 8–6). It is rather unusual not to observe AV JEBs in spite of an extremely slow ventricular rhythm. In this circumstance, concealed AV conduction is considered to be responsible, that is, the AV JEBs fails to appear because the AV junctional pacemaker is passively discharged by the atrial impulse that penetrated deeply into the AV junction. Ventricular escape beats rarely appear in high degree AV block when the AV junction is unable to function as a secondary pacemaker or when the block is distal to the AV node.

**P-P and R-R Intervals:** The P-P intervals in high degree AV block are generally regular, but they may vary when ordinary sinus arrhythmia, SA block, or ventriculophasic sinus arrhythmia is present.

The R-R intervals are almost always irregular in high degree AV block because of the frequent occurrence of AV JEBs in addition to the conducted beats. The R-R intervals become unexpectedly irregular when concealed AV conduction and/or supernormal AV conduction occurs. When the AV conduction ratio is constant, without AV JEBs, the R-R intervals are regular, but the R-R intervals become irregular when the AV conduction ratios are inconstant. When the AV conduction ratio alternates (e.g., 2:1 alternating with 4:1 AV conduction), ventricular pseudo bigeminy results.

**Configuration of QRS Complex:** The configuration of the QRS complex depends greatly upon the origin of the QRS complex. Conducted beats are usually normal in configuration (Fig. 8–6) unless LBBB or RBBB is present. The QRS complex of a VEB is, needless to say, wide and bizarre. Various QRS configurations may be observed when ventricular fusion beats of varying degrees occur.

### Mechanism

High degree (advanced) AV block may be due to various fundamental mechanisms. As in second degree AV block, the same mechanism responsible for the production of Mobitz type I (Wenckebach AV block) or II AV block may induce high degree AV block.

As seen in second degree or complete AV block, high degree AV may be due to a block in the AV node (AV nodal block), within the His bundle (intra-His block), or below the His bundle (infra-His block). When advanced AV block is due to infra-His block, the finding represents incomplete BBBB (partial TFB).

### Clinical Significance

The clinical significance of high degree AV block is very similar to that of complete AV block and is discussed later in this chapter.

## COMPLETE (THIRD DEGREE) ATRIOVENTRICULAR BLOCK

Complete (third degree) AV block is characterized by independent atrial and ventricular activities resulting from complete block at the

AV junctional tissues, AV (common) bundle, and bilateral bundle branches. When atrial impulses fail to conduct to the ventricles, due to complete AV block, a subsidiary pacemaker located anywhere distal to the site of block takes over ventricular activity. Among the many potential pacemakers located below the site of the block, the pacemaker with the fastest inherent rate will take over control of ventricular activity. In general, the AV junction acts as a pacemaker when the block occurs in the AV junction, and the block in this case is usually due to drug toxicity (e.g., DI) or vagal influence. In contrast to this, a pacemaker located in the AV (common) bundle, bundle branches, or ventricles often takes over ventricular activity when the block is distal to the AV node. In complete AV block, the atrial rate is usually faster than the ventricular rate. Because of the independence of atrial and ventricular activities in complete AV block, complete AV dissociation always occurs. As described previously, complete AV block is 1 of the 3 major basic rhythm disturbances responsible for the production of AV dissociation (Chapter 6).

Complete AV block is considered to be due to a prolongation of the absolute refractory period so that it occupies the entire cardiac cycle. As a result, no relative refractory phase is present. Complete AV block may be observed in various organic heart diseases, but the most common cause is a degenerative-sclerotic process in the conduction system with or without definite evidence of CAD. The next most common cause is DI, in which the site of block is always within the AV node (AV nodal block).

## Diagnostic Criteria

**Relationship Between Atrial and Ventricular Activities:** In complete (third degree) AV block, atrial and ventricular activities must be independent throughout the tracing because of the complete blocking of the atrial impulses at the AV junction, AV (common) bundle, or bilateral bundle branches (Figs. 2–4 and 6–3). By definition, complete AV block cannot be diagnosed even if there is only a single ventricular captured beat. In complete AV block, the atrial rate is always faster than the ventricular rate. The fact that complete AV block is 1 of the 3 major underlying rhythm disorders producing AV dissociation has been repeatedly emphasized (Chapter 6).

**Atrial Mechanism:** The atria may be controlled by the sinus node (Fig. 2–4), but they may be controlled by any ectopic focus in the atria. Thus, ectopic atrial mechanisms may include AF, atrial flutter, or AT (Fig. 6–3). Extremely rarely, the atria and ventricles may be independently controlled by 2 different pacemakers in the AV junction to produce double AV junctional rhythm. In this case, the atrial rate is, of course, faster than the ventricular rate. Double AV junctional rhythm is 1 of the rarer causes of AV dissociation.

**Ventricular Mechanism:** Since none of the atrial impulses reach the ventricles due to a block at the site mentioned before, AV JER or, less commonly, VER develops to control the ventricles as a physiologic mechanism. When the subsidiary pacemaker is located above the bifurcation of the common bundle and in the AV junctional tissue below the blocked zone, the QRS complex is usually normal in configuration (Figs. 2–4 and 6–3). This type of ectopic rhythm is termed "A-V JER." In general, the ventricular rate in AV JER is between 40 and 60 beats/min, but it may be slower than 40 beats/min. In the latter case, an ectopic pacemaker is assumed to be located in the common bundle (His bundle).

When the ectopic pacemaker is located below the bifurcation of the AV (common) bundle, the configuration of the QRS complex is wide and bizarre because the propagation of the impulses in the ventricles occurs in an abnormal fashion (Fig. 2–4). This type of ectopic rhythm is termed "ventricular escape (idioventricular) rhythm" and its usual rate is between 30 and 40 beats/min. Occasionally, the ventricular rate may be slower than 30 beats/min, and it may be as slow as 15–20 beats/min, particularly in elderly individuals.

**P-P and R-R Intervals:** When the atrial mechanism is sinus, the P-P intervals are often regular, unless ordinary sinus arrhythmia or intermittent SA block is present. In approximately

30% of cases of complete AV block, the P-P interval that contains the QRS complex is shorter than the P-P interval without the QRS complex, in spite of the independence of the atrial and ventricular activities (Fig. 4–1). This is termed "ventriculophasic sinus arrhythmia." Extremely rarely, the reverse phenomenon may occur. Ventriculophasic sinus arrhythmia is discussed in detail in Chapter 4.

The R-R intervals in AV JER or VER are usually regular (Figs. 2–4 and 6–3). However, not uncommonly, the R-R intervals in complete AV block may be irregular due to various causes, including:

1. Multiple pacemakers in the AV junction and/or in the ventricles
2. Irregular discharge of a single pacemaker in the AV junction or ventricles
3. Exit block of varying degrees

**Atrioventricular Dissociation:** As repeatedly emphasized, complete AV block is 1 of the commonest causes of complete AV dissociation (Chapter 6).

Diagnostic criteria of complete AV block are summarized as follows:

1. Independent atrial and ventricular activities producing AV dissociation
2. Atrial mechanism may be sinus or ectopic (AF, atrial flutter, or AT and rarely AV junctional)
3. Ventricular mechanism may be JER or VER (regular and slow ventricular cycle, slower than 60 beats/min)
4. Ventriculophasic sinus arrhythmia in 30%

## Mechanism

Complete AV block is commonly due to block at the AV junction and not uncommonly due to block at the AV (common) bundle (His bundle) or bilateral bundle branches.

Depending upon the etiologic factors, complete AV block may be transient or permanent. For example, complete AV block due to acute diaphragmatic MI, DI, or acute myocarditis is usually transient, whereas anterior MI often produces a permanent complete AV block. In addition, AV JER is almost always produced in the former because of reversible changes that occur at the AV junction (AV nodal block). In contrast to this, VER is often produced in the latter because of irreversible damage occurring below the bifurcation of the AV bundle (infranodal block). Chronic degenerative-sclerotic change in the AV conduction system in elderly individuals likewise produces a permanent complete AV block. It has been shown that approximately 30–40% of all cases of complete AV block are actually due to BBBB (complete TFB). BBBB is discussed in detail in Chapter 9.

In complete AV block, the absolute refractory period is maximally prolonged in the AV conduction system and occupies the entire cardiac cycle, leaving no time for a relative refractory period.

It is interesting to note that complete AV block may be only unidirectional, particularly in the AV junction. That is, complete antegrade AV block may exist in the presence of unimpaired retrograde VA conduction, or vice versa. Thus, it is not uncommon to observe 1 or more atrial captured beats in the presence of complete antegrade AV block. Furthermore, artificial pacemaker-induced ventricular rhythm, with occasional or even continuous atrial captured beats, is not uncommon, in spite of the fact that the artificial pacemaker was used for the treatment of complete AV block.

## Clinical Significance

The various causes of first, second, and high degree AV block, described previously in this chapter, may also induce complete AV block when the severity of the various causes is far advanced. The causes include intoxication by various drugs (e.g., DI), acute infections (rheumatic fever, diphtheria, various viral, bacterial, and fungal infections), electrolyte imbalances, and CAD. Complete AV block produced by these factors is often transient. For example, complete AV block of acute onset, which is most commonly due to acute diaphragmatic MI or DI, is often transient because the damage in the AV junction is usually reversible. On the other hand, complete AV block due to an anterior MI is frequently permanent because of irreversible damage occurring in the common bundle and/or both bundle branches.

In chronic acquired complete AV block, the most common cause is a degenerative-sclerotic process in the AV conduction systems with or without any evidence of CAD, especially in elderly persons. Less commonly, chronic acquired complete AV block may be due to a chronic inflammatory process, such as RHD, diphtheria, syphilitic heart disease, and Chagas' heart disease. Rarely, tumors or a granulomatous lesion may produce complete AV block, and complete AV block is occasionally induced by cardiac surgery or other traumas.

Congenital complete AV block may or may not be associated with other congenital cardiac anomalies. Common cardiac anomalies associated with congenital complete AV block include Ebstein's disease and ventricular septal defect.

Various symptoms and signs may be observed in complete AV block, and the symptoms and signs due to the underlying heart disease will be observed accordingly. The symptoms, in general, in complete AV block are markedly different in the congenital and acquired forms. Congenital complete AV block without other cardiac anomalies is usually asymptomatic until the ventricular rate slows down markedly when the individual gets older. Conversely, acquired complete AV block nearly always produces various symptoms. This discrepancy is attributed to a higher incidence of advanced heart disease in older people in acquired complete AV block as compared with the congenital form. In addition, various symptoms in complete AV block are greatly influenced by the site of AV block, the ventricular rate, and the underlying causes, especially the severity of the heart disease. When the ventricular mechanism is AV JER, complete AV block per se may not produce any significant symptoms because of a relatively rapid ventricular rate in addition to normal intraventricular conduction. In congenital complete AV block, AV JER is nearly always present because the block occurs above the bifurcation of the AV (common) bundle.

Severe CHF and/or Adams-Stokes syndrome frequently occurs in acquired complete AV block, particularly when the ventricular rate is slow and advanced heart disease exists. This is observed because the cardiac output is further reduced when the ventricular mechanism is VER, since the ventricles are activated in an abnormal fashion in addition to the markedly slow ventricular rate.

Implantation of a permanent artificial pacemaker is almost always necessary for the treatment of chronic complete AV block, especially when dealing with infranodal complete AV block. Transient complete AV block (e.g., in acute diaphragmatic MI) may not require active treatment. Digitalis should be discontinued immediately when complete AV block is considered to be due to DI. Permanent artificial pacemaker implantation is recommended in congenital complete AV block even if the individual is asymptomatic because the block is permanent and various symptoms as a result of slow ventricular rate eventually occur as the patient gets older.

# Chapter 9

# Intraventricular Conduction Disturbances

Various forms of intraventricular conduction disturbances may occur under different clinical circumstances. The most common and well-recognized forms of intraventricular conduction disturbances are RBBB and LBBB. In BBB, the impulse will be conducted via an intact bundle branch so that the ventricle with a blocked bundle branch will be activated later than the ventricle with an intact bundle branch. Therefore, instead of the simultaneous activation of both ventricles that occurs under normal circumstances, BBB produces asynchronous activation of the 2 ventricles. The incidence of LBBB and the incidence of RBBB are considered to be almost equal.

Although it is less well recognized, some intraventricular conduction disturbances are due to a conduction delay involving both ventricles diffusely. This type of conduction delay is termed "nonspecific" or "diffuse" intraventricular conduction disturbance. As a rule, intraventricular conduction disturbances are recognized by a prolongation of the QRS interval, but some intraventricular conduction disturbances produce little or no prolongation of the QRS interval. For example, a block at 1 of the subdivisions of the left bundle branch system (hemiblock) causes an abnormal QRS axis deviation without significant alteration in the QRS interval.

Bundle branch block has a close relationship to ventricular hypertrophy. This is more so in LBBB because the underlying process of LBBB is almost always LVH, particularly in adults. In addition, some cardiac lesions, such as an atrial septal defect, are almost always associated with an RBBB pattern (Fig. 9–1). The configuration of BBB commonly demonstrates an exaggerated form of corresponding ventricular hypertrophy in both the QRS complex and ST, T waves.

Left bundle branch block tends to produce more widening of the QRS complex than does RBBB. Bundle branch block (either right or left) generally is said to be complete when the QRS interval is 0.12 second or wider (in limb leads). Incomplete BBB is diagnosed when the QRS interval is between 0.10 and 0.11 second (0.09 second in some cases). Customarily the term "complete" is omitted in the actual ECG interpretation; thus, BBB without specifying complete or incomplete automatically means "complete." The term "incomplete" should always be added in the actual interpretation when applicable. It is not uncommon to observe a relatively narrow QRS interval (less than 0.10 second), especially when dealing with incomplete RBBB.

Bundle branch block (either right or left) is commonly chronic and permanent, but it may occur intermittently. Intermittent BBB may occur depending upon the heart rate (rate dependent) or it may be unrelated to the heart rate (rate independent).

When the conduction disturbances involve both right and left bundle branches, various ECG abnormalities are produced. Bilateral bundle branch block (BBBB) includes BFB and TFB. Complete AV block is produced when the block in both bundle branches is complete (complete TFB). Various complex arrhythmias may be observed, however, if the BBBB is incomplete (BBBB is discussed in detail in this chapter).

Bundle branch block can be encountered in normal as well as in diseased hearts, but the presence of LBBB nearly always indicates a diseased heart.

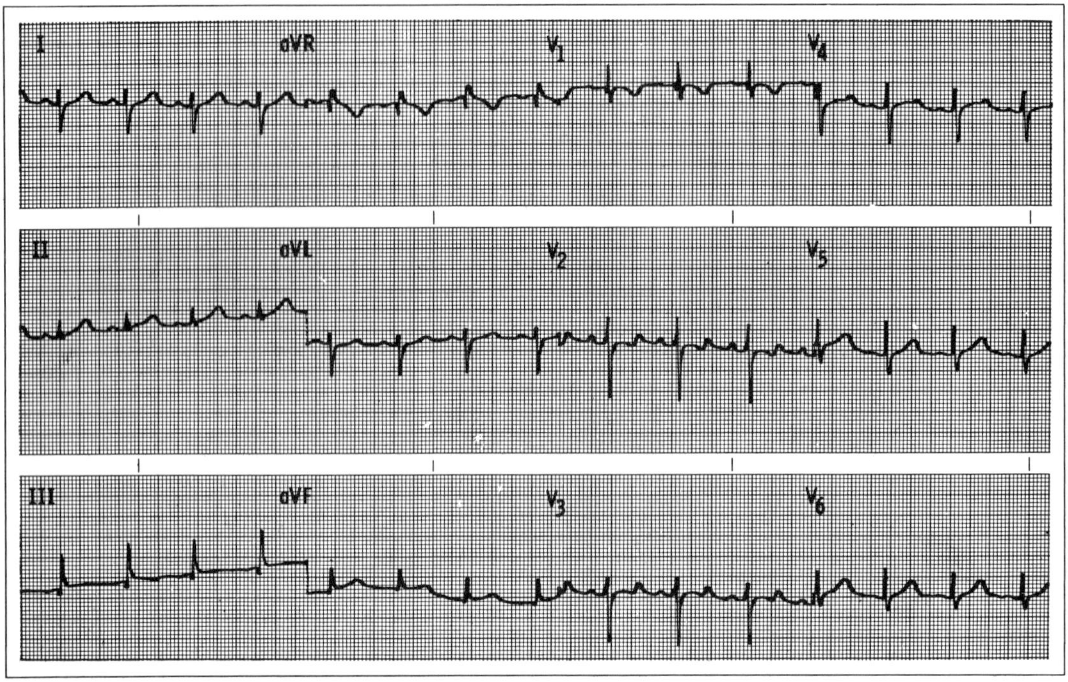


**Fig. 9–1.** This ECG tracing was obtained from a patient with atrial septal defect, ostium secundum type. The ECG abnormalities include incomplete RBBB pattern and right axis deviation of the QRS complexes, suggestive of right ventricular hypertrophy (RVH).

## RIGHT BUNDLE BRANCH BLOCK

### Diagnostic Criteria

Right bundle branch block typically produces an rSR′ or M pattern in the right precordial leads (leads $V_{1-3}$) and slurred and deep S waves in the left precordial leads (leads I, aVL, and $V_{4-6}$). This finding is observed because of a delayed activation of the right ventricle (Fig. 9–2)—that is, the right ventricle is activated following the completion of LV activation through the ventricular myocardium rather than the right bundle branch system. This abnormal activation of the right ventricle is primarily responsible for wide and slurred R′ waves (second R waves of the QRS complexes) in the right precordial leads and wide and slurred S waves in the left precordial leads (Fig. 9–2). Leads I and aVL usually show similar findings to those in leads $V_{4-6}$. The QRS interval is 0.12 second or more in complete (Fig. 9–2) and 0.10 to 0.11 second in incomplete RBBB (Fig. 9–1). The initial vector during ventricular septal activation remains normal. In addition, the first half of the QRS complex in RBBB is usually not altered significantly. Vectorcardiographically, the conduction delay primarily involves the last 0.04 second vectors during ventricular activation.

The QRS axis in uncomplicated RBBB is expected to be normal, although it is often difficult to determine a precise electrical axis. When RBBB is associated with abnormal axis deviation, BFB is usually considered to be present. For example, left axis deviation in the presence of RBBB often indicates coexisting left anterior hemiblock (Fig. 9–3). On the other hand, right axis deviation in the presence of RBBB usually indicates coexisting left posterior hemiblock (Fig. 9–4).

In pure RBBB, T waves in the right precordial leads are inverted (sometimes biphasic) because of the secondary T wave change (Fig. 9–2). In

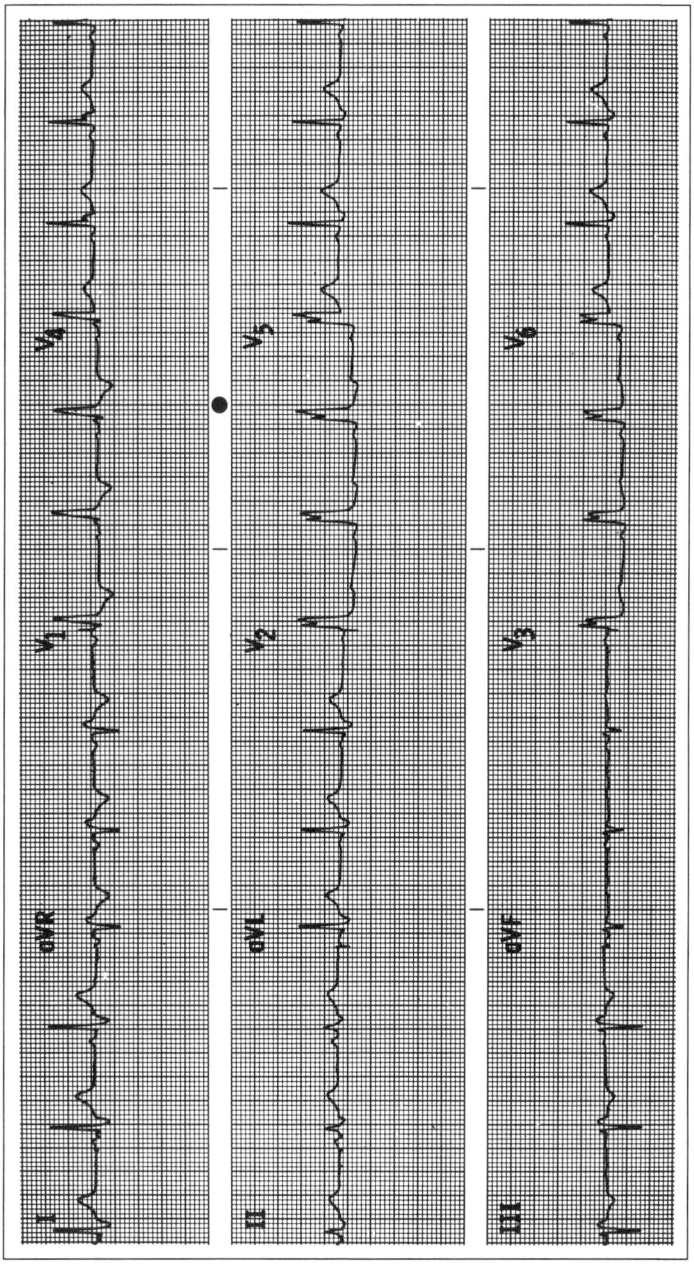


**Fig. 9–2.** Sinus rhythm with RBBB.

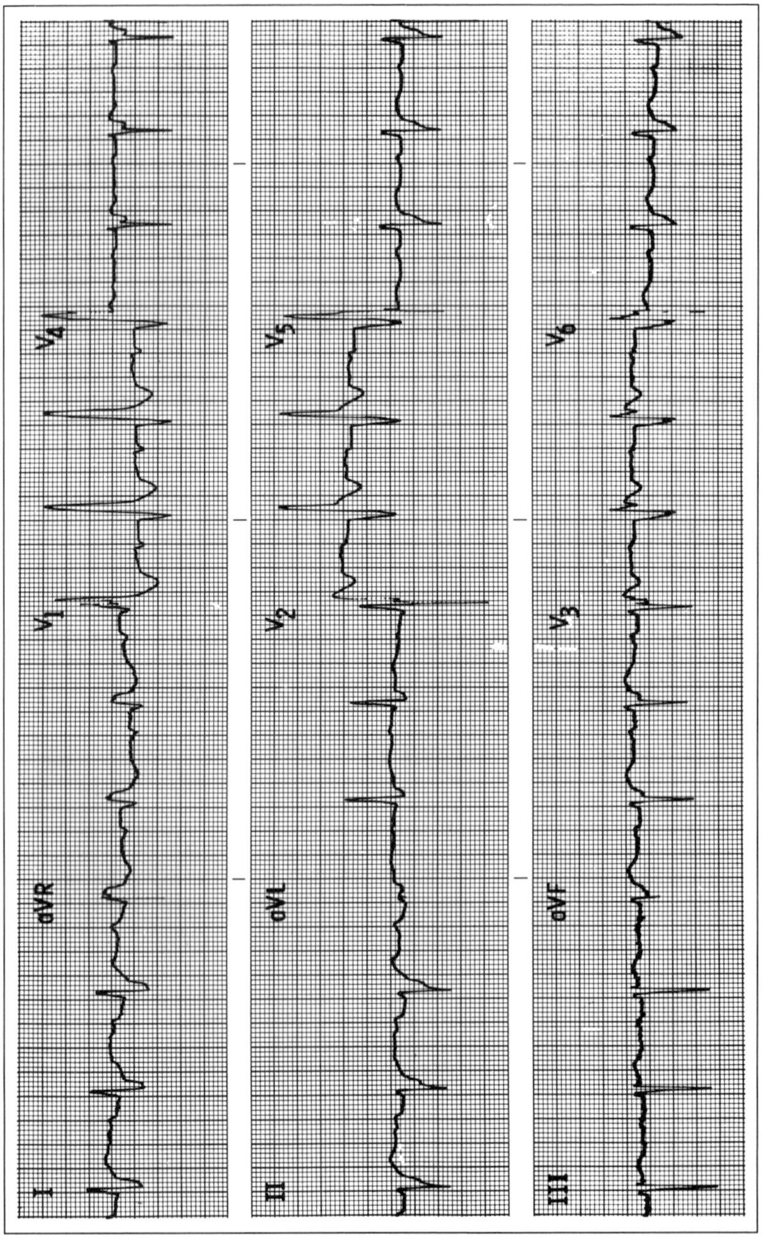


**Fig. 9–3.** Sinus rhythm with first degree AV block and BFB (RBBB with left anterior hemiblock) due to acute anteroseptal MI. The prophylactic artificial pacing is indicated.

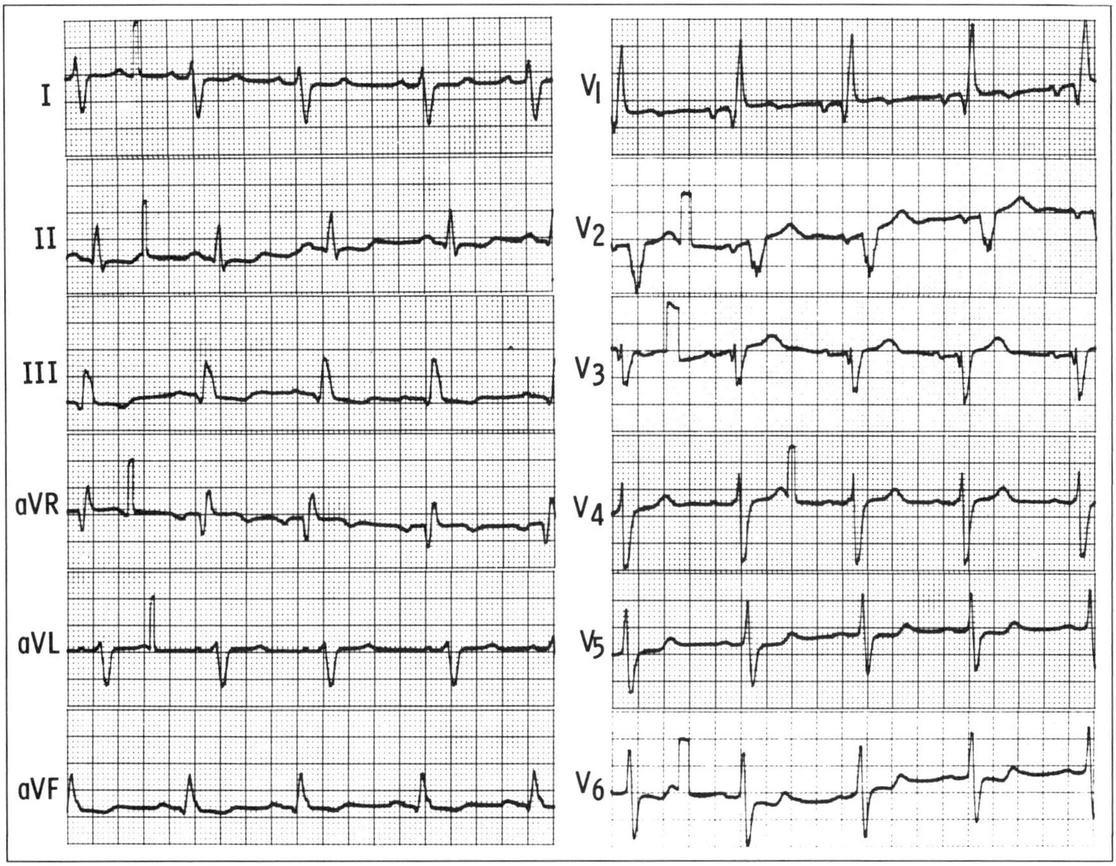


**Fig. 9–4.** Sinus rhythm with BFB (RBBB with left posterior hemiblock) due to recent anteroseptal MI. The prophylactic pacing is indicated. In addition, old diaphragmatic MI is suggested.

general, the T axis and the QRS axis are almost 180° discordant. When other abnormalities, such as myocardial ischemia, coexist, the primary T wave change replaces the secondary T wave change.

The diagnostic criteria of RBBB are summarized as follows:

1. QRS interval ≥ 0.12 second
2. rSR′ or M pattern of QRS complex in leads $V_{1-3}$
3. Deep and slurred S waves in leads I, aVL, and $V_{4-6}$
4. Secondary ST, T wave change in leads $V_{1-3}$

## Intermittent Right Bundle Branch Block

Right bundle branch block is usually fixed and permanent, but it may occur intermittently (Fig. 9–5). Intermittent RBBB is often related to the ventricular rate. Right BBB develops as the ventricular rate increases because the impulse will find the right bundle branch still in the refractory period. On the other hand, the impulse will be conducted normally during slower ventricular rate because the refractory period in the right bundle branch is over. The ventricular rate at which the intraventricular conduction

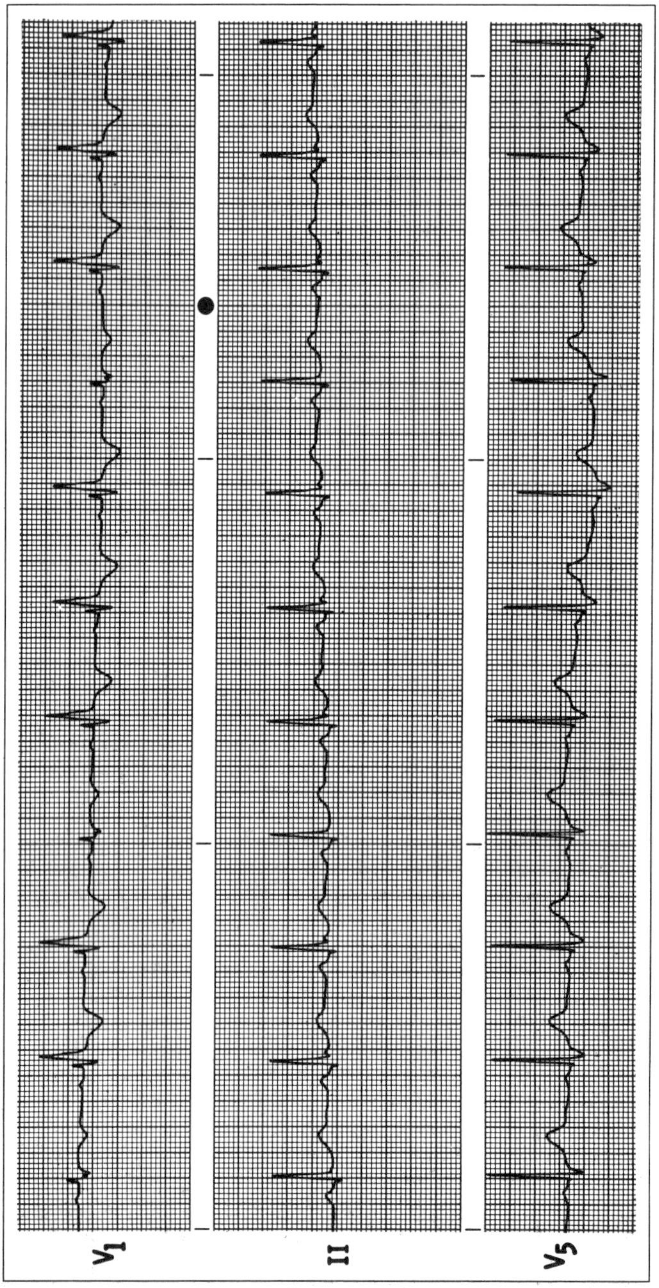


Fig. 9–5. Sinus rhythm with intermittent RBBB (rate independent).

changes is called the "critical rate." This type of conduction disturbance is termed "rate-dependent RBBB." Right BBB occurring regularly on every other or every third beat is also a form of rate-dependent RBBB. On rare occasions, RBBB may develop as the ventricular rate slows as a paradoxical phenomenon. This finding has been termed "bradycardia-dependent RBBB." Not uncommonly, intermittent RBBB may develop unrelated to the ventricular rate. This is termed "rate-independent RBBB." Intermittent RBBB superficially resembles VPCs or a short run of VT.

### Clinical Significance

Not uncommonly, RBBB may be observed in apparently healthy individuals. On the other hand, RBBB may be encountered in such conditions as coronary or hypertensive heart disease, cardiac tumors, cardiomyopathies, myocarditis, and syphilitic, rheumatic, and congenital heart diseases. In particular, atrial septal defect is almost always associated with an RBBB pattern (Fig. 9–1). Tetralogy of Fallot commonly produces a BFB that consists of RBBB and left posterior hemiblock. Right BBB of sudden onset is frequently due to acute pulmonary embolism or infarction. Intermittent RBBB may be found in acute CHF, acute MI, acute pericarditis, or myocarditis. In central South America, the most common cause of RBBB is reported to be Chagas' heart disease.

## LEFT BUNDLE BRANCH BLOCK

### Diagnostic Criteria

The most important ECG finding in LBBB is an alteration of the initial vector during ventricular septal activation, wherein the initial septal activation begins from right to left (Fig. 9–6) instead of the normal direction of left to right. This reversed ventricular septal vector is responsible for the absence of a physiologic (septal) q wave in leads $V_{4-6}$ (Fig. 9–6). In approximately two thirds of LBBB, the initial vector is

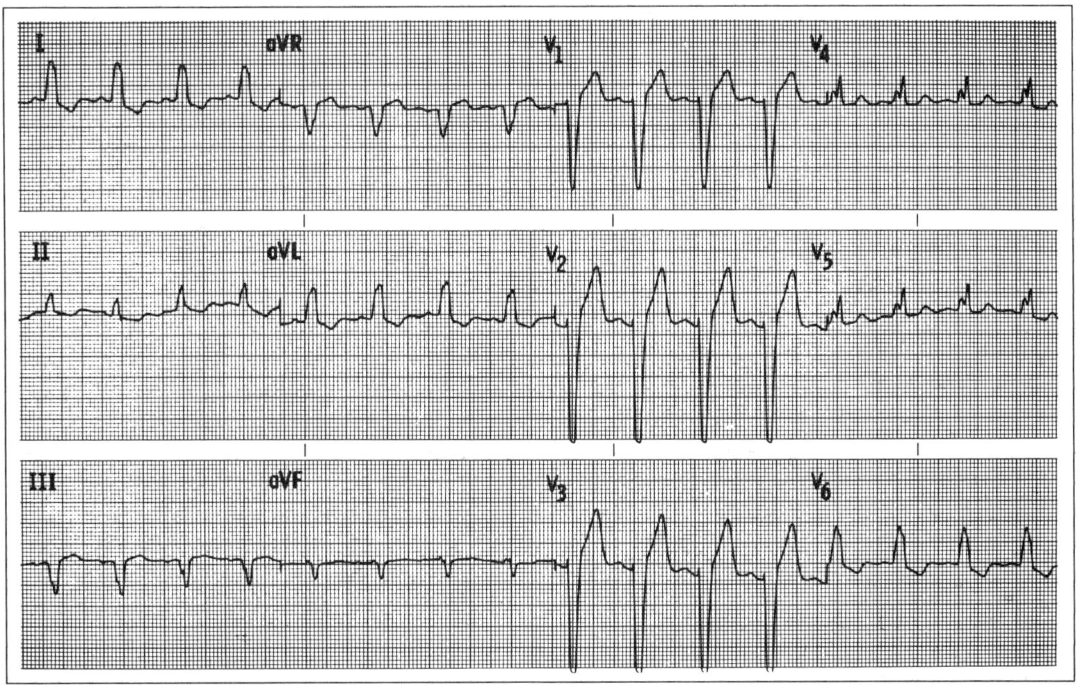


**Fig. 9–6.** Sinus rhythm with LBBB.

directed from right to left and anteriorly. In the remaining one third of LBBB, the initial vector is directed from right to left and posteriorly. Depending upon the direction of the initial vector, the amplitude of the R waves in leads $V_{1-3}$ may be almost or even completely absent, or they may be relatively tall. After the ventricular septal activation, the right ventricle is activated followed by LV activation (Fig. 9–6). Instead of simultaneous activation of both ventricles, the LV activation is delayed in LBBB. Thus, the left ventricle is activated via ordinary ventricular myocardium rather than the left bundle branch system. The abnormal and slow LV activation is responsible for the R′ waves (the second R waves of the QRS) in the left precordial leads (Fig. 9–6), and consequently, LBBB characteristically produces wide QS or rS waves in the right precordial leads (leads $V_{1-3}$) and rsR′ pattern or broad R waves in the left precordial leads (leads $V_{4-6}$). Leads I and aVL have similar ECG findings as shown in leads $V_{4-6}$. The QRS axis may be normal, but it commonly shows left axis deviation. When right axis deviation is present in LBBB, coexisting RVH is strongly suggested.

The secondary T wave change is always present in the left precordial leads in uncomplicated LBBB (Fig. 9–6). The secondary T wave change is characterized by biphasic or inverted (not symmetric nor deep) T waves in leads $V_{4-6}$, and the direction of the T waves is almost 180° discordant to the direction of the QRS complexes (Fig. 9–6). When myocardial ischemia or acute MI is superimposed on the LBBB, the primary T wave change (deeply and symmetrically inverted T waves) replaces the secondary T wave change (Fig. 9–7). As in RBBB, LBBB is said to be complete when the QRS interval is 0.12 second or wider (Fig. 9–6) and incomplete when the QRS interval is between 0.10 and 0.11 second. Vectorcardiographically, the conduction delay involves primarily the midportion or the terminal 0.04 second vectors of the QRS loop.

The diagnostic criteria of LBBB are summarized as follows:

1. QRS interval $\geq$ 0.12 second
2. Absence of septal q waves in leads I, aVL, and $V_{4-6}$
3. rsR′, M pattern or broad R waves in leads I, aVL, and $V_{4-6}$
4. Broad QS or rS waves in leads $V_{1-3}$
5. Secondary, ST, T wave change in leads I, aVL, and $V_{4-6}$

## Intermittent Left Bundle Branch Block

As in RBBB, LBBB may appear intermittently (Fig. 9–8). Intermittent LBBB may or may not be related to the ventricular rate. The term "rate-dependent LBBB" is applied when LBBB develops as the ventricular rate accelerates. This is observed when the impulse finds the left bundle branch system in its refractory period during the faster rate. When the rate becomes slow enough for the left bundle branch system to recover its refractory period, a normal ventricular activation ensues. The ventricular rate at which intraventricular conduction changes is termed the "critical rate." Left BBB occurring every other or every third beat is also a form of rate-dependent LBBB. On rare occasions, LBBB develops paradoxically as the ventricular rate slows. This is termed "bradycardia-dependent LBBB." When LBBB occurs intermittently but unrelated to the ventricular rate, the term "rate-independent LBBB" is used.

## Clinical Significance

The presence of LBBB almost always indicates a diseased heart, particularly coronary and hypertensive heart diseases. Less commonly, LBBB may be encountered in aortic stenosis, cardiomyopathy, myocarditis, and congenital heart diseases. Rarely, LBBB may occur in syphilitic, traumatic, or rheumatic heart diseases and cardiac tumors. Left BBB in an apparently healthy heart is extremely unusual. Intermittent LBBB usually becomes fixed and permanent as time goes by. In general, LBBB is much more common in elderly individuals with diseased hearts than is RBBB. The prognosis is extremely grave when acute MI is superimposed on the preexisting LBBB or when LBBB is produced by anteroseptal MI.

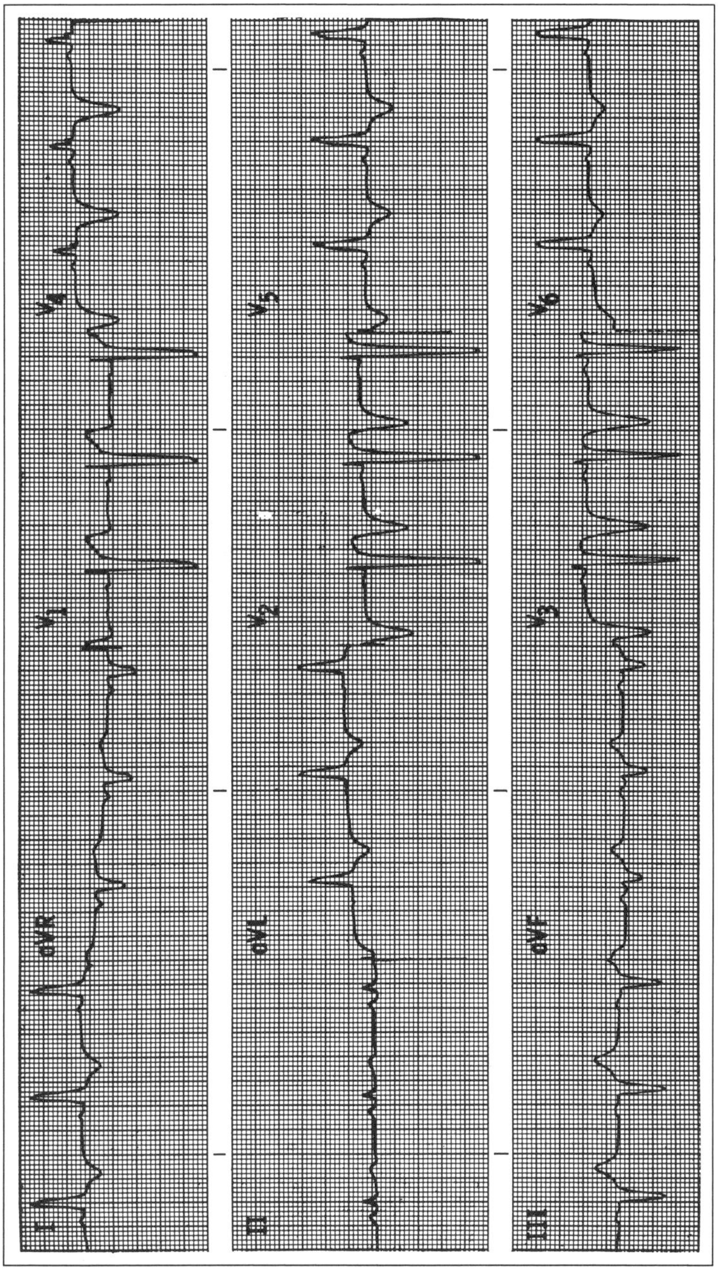


**Fig. 9–7.** Sinus rhythm and LBBB associated with primary T wave change (deeply and symmetrically inverted T waves in leads $V_{1-6}$) strongly suggestive of acute anterior MI.

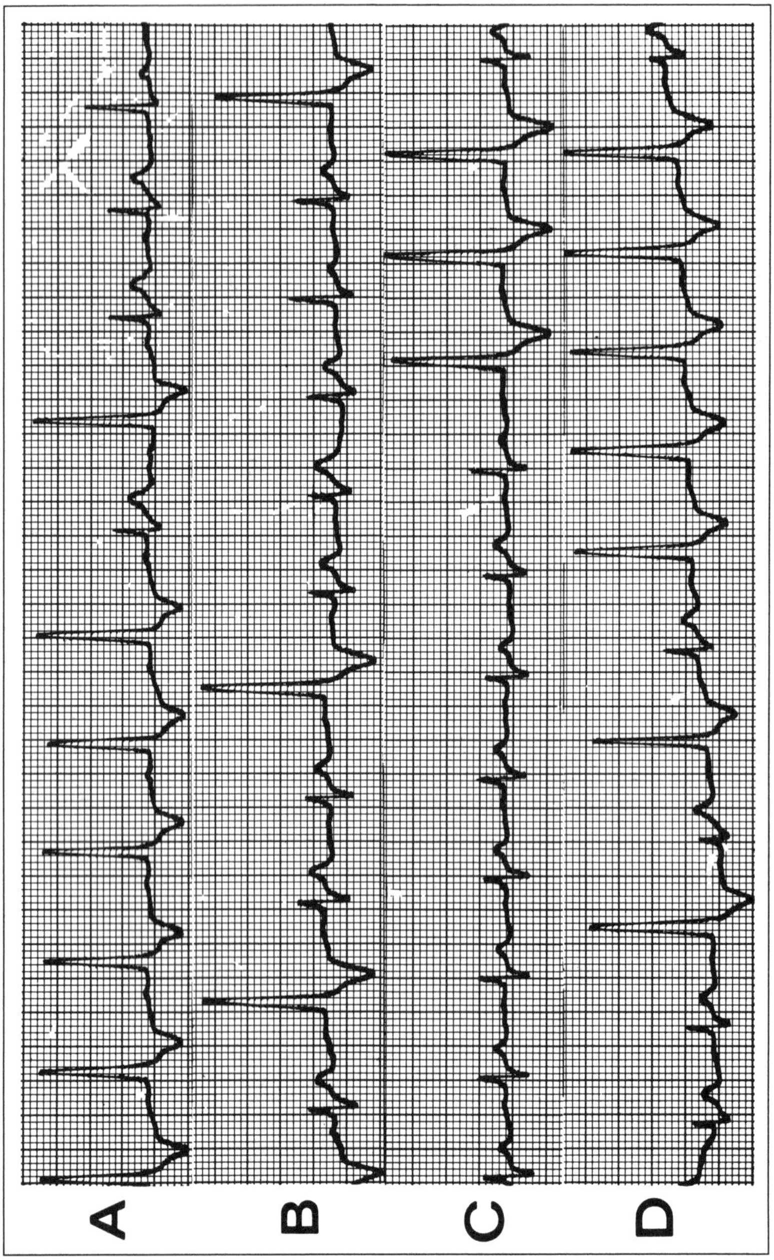


**Fig. 9–8.** Sinus rhythm with intermittent LBBB (rate independent). The Holter monitor ECG rhythm strips A, B, C, and D are not continuous.

## NONSPECIFIC (DIFFUSE) INTRAVENTRICULAR CONDUCTION DISTURBANCE

A prolonged QRS interval (0.12 second or more) may develop because of a diffuse conduction delay during the entire ventricular depolarization rather than because of a localized block at 1 of the bundle branches. Thus, the configuration of the QRS complex is an exaggerated form of the underlying QRS complex (Fig. 9–9). This type of intraventricular conduction delay is termed a "nonspecific" or "diffuse" intraventricular conduction defect. The nonspecific intraventricular conduction defect superficially resembles LBBB, but characteristic features of the latter are lacking in the former. The nonspecific intraventricular conduction defect is not uncommonly encountered in elderly individuals even without significant heart disease. Although MI often produces hemiblocks, RBBB, LBBB, BFB, and TFB, diffuse intraventricular block is also frequently caused by MI. Less commonly, the underlying causes for the nonspecific intraventricular conduction defect may be quinidine or procainamide toxicity and hyperkalemia. In addition, cardiomyopathies are often associated with a nonspecific intraventricular conduction defect.

Various factors and clinical circumstances that may cause diffuse (nonspecific) intraventricular block are summarized in Table 9–1.

**TABLE 9–1. Factors that may cause diffuse (nonspecific) intraventricular block**

A. Drugs
   1. Quinidine, procainamide (Pronestyl)
B. Electrolyte imbalance
   1. Advanced hyperkalemia
C. Heart diseases
   1. Advanced underlying heart disease
   2. Cardiomyopathies
   3. Myocardial infarction
D. Following cardiac arrest
   1. Either cardiac or noncardiac patients
E. Miscellaneous
   1. Elderly individuals
   2. Hypothermia

## HEMIBLOCKS

Left bundle branch consists of 2 subdivisions, anterior (superior) and posterior (inferior). The anterior division of the left bundle branch traverses the base of the anterior papillary muscle of the left ventricle, whereas the posterior division runs toward the posterior papillary muscle. Anatomically, the anterior division is located superiorly, while the posterior division is situated inferiorly (Fig. 1–1).

When these 2 subdivisions are intact, the impulse is transmitted to the left ventricle via anterior and posterior divisions simultaneously (Fig. 9–10). The term "hemiblock" is used when 1 of the subdivisions of the left bundle branch is blocked. In left anterior (superior) hemiblock, the impulse is transmitted through the intact posterior division to activate the left ventricle. Since the impulse conducted via the posterior division is directed superiorly and to the left (Fig. 9–10), marked left axis deviation is observed in left anterior hemiblock. In addition, a small q wave in lead I with a small r wave in lead III is usually observed in left anterior hemiblock because of downward and rightward initial septal activation (Fig. 9–11). The above findings are observed in left anterior hemiblock specifically because the posterior papillary muscle is located not only inferiorly but also medial to the anterior papillary muscle. Following septal activation, major ventricular forces are directed superiorly and to the left, leading to marked left axis deviation (more than −45°) in left anterior hemiblock (Fig. 9–11).

Conversely, in left posterior hemiblock, the left ventricle is activated via an intact anterior division (Fig. 9–10). Since the impulse conducted through the anterior division is directed inferiorly and to the right, right axis deviation is produced in left posterior hemiblock (Fig. 9–12). A small r wave in lead I with a small q wave in lead III is observed in left posterior hemiblock because the initial vector is directed superiorly and to the left (Fig. 9–12).

There is usually little (0.01–0.02 second) or no prolongation of the QRS interval in hemiblocks because the Purkinje fibers in terri-

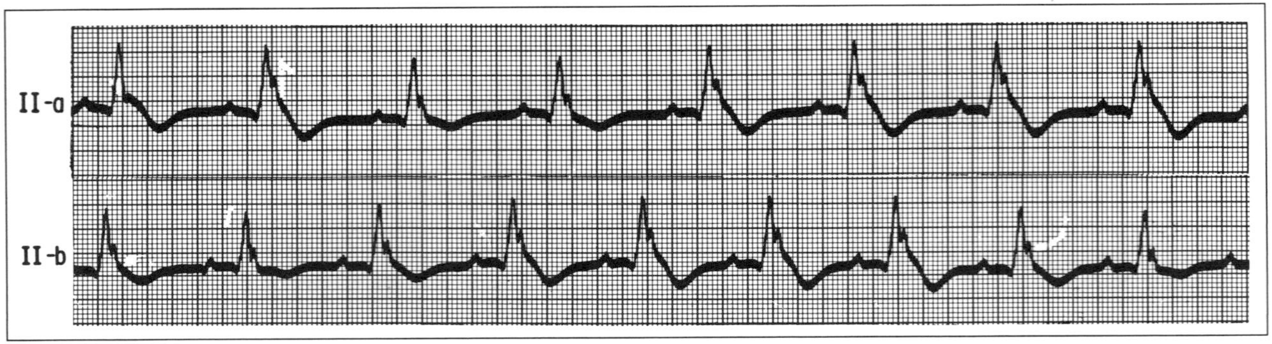


**Fig. 9–9.** Sinus arrhythmia with first degree AV block and diffuse (nonspecific) intraventricular block. Diaphragmatic MI is a possibility. Leads II-a and II-b are not continuous.

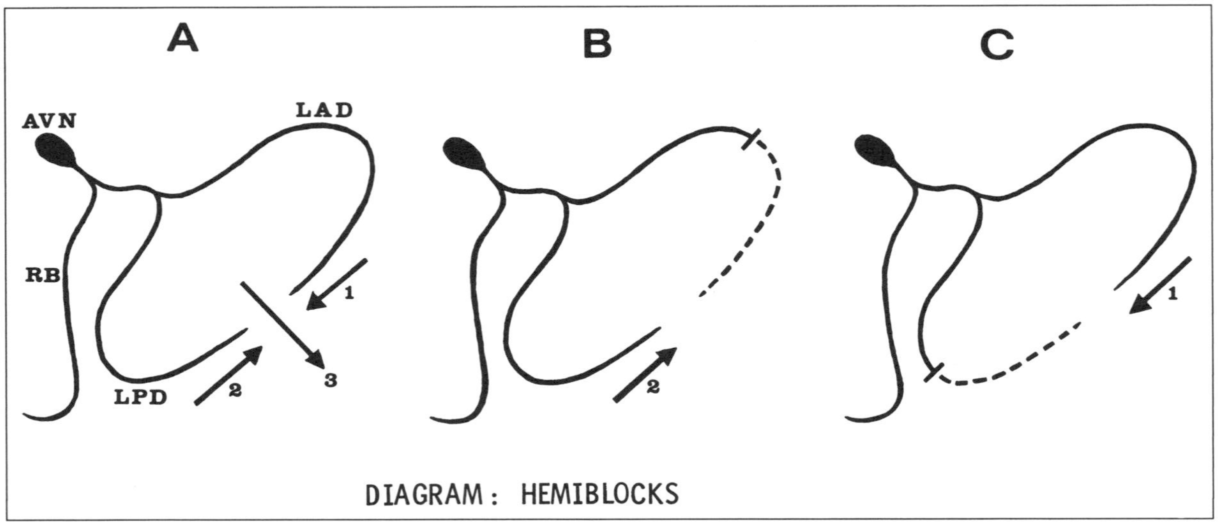


**Fig. 9–10.** Hemiblocks. **A.** When both anterior and posterior divisions of the left bundle branch system are intact, the left ventricle is activated via both divisions (vectors 1 and 2) so that the resultant forces of vectors 1 and 2 produce vector 3. **B.** When 1 of 2 divisions of the left bundle branch system is blocked, however, the impulses must travel through the intact division only. That is, in anterior hemiblock, vector 1 is no longer present, and, as a result, the left ventricle is activated via the intact posterior division (vector 2). In this case, the electrical axis shifts to the left and superiorly, creating marked left axis deviation. **C.** For the same reason, posterior hemiblock produces right axis deviation because the left ventricle is activated via the intact anterior division (vector 1). AVN = AV node; LAD = left anterior division; LPD = left posterior division; RB = right bundle branch.

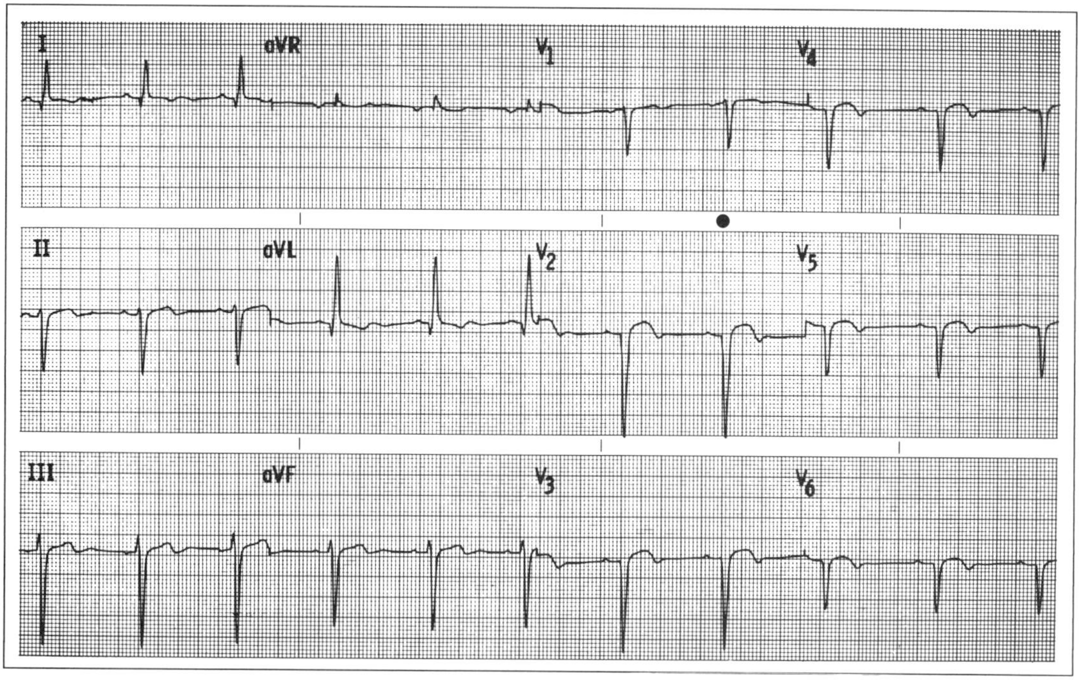


**Fig. 9–11.** Sinus rhythm with left anterior hemiblock (QRS axis: −65°) associated with acute extensive anterior MI.

tories of left anterior and posterior divisions are richly confluent. In other words, marked left axis deviation and right axis deviation are manifestations of left anterior and posterior hemiblock, respectively (Figs. 9–11 and 9–12). Hemiblocks may occur intermittently (Fig. 9–13), which is analogous to intermittent BBB. It should be pointed out, however, that abnormal QRS axis deviation is not necessarily due to hemiblocks. Right axis deviation, for example, is commonly due to RVH or acute pulmonary embolism. In addition, left axis deviation can be found in various circumstances; for example, LVH is often associated with left axis deviation. Furthermore, diaphragmatic MI frequently causes a marked leftward and superior shift of the QRS axis (pseudoleft axis deviation). Similarly, high lateral MI often produces pseudoright axis deviation. Marked left or right axis deviation is frequently encountered in advanced obstructive lung disease. Therefore, the hemiblocks should be diagnosed by evaluating the total clinical picture. The diagnosis of hemiblocks is generally almost certain when marked left or right axis deviation occurs suddenly, particularly in acute MI.

The diagnostic criteria of the hemiblocks are summarized as follows:

*Diagnostic Criteria of Left Anterior Hemiblock*

1. Marked left axis deviation (−45 to −90°) of QRS complexes
2. Small q wave in lead I and small r wave in lead III
3. Little or no prolongation of QRS interval
4. No evidence of other factors responsible for left axis deviation (true or pseudo).

*Diagnostic Criteria of Left Posterior Hemiblock*

1. Marked right axis deviation (+105 to +180°) of QRS complexes
2. Small r wave in lead I and small q wave in lead III
3. No evidence of other factors responsible for right axis deviation (true or pseudo)

A pure form of hemiblock is not uncommon, especially during acute anterior MI (Fig. 9–11), but RBBB often coexists with hemiblock (Fig. 9–3). A pure form of left anterior hemiblock is much more common than of left posterior hemiblock. Left posterior hemiblock frequently coexists with RBBB as a manifestation of BBBB (Fig. 9–4). Why the incidence of left posterior hemiblock is much lower than that of left anterior hemiblock can be explained as follows. The posterior division is shorter and thicker and less influenced by the stresses of outflow pressure because of its inflow tract structure. It also has a double blood supply as compared with the anterior division.

Chronic hemiblocks are often found in individuals without demonstrable heart disease, especially in elderly people. On the other hand, acute hemiblocks are nearly always due to acute anteroseptal MI (Fig. 9–11). Less commonly, hemiblocks may be encountered in cardiomyopathies, calcified aortic disease, and hyperkalemia.

## BIFASCICULAR BLOCK AND TRIFASCICULAR BLOCK

### Diagnostic Criteria

Bifascicular block (BFB) exists when 2 fascicles are blocked simultaneously. Bifascicular block is a form of incomplete BBBB (Table 9–2). The most common BFB is a combination of RBBB and left anterior hemiblock (Fig. 9–3).

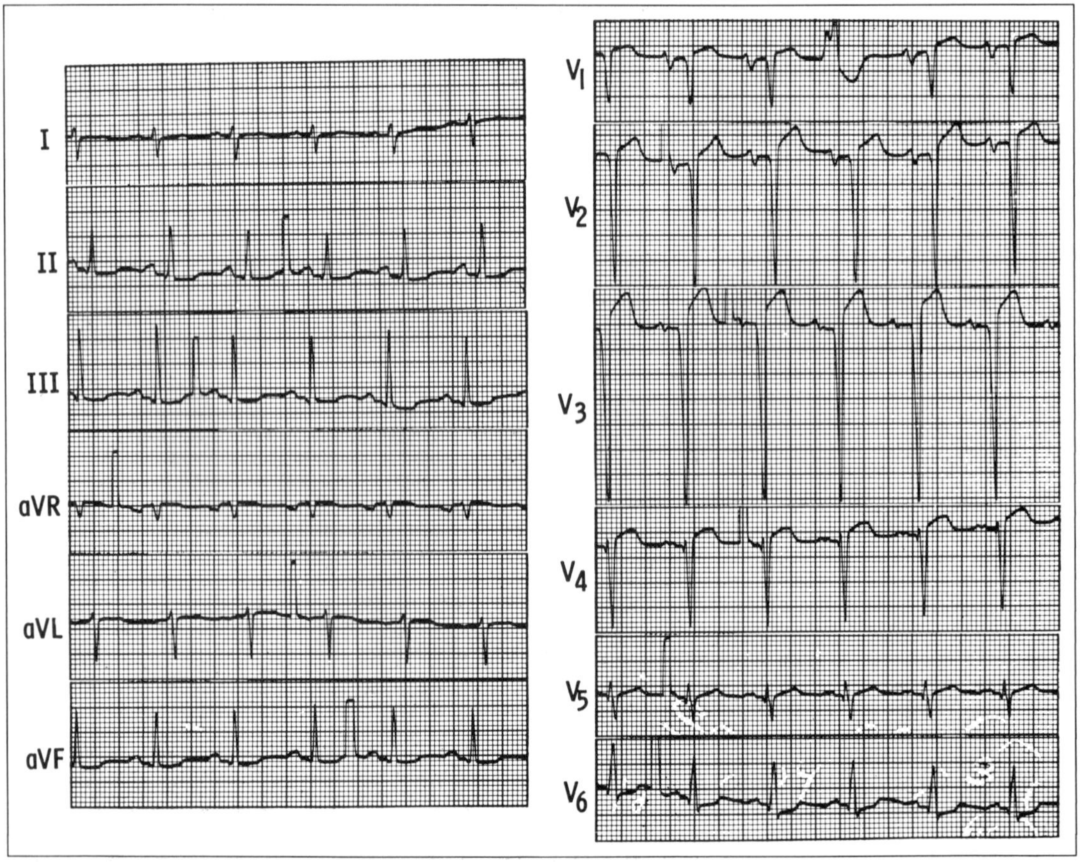


**Fig. 9–12.** Sinus rhythm with left posterior hemiblock (QRS axis: +105°) associated with recent extensive anterior MI. Note a VPC (lead $V_1$).

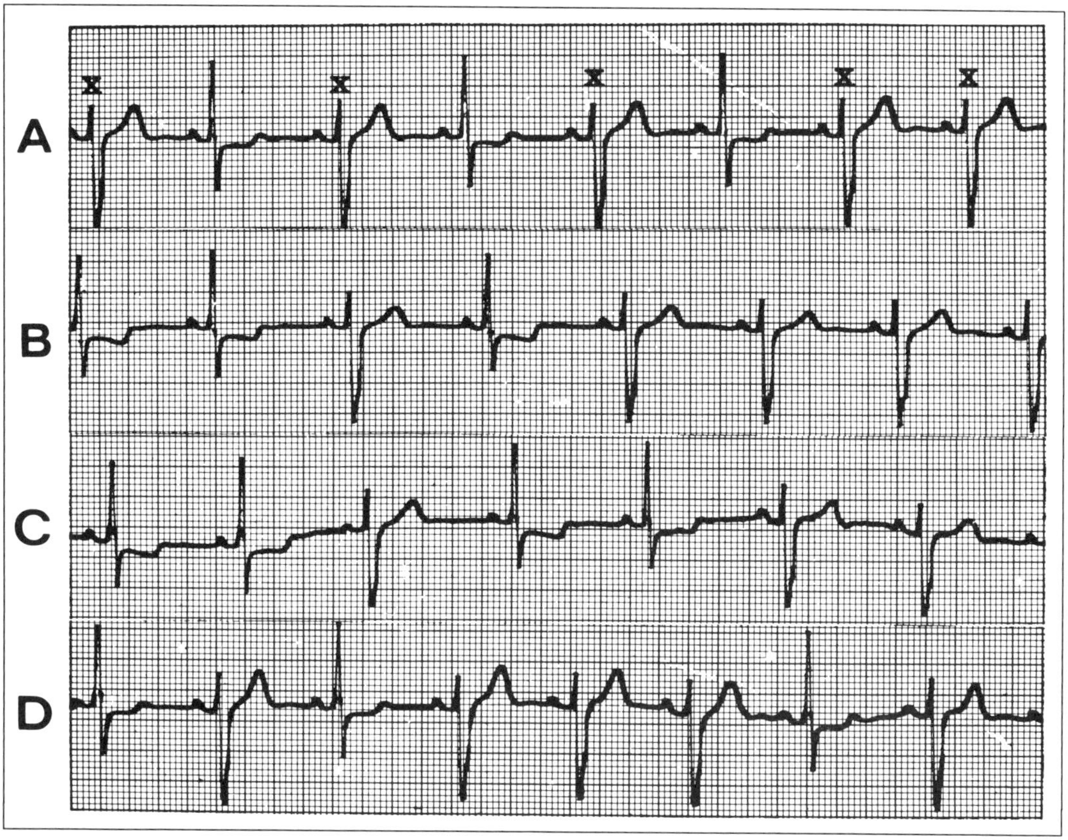


**Fig. 9–13.** Sinus rhythm with intermittent left anterior hemiblock (rate independent, marked X). The Holter monitor ECG rhythm strips A, B, C, and D are not continuous.

**TABLE 9–2. Diagnostic criteria of bilateral bundle branch block (Bifascicular Block and Trifascicular Block)**

1. Right bundle branch block with left anterior hemiblock
2. Right bundle branch block with left posterior hemiblock
3. Alternating left and right bundle branch block
4. Left or right bundle branch block with first degree or second degree AV block
5. Left or right bundle branch block with prolonged H-V interval > 55 milliseconds
6. Left bundle branch block on one occasion and right bundle branch block on another occasion
7. Mobitz type II AV block
8. Any combination of the above findings
9. Complete AV block with ventricular escape (idioventricular) rhythm

Bifascicular block consisting of RBBB and left posterior hemiblock (Fig. 9–4) is an uncommon occurrence.

In broad terms, the TFB can be defined as simultaneous block (complete or incomplete) in any 3 of 5 ventricular conducting fascicles, including the His bundle, the right bundle branch, the left bundle branch, and the anterior and posterior divisions of the left bundle branch. However, TFB is used specifically when a block involves simultaneously the 3 peripheral fascicles, namely, the right bundle branch, and the anterior and posterior divisions of the left bundle branch. Thus, TFB is an expression of BBBB (Table 9–2).

When all of the 3 peripheral fascicles are completely blocked, complete AV block (complete TFB) is the end result. In this case, ventricular escape (idioventricular) rhythm with very slow ventricular rate is produced (Chapter 8). The diagnosis of TFB is certain when the same patient exhibits a combination of RBBB and left posterior hemiblock on one occasion and RBBB with left anterior hemiblock on another occasion. However, various ECG manifestations will be produced when 1 or more of the 3 fascicles are incompletely and/or intermittently blocked. Extremely complicated ECG findings can result when the degree of incomplete block is different in the 3 fascicles (Fig. 9–14). Atrioventricular block of varying degrees associated with RBBB or LBBB and/or anterior or posterior hemiblock is usually a typical example of incomplete TFB (Fig. 9–14).

Mobitz type II AV block is an expression of incomplete TFB in which the QRS complexes nearly always disclose RBBB or LBBB, hemiblocks, or BFB (Fig. 8–3). When 2:1 AV block is associated with RBBB or LBBB or BFB, the block represents Mobitz type II AV block in nearly all cases (Chapter 8).

Various ECG manifestations of BBBB are summarized in Table 9–2.

## Clinical Significance and Therapeutic Approach

The clinical significance of BFB or TFB varies markedly depending upon the onset and progress of the block. For example, chronic BFB or incomplete TFB (chronic) is often asymptomatic, and no particular treatment is indicated as long as the patient is asymptomatic. On the other hand, a prophylactic artificial pacing is required when the patient develops BFB or TFB acutely as a result of acute anterior MI (Fig. 9–3). The artificial pacemaker is recommended in this case regardless of symptoms because complete AV block may soon follow. In addition, acute hemiblock, BFB, or TFB may be observed in marked hyperkalemia and myocarditis. These intraventricular conduction disturbances are also not uncommon during the post operative period for various cardiac lesions and during cardiac catheterization. Among congenital heart diseases, atrial septal defect of the ostium secundum type is frequently associated with RBBB pattern with normal or right axis deviation of the QRS complexes. On the other hand, BFB consisting of RBBB and left anterior hemiblock is often observed in patients with atrial septal defect, ostium primum type. Another example is that tetralogy of Fallot is commonly associated with RBBB and left posterior hemiblock causing BFB. Under these circumstances, congenital BFB does not seem to progress to higher degree BBBB, and an artificial pacemaker is not indicated.

Chronic BFB or chronic incomplete TFB may lead to complete AV block at some time in the future, but it is impossible to predict the exact time when complete AV block will be produced. There are numerous elderly individuals with chronic BFB or incomplete TFB who are completely asymptomatic.

Two major factors will primarily determine the indications for permanent artificial cardiac pacing. The first and the most important factor is the presence of symptoms (e.g., dizziness, near-syncope, syncope, hypotension, and CHF) directly due to slow ventricular rate (usually slower than 40 beats/min). Needless to say, permanent artificial pacing is urgently needed for complete AV block due to complete TFB leading to very slow VER (Chapter 8). Another factor is the ventricular rate itself. When the ventricular rate is slower than 40 beats/min in chronic BFB or TFB, permanent artificial pacing is considered to be indicated even if the patient may be asymptomatic. Permanent pacing is also indicated when advanced BBBB is associated with frequent VPCs or ectopic tachyarrhythmia causing bradytachyarrhythmia syndrome (BTS). At times, after the termination of ectopic tachyarrhythmia (e.g., VT or VF) either spontaneously, by drugs, or by DC shock, slow and unstable VER may be produced (often in the presence of AF). This is also a form of BTS, and the bradyarrhythmia component in this case is an expression of BBBB. Again, permanent artificial pacing is indicated under this circumstance.

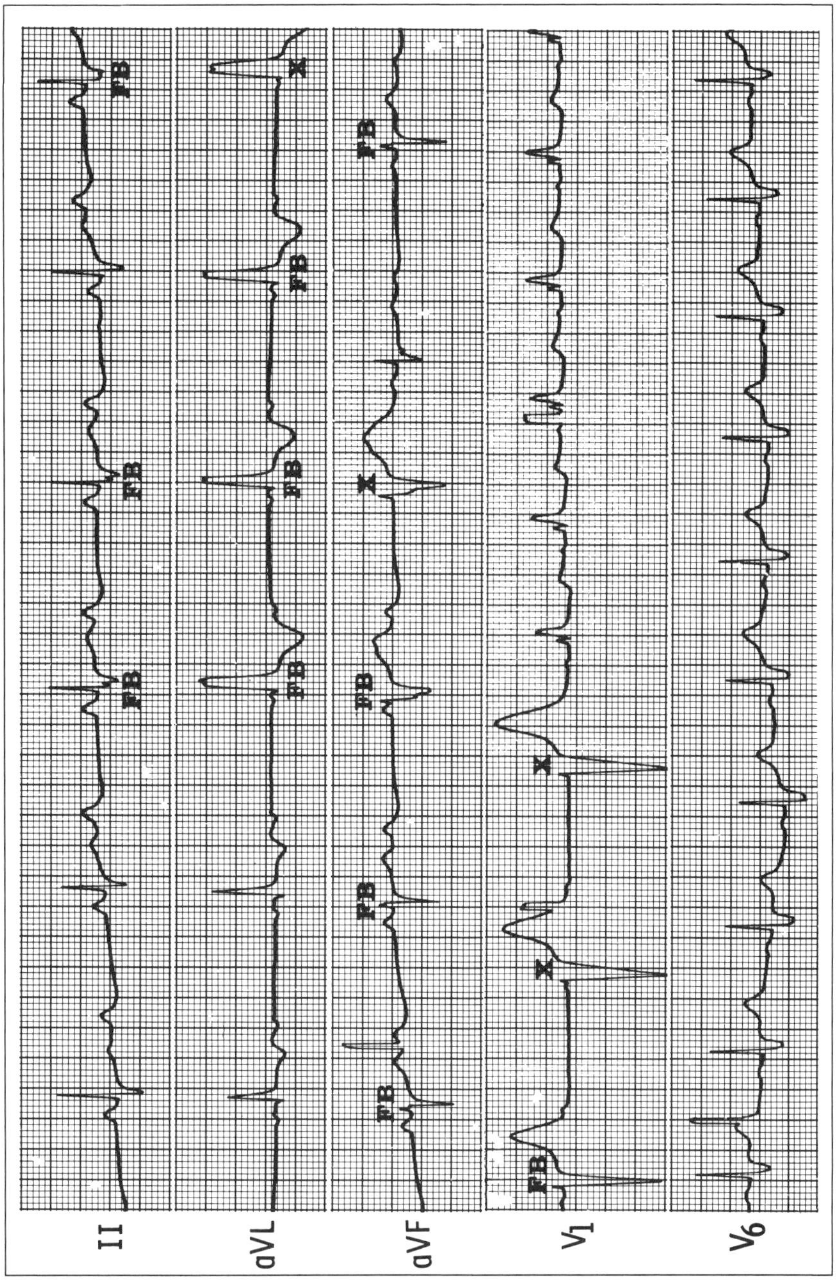


**Fig. 9–14.** This ECG tracing is an example of advanced BBBB (advanced incomplete TFB). It reveals sinus rhythm with advanced AV block (infranodal block) producing intermittent VER (X) and intermittent 2:1 AV block associated with RBBB. Note frequent ventricular fusion beats (FB).

Mobitz type II AV block (Fig. 8–3) is an expression of incomplete BBBB for which permanent cardiac pacing is recommended by most investigators. When 2:1 AV block is associated with bundle branch block (either left or right), or BFB (e.g., a combination of RBBB and left anterior hemiblock), it is considered to be a variant of Mobitz type II AV block (Fig. 8–4). Permanent cardiac pacing is indicated in these cases.

When BBBB is further advanced, complex rhythm abnormalities will be produced (Fig. 9–14). For example, advanced incomplete BBBB may be manifested by RBBB or LBBB with 2:1 or Mobitz type II AV block, with areas of complete AV block as a result of complete TFB producing VER. Another example may be manifested by varying degree advanced AV block (e.g., 3:1 or 4:1 AV block) associated with RBBB or LBBB (or alternating bundle branch block) and intermittent complete AV block. Eventually, advanced incomplete BBBB leads to complete BBBB complete AV block as a result of complete TFB (Chapter 8).

*Chapter 10*

# Differential Diagnosis of Tachyarrhythmias

Because of the ready availability of direct current (DC) shock for treatment of various ectopic tachyarrhythmias, there has been a tendency to oversimplify the diagnosis of various tachyarrhythmias. However, it should be emphasized that DC shock is not only ineffective but also hazardous in the treatment of digitalis-induced tachyarrhythmias, particularly those of ventricular origin. Furthermore, the precise diagnosis of a given tachyarrhythmia enables one to employ the proper drug therapy. For example, digitalis is often the drug of choice in the treatment of various supraventricular tachyarrhythmias, regardless of the configuration of the QRS complex, whereas the drug is either ineffective or even contraindicated in the treatment of ventricular tachyarrhythmias. In addition, a correct and precise diagnosis of the tachyarrhythmia is important when evaluating the total clinical picture of a given patient because certain arrhythmias are almost pathognomonic features of certain clinical entities, e.g., AT with varying AV block (Fig. 5–8) and nonparoxysmal AV JT in the presence of AF (Fig. 6–4) during digitalization are almost pathognomonic features of DI.

As described in Chapter 1, rapid heart action may originate from any portion of the heart. Thus, rapid heart action may be sinus in origin, or it may be ectopic in origin. In addition, tachyarrhythmias may occur in paroxysmal and nonparoxysmal forms. The nonparoxysmal form may originate from a primary (sinus) or ectopic pacemaker, while paroxysmal tachyarrhythmias are always ectopic in origin. Since sinus tachycardia can be diagnosed without any difficulty in most instances, primarily ectopic tachyarrhythmias are discussed, and the main discussion is focused on differential diagnosis among various supraventricular tachyarrhythmias with wide QRS complexes and ventricular tachyarrhythmias because of their practical importance.

It should be pointed out that any supraventricular tachyarrhythmias may coexist with any ventricular tachyarrhythmias, leading to double or even triple ectopic tachyarrhythmias. On the other hand, multifocal supraventricular tachyarrhythmias, such as a combination of AF or atrial flutter with independent AV JT or double AV JT, may occur. These multifocal tachyarrhythmias are rare forms of AV dissociation.

Although it has been known for many years that the differential diagnosis between supraventricular and ventricular tachyarrhythmias is extremely important in view of their management and prognosis, it is often difficult or, at times, impossible to distinguish between them. The reason for this is that supraventricular tachyarrhythmias, regardless of the fundamental mechanism involved, may closely resemble ventricular tachyarrhythmias when the QRS complex is wide in the former. Because of the difficulty in distinguishing them, various additional studies, such as esophageal and intracardiac ECGs including His bundle recording, have been utilized recently in order to identify the atrial activity in relation to the His bundle potential and ventricular activity (Fig. 2–5).

Although differential diagnosis between supraventricular and ventricular tachyarrhythmias is not always possible in every instance, the following outline may be used to distinguish them.

I. Identification of the atrial activity
   A. Determination of the relationship between atrial and ventricular activities

    B. Comparison between atrial and ventricular cycles
II. Evaluation of the configuration of the QRS complexes during the tachyarrhythmia
    A. Comparison of the QRS complexes during the tachyarrhythmia and isolated ectopic beats preceding or following the rapid heart action
    B. Comparison of the QRS complexes during the tachyarrhythmia and ventricular captured beats
    C. Determination of preexisting LBBB or RBBB
    D. Determination of preexisting WPW syndrome
    E. Determination of aberrant ventricular conduction
III. Evaluation of the response to CSS
IV. Determination of the regularity of R-R cycles (ventricular cycle)
V. Evaluation of the coupling intervals and the posttachyarrhythmia pause
VI. Determination of the heart rate
VII. Identification of the His bundle potential in relation to the ventricular activity

## IDENTIFICATION OF ATRIAL ACTIVITY

Identification of the atrial activity is the first step in the determination of the origin of the tachyarrhythmia. When the P wave is definitely present, the relationship between the P wave and the QRS complex must be determined. When the ectopic P waves precede the QRS complex, regardless of the configuration of the latter, the tachycardia is supraventricular in origin. In this circumstance, the tachycardia is atrial in origin if the axis of the ectopic P wave is similar to that of the sinus P wave (Fig. 5–7). On the other hand, AV junctional or reciprocating tachycardia can be diagnosed when the retrograde P wave (inverted P wave in lead II and upright P wave in lead aVR) precedes the QRS complex, regardless of its configuration. When the QRS complex is wide and/or bizarre, either because of preexisting or rate-dependent BBB or because of aberrant ventricular conduction, it closely mimics VT even if there are P waves preceding the QRS complexes (Figs. 5–7, 5–16, and 5–17). Ventricular tachycardia may be closely simulated even in sinus tachycardia when there is BBB.

When the ectopic P waves, which are conducted in a retrograde fashion, follow the QRS complexes, the origin of the ectopic impulses may be either in the AV junction or in the ventricles. In this circumstance, AV JT is probably present when the QRS complex is narrow. However, VT may produce retrograde P waves that may resemble AV JT.

Comparison between atrial and ventricular cycles is important because the atrial to ventricular conduction ratio may be 1:1, or it may be any multiple one of the other, or it may show Wenckebach phenomenon (Figs. 5–7, 5–8, and 5–11).

In the presence of regularly occurring P waves (either sinus or ectopic), the QRS complexes may independently originate from either the AV junction or the ventricles, leading to complete or incomplete AV dissociation. Thus, the presence of AV dissociation does not favor or exclude the diagnosis of AV JT or VT. In addition, AV JT or VT may develop in the presence of atrial tachyarrhythmias, including AF, atrial flutter, and AT, leading to AV dissociation (Fig. 6–4). In these circumstances, the comparison of the configuration of the QRS complex during the tachycardia and of a ventricular captured beat is often the only clue to distinguish between them. This aspect of the differential diagnosis is discussed later in this chapter. The differential diagnosis between AV JT with a wide QRS complex and VT is one of the most difficult problems in the interpretation of cardiac arrhythmias because each may closely simulate the other. The most common cause of a wide QRS complex in AV JT is preexisting BBB.

## EVALUATION OF CONFIGURATION OF QRS COMPLEX DURING TACHYARRHYTHMIAS

Evaluation of the configuration of the QRS complexes during the tachycardia and comparison with that of isolated ectopic beats preceding or following the rapid heart action are often the only clue to identifying the exact location of the ectopic impulse formation. This is true because the same ectopic focus is believed to be capable of producing isolated ectopic beats as well as tachyarrhythmias. For example, isolated APCs often lead to atrial group beats, AT, AF, or atrial flutter, and these atrial tachyarrhythmias are often followed by isolated APCs upon termination of the rapid heart action (Fig. 5–7). This information is extremely valuable when the QRS complex is wide and/or bizarre during the tachyarrhythmia and isolated APCs resulting either from preexisting or rate-dependent BBB or from aberrant ventricular conduction (Fig. 5–7).

The most practical point in the differential diagnosis is to compare the configuration of the QRS complex during the tachycardia with isolated VPCs before and after the tachycardia. When the configurations of the QRS complexes of the isolated VPCs and tachycardia are identical, the diagnosis of VT is certain (Fig. 7–10).

Comparison of QRS configurations during the tachycardia and ventricular captured beats (or reciprocal beats) is another important aspect of the differential diagnosis in the presence of incomplete AV dissociation. When the QRS complexes of ventricular captured beats or reciprocal beats have the same configuration as that of the tachycardia, regardless of whether the QRS complex is narrow or wide, the tachycardia is AV junctional in origin. Conversely, if the contours of the QRS complexes in the ventricular captured beats or reciprocal beats and the tachycardia are different, the diagnosis of VT can be made.

It should be emphasized that the presence of ventricular fusion beats favors VT.

Determination of preexisting LBBB or RBBB is, at times, the only clue to distinguish between supraventricular and ventricular tachyarrhythmias, particularly when the atrial activity is not discernible or is independent of the QRS complex and the QRS complex is wide and/or bizarre. Thus, when the ECG that was taken preceding or following an episode of rapid heart action shows LBBB or RBBB and when the QRS contour is identical to that seen during the tachyarrhythmia, the diagnosis of VT is definitely excluded (Figs. 10–1 and 10–2). Similarly, AF or atrial flutter with preexisting or rate-dependent LBBB or RBBB also closely mimics VT (Fig. 5–17). In these circumstances, grossly irregular R-R cycles and identification of fibrillation or flutter waves exclude VT.

Knowledge of a preexisting WPW syndrome is also very helpful in differentiating various rapid heart actions. This syndrome is known to be associated with various supraventricular tachyarrhythmias with wide QRS complexes due to anomalous AV conduction, thus closely resembling ventricular tachyarrhythmias (Figs. 10–3 and 10–4). A detailed description of the various supraventricular tachyarrhythmias associated with the WPW syndrome is found in Chapter 13.

Recognition of aberrant ventricular conduction in supraventricular tachyarrhythmias is extremely important in order to distinguish them from ventricular tachyarrhythmias. Aberrant ventricular conduction is favored by the following findings: RBBB pattern, absence of the posttachyarrhythmia pause, varying coupling intervals, a long cycle preceding the coupling interval (Ashman's phenomenon), identical or similar initial vectors between the abnormal beat and the normally conducted beat, and so on (Figs. 5–5, 5–7, and 5–16).

It is extremely important to identify various artifacts because various tachyarrhythmias can be closely simulated by the artifacts (Figs. 3–1 and 3–2).

## Ashman's Phenomenon

The most important factor for the production of aberrant ventricular conduction is Ashman's phenomenon (Figs. 5–5 and 5–16). In 1945, Ashman had described the ECG finding that aberrant ventricular conduction tends to occur following a long ventricular cycle (R-R interval) preceding the coupling interval (the interval from a bizarre beat to the normal beat of the basic rhythm). It can be said that the longer the ventricular cycle (R-R interval), the longer is the refractory period following it; the shorter the ventricular cycle, the shorter is the refractory period.

Diagnostic criteria of Ashman's phenomenon are as follows:

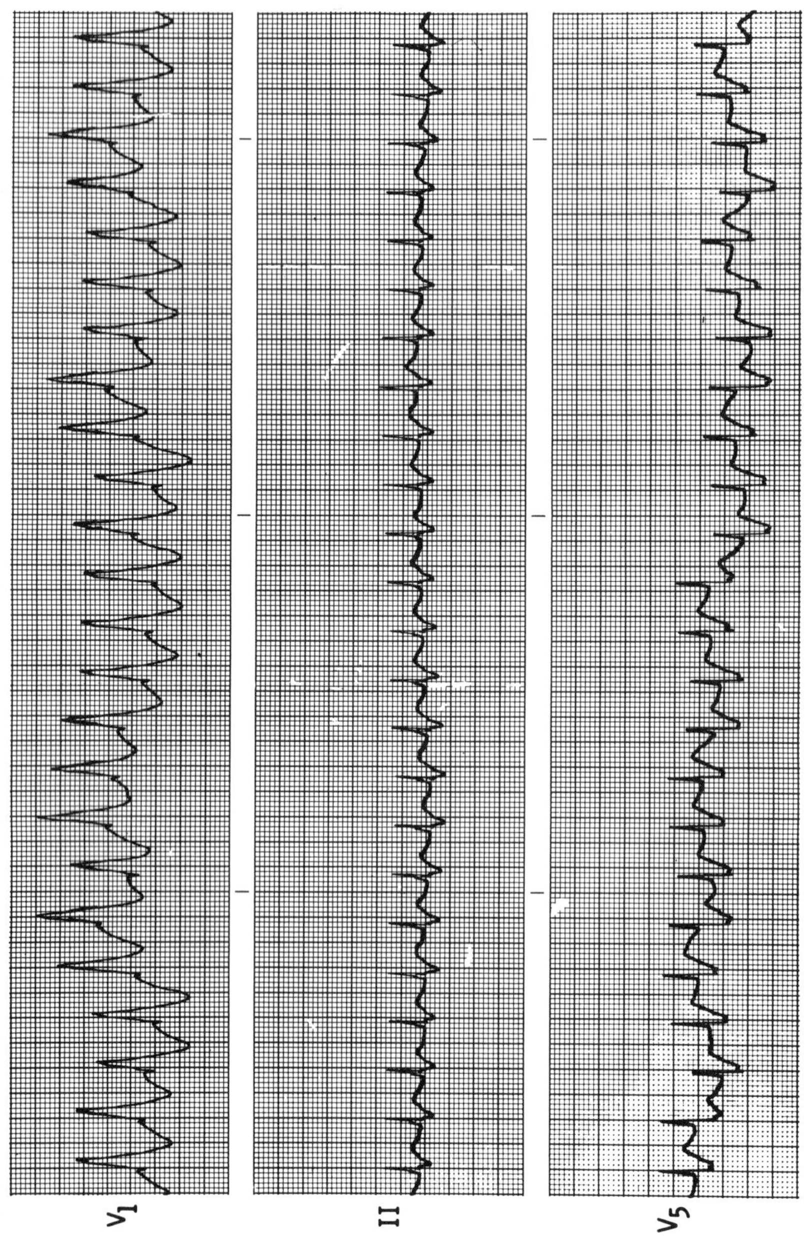


**Fig. 10–1.** Figures 10–1 and 10–2 were obtained from the same patient. A regular tachycardia with broad QRS complexes (rate: 150 beats/min). Since the QRS configuration during the tachycardia is identical to that of sinus rhythm (Fig. 10–2), the tachycardia is proven to be supraventricular tachycardia with RBBB.

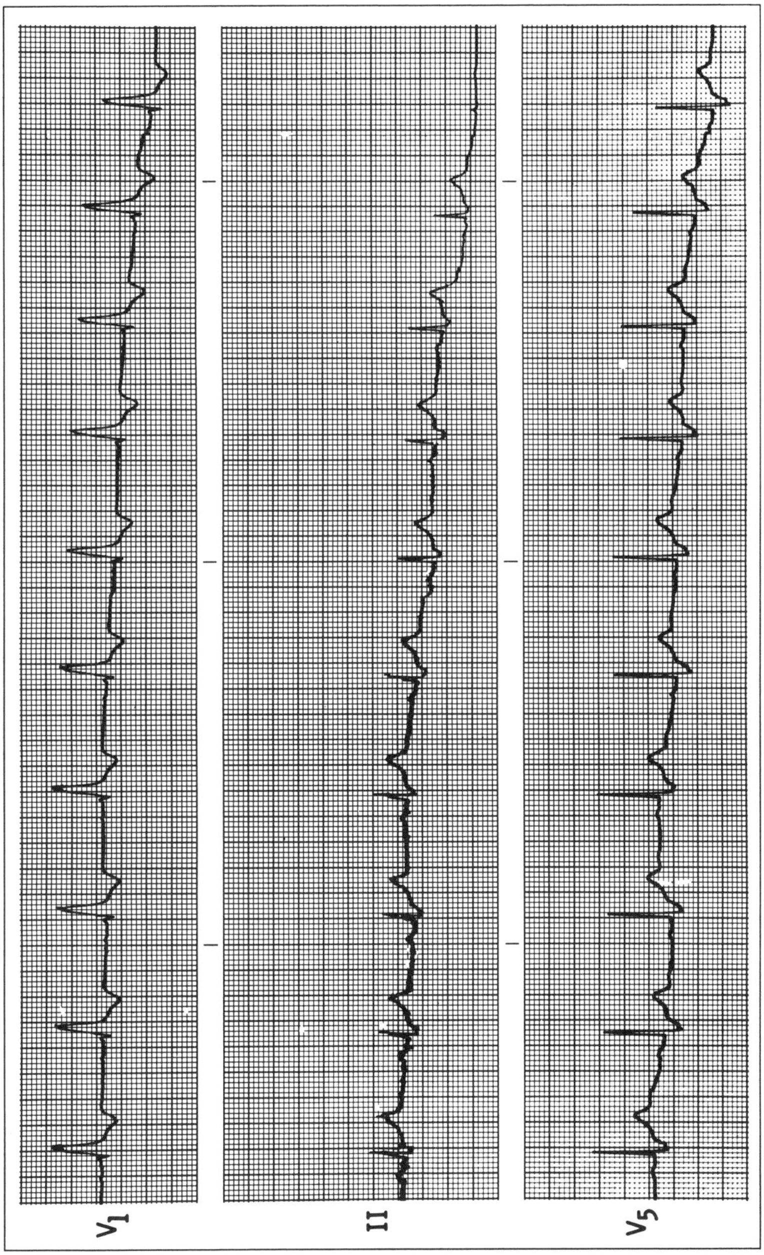


**Fig. 10–2.** Sinus rhythm with RBBB (same patient as in Fig. 10–1).

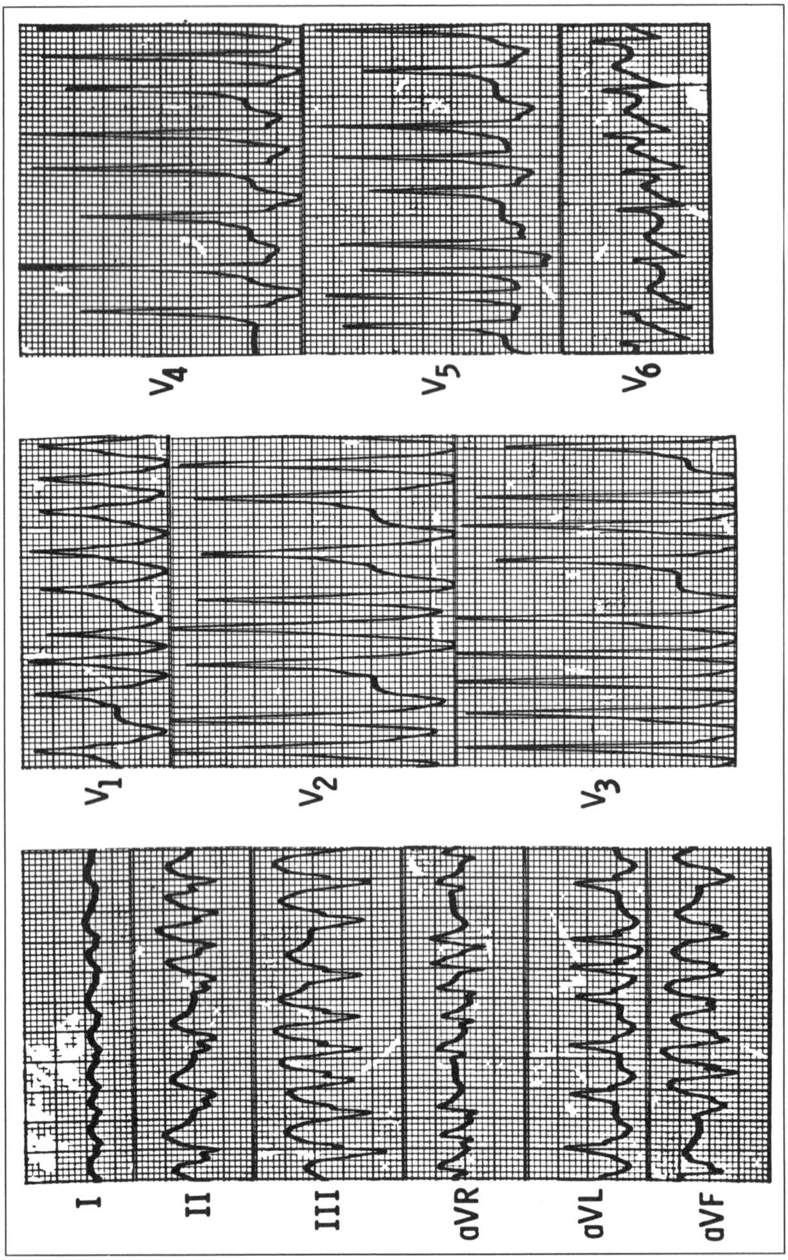


Fig. 10–3. Fig. 10–3 and 10–4 were taken on the same 24-year-old man. Atrial fibrillation with anomalous AV conduction because of WPW syndrome, type A (proven in Fig. 10–4). Ventricular tachycardia is closely simulated.

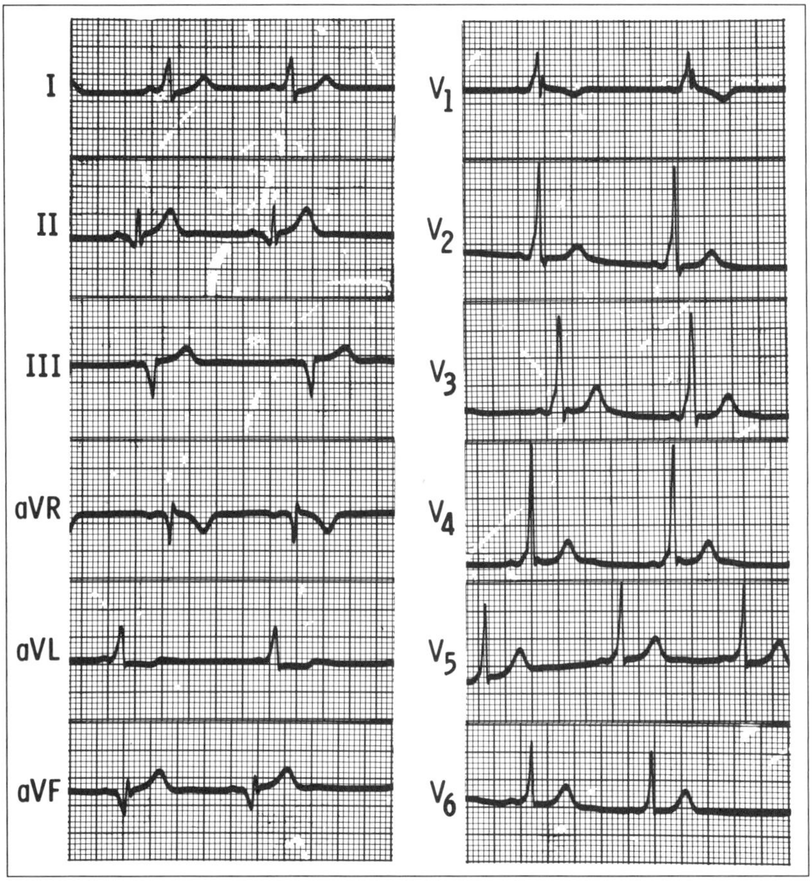


**Fig. 10–4.** Sinus arrhythmia with WPW syndrome, type A (same patient as in Fig. 10–3). Pseudodiaphragmatic MI is shown in this tracing because the delta wave is directed superiorly, a common occurrence.

1. Ashman's phenomenon may be recognized in any cardiac rhythm when aberrant ventricular conduction occurs following a long ventricular cycle (Figs. 5–5 and 5–16).
2. The aberrant ventricular conduction is more pronounced in a ventricular complex following the longest ventricular cycle as a result of marked Ashman's phenomenon (Fig. 5–16).
3. Atrial or AV junctional bigeminy nearly always shows aberrant ventricular conduction in atrial or AV junctional premature beats because of Ashman's phenomenon (Fig. 5–5). This is observed because atrial or AV junctional premature beats must follow a long ventricular cycle (postectopic pause) during atrial or AV junctional bigeminy (Fig. 5–5).
4. The P-R interval of atrial or AV junctional premature beat is often long during bigeminy, again as a result of Ashman's phenomenon. For the same reason, blocked APCs are common during atrial bigeminy (blocked atrial bigeminy).
5. Ashman's phenomenon is pronounced when the ventricular cycle becomes suddenly shortened following a long ventricular cycle, particularly in AF. As a result, aberrant ventricular conduction occurs. It is not uncommon to observe consecutively occurring aberrant ventricular conduction

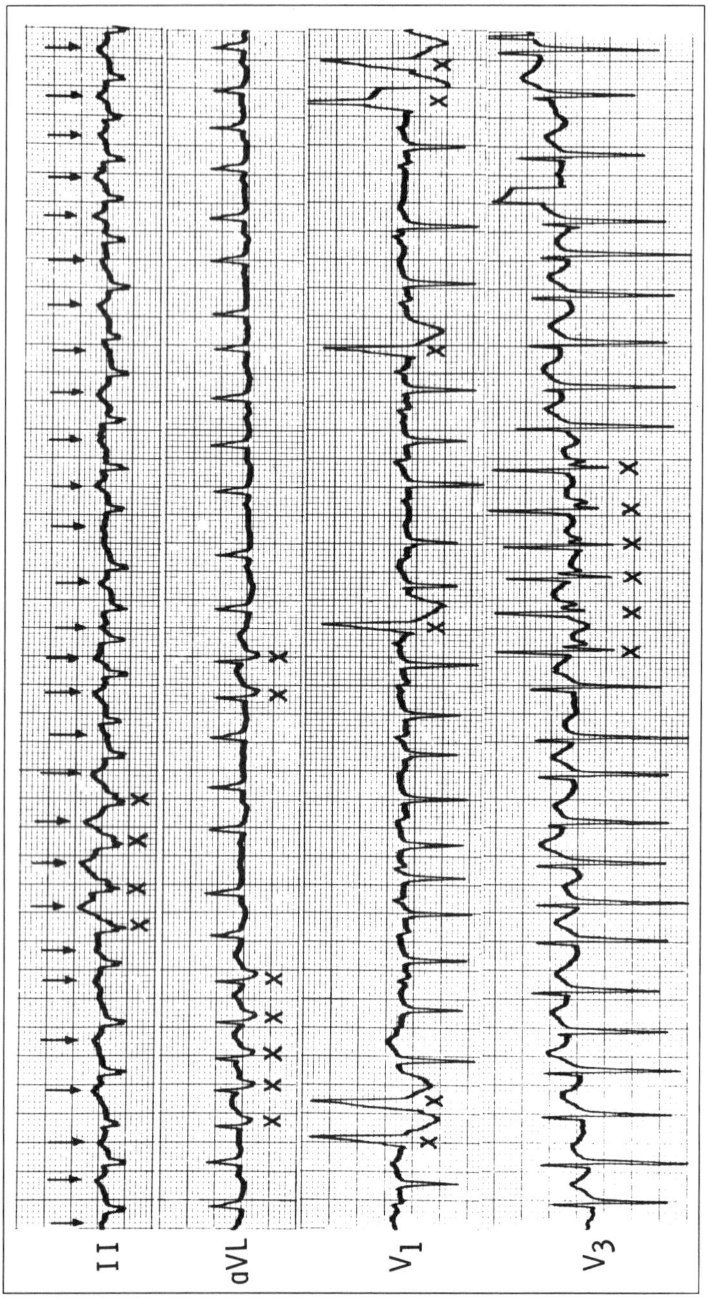


Fig. 10–5. Multifocal atrial tachycardia (MAT) with frequent aberrant ventricular conduction (X) initiated by Ashman's phenomenon. Arrows indicate ectopic P waves.

once it is initiated by Ashman's phenomenon (Fig. 5–16). This ECG finding closely simulates VT.

6. Ashman's phenomenon may be encountered in MAT, which leads to aberrant ventricular conduction (Fig. 10–5).
7. Occasionally, a sinus beat (ventricular captured beat) during incomplete AV dissociation may show aberrant ventricular conduction as a result of Ashman's phenomenon.
8. The configuration of the QRS complex during aberrant ventricular conduction as a result of Ashman's phenomenon is commonly (about 80–85%) that of an RBBB pattern (Figs. 5–16 and 10–5), and only 15–20% may show an LBBB pattern. Not uncommonly, aberrantly conducted beats may reveal an ECG finding of BFB pattern consisting of RBBB pattern and left anterior or posterior hemiblock pattern. At times, aberrantly conducted beats may show both LBBB pattern and RBBB pattern in the same ECG tracing. The alteration of the QRS contour in aberrant ventricular conduction represents functional (not true) BBB and/or hemiblock.
9. The secondary T wave change is observed in aberrantly conducted QRS complex. The T wave alteration in this circumstance is analogous to that of VPCs or LBBB or RBBB.

**TABLE 10–1. ECG findings causing broad (bizarre) QRS complexes**

A. Ventricular ectopy
   1. Ventricular premature contractions
   2. Ventricular parasystole
   3. Ventricular tachycardia
   4. Ventricular escape beats or rhythm
   5. Ventricular fibrillation or flutter
B. Intraventricular block
   1. Right bundle branch block
   2. Left bundle branch block
   3. Bifascicular or trifascicular block
   4. Diffuse (nonspecific) intraventricular block
C. Aberrant ventricular conduction
   1. Ashman's phenomenon
   2. Short coupling interval
   3. Very rapid supraventricular tachyarrhythmias of various origins or mechanisms
D. Wolff-Parkinson-White syndrome
E. Artificial pacemaker-induced ventricular beats or rhythm

Reproduced with permission from Chung: Principles of Cardiac Arrhythmias, 3rd ed. Baltimore, Williams & Wilkins, 1983.

**TABLE 10–2. ECG findings supporting (or favoring) ventricular ectopy**

A. Full compensatory pause during sinus rhythm (occasionally interpolated)—no disturbance on the sinus P-P cycle
B. Significant pause after a bizarre QRS complex in atrial fibrillation or flutter
C. No premature P wave preceding a bizarre QRS complex
D. Extremely broad and bizarre QRS complex
E. No evidence of Ashman's phenomenon
F. Left bundle branch block pattern or multiformed
G. Bizarre QRS complex in elderly or cardiac patients and/or in digitalis toxicity

Reproduced with permission from Chung: Principles of Cardiac Arrhythmias, 3rd ed. Baltimore, Williams & Wilkins, 1983.

Various ECG findings causing broad (bizarre) QRS complexes are summarized in Table 10–1, and various ECG findings that support (or favor) ventricular ectopy are summarized in Table 10–2.

## EVALUATION OF RESPONSE TO CAROTID SINUS STIMULATION

The response to CSS is different depending upon the nature and origin of the various tachyarrhythmias (Table 10–3). Sinus tachycardia is only transiently slowed by CSS, and the original sinus rate returns soon after the procedure is over. At times, however, varying degree AV block may be produced by CSS in sinus tachycardia.

When CSS is applied for AT, there may be 3 different responses: no response at all, restoration of sinus rhythm (Fig. 5–9), or a slowing of the ventricular rate resulting from increased AV block, especially when the underlying cause is DI. The response of AV JT to CSS is similar to

**TABLE 10–3. Cardiac arrhythmias: various responses to carotid sinus stimulation***

| Arrhythmias | Responses |
|---|---|
| Sinus tachycardia | 1. Transient slowing of sinus (atrial) rate |
| | 2. Varying degree AV block (less common) |
| Atrial tachycardia | 1. Termination |
| | 2. No response |
| | 3. Slowing of ventricular rate due to increased AV block (less common) |
| | 4. Increased atrial rate (less common) |
| Atrial fibrillation or flutter | 1. Slowing of ventricular rate due to increased AV block |
| AV junctional tachycardia | |
| Paroxysmal | 1. Termination |
| | 2. No response |
| Nonparoxysmal | No response |
| Ventricular tachyarrhythmias | No response (rare exceptions) |
| WPW syndrome | Vary |
| Parasystole | Vary |

*Carotid sinus stimulation is not recommended in digitalis intoxication or in hypersensitive individuals.
Reproduced with permission from Chung: Principles of Cardiac Arrhythmias, 3rd ed. Baltimore, Williams & Wilkins, 1983.

that of AT. That is, AV JT (usually paroxysmal) may convert to sinus rhythm, or it may not be influenced by the procedure. In reciprocating tachycardia, slowing of the ventricular rate may be produced as a result of increased AV block by CSS.

When CSS is applied to AF or atrial flutter, a slowing of the ventricular rate is invariably produced because of the increased AV block. Occasionally, a long ventricular standstill may result when CSS is applied to elderly patients with AF or atrial flutter. In contrast to supraventricular tachyarrhythmias, VT, as a rule, does not respond to CSS. Thus, no response to the procedure does not diagnose or exclude supraventricular tachycardia or VT, but VT is excluded if there is any response to CSS.

## DETERMINATION OF REGULARITY OF R-R CYCLES

Although it has been said that VT often shows a slight irregularity of the R-R cycles, it is rather uncommon to recognize any appreciable irregularity except when VT transforms to VF. Conversely, supraventricular (atrial or AV junctional) tachycardia may produce a slight irregularity of the cardiac cycle, particularly in the initial portion of the paroxysm. Thus, slight irregularity of the R-R cycles is not a useful criterion for the differential diagnosis of supraventricular tachycardia and VT.

Grossly irregular R-R cycles, regardless of the configuration of the QRS complex, are nearly always due to AF and, less commonly, may be due to atrial flutter or AT with varying AV response or VF. When the QRS complex is wide and/or bizarre, owing to preexisting or rate-dependent BBB (Figs. 5–17, 10–1, and 10–2), aberrant ventricular conduction (Figs. 5–7, 5–16, and 10–5), or anomalous AV conduction in the WPW syndrome (Fig. 10–3), VT is closely simulated. On the other hand, when the R-R cycles show a regular irregularity, the tachycardia often arises from the AV junction, and the irregularity is often due to Wenckebach exit block or the periodic occurrence of reciprocal beats.

## EVALUATION OF COUPLING INTERVALS AND POSTTACHYARRHYTHMIA PAUSE

In general, the coupling intervals are constant in VT or VPCs (Fig. 7–10). Conversely, wide and/or bizarre QRS complexes due to aberrant ventricular conduction in AF always have varying coupling intervals (Fig. 5–16). In addition, VT is always followed by a posttachycardia pause, and aberrantly conducted beats in AF are not followed by a long pause (Fig. 5–16).

## DETERMINATION OF HEART RATE

Although various tachyarrhythmias produce different rate ranges (Chapter 1), the heart rate is not a reliable index to use for the differential diagnosis of supraventricular and ventricular tachyarrhythmias because of the overlap of the heart rates. Nevertheless, a ventricular rate beyond 200 beats/min usually favors supraventricular tachyarrhythmias, and a ventricular rate faster than 250 beats/min nearly always indicates AF or atrial flutter, regardless of the width of the complex.

## IDENTIFICATION OF HIS BUNDLE POTENTIAL IN RELATION TO VENTRICULAR ACTIVITY

Recently, study of the His bundle potential has been utilized in order to locate the precise origin of the ectopic focus or conduction defect. When the ventricular activity is preceded by a His bundle potential, the rapid heart action is due to a supraventricular tachycardia (Fig. 2–5). Conversely, in VT the QRS complex is not preceded by the His bundle potential (Fig. 2–5).

## CONCLUSION

The differential diagnosis between supraventricular and ventricular tachyarrhythmias is often difficult and at times impossible because many features mimic each other. Yet, it is extremely important to distinguish the two because their management and prognosis are different.

When the QRS complexes of supraventricular tachyarrhythmias are wide and/or bizarre, the following may be used to distinguish them from VT:

1. Determination of the relationship between atrial and ventricular activities
2. Comparison of the QRS complexes during tachyarrhythmias with those of ventricular captured beats
3. Comparison of the QRS complexes during tachyarrhythmias with those of isolated ectopic beats before or after the episode of rapid heart action
4. Recognition of a preexisting or rate-dependent LBBB or RBBB
5. Recognition of a preexisting WPW syndrome
6. Recognition of aberrant ventricular conduction and Ashman's phenomenon
7. Evaluation of the response to CSS
8. Determination of the regularity of the R-R cycles
9. Identification of the His bundle potential in relationship to ventricular activity

# Chapter 11

# Aberrant Ventricular Conduction

The term "aberrant ventricular conduction" is used when an alteration of the supraventricular impulse occurs regardless of the fundamental mechanism of the arrhythmia, thus producing an alteration of the QRS complex on the ECG. This is observed when the supraventricular impulses are propagated through the ventricles during the partial refractory phase. Thus, aberrant ventricular conduction tends to occur in supraventricular impulses (either isolated beat, group beats, or tachycardia) when the coupling interval is very short, when Ashman's phenomenon is present, and when the ventricular rate of the tachycardia is very fast. The degree of the aberrant ventricular conduction varies markedly depending upon the degree of the refractory period in the ventricles when the supraventricular impulses are conducted to the ventricles. Therefore, the configuration of the aberrantly conducted QRS complex may be slightly different from that of the normally conducted beat, or the QRS complex may be extremely bizarre.

In general, the configuration of the aberrantly conducted beats may show RBBB pattern (Figs. 5–16 and 10–5), LBBB pattern, and left anterior or posterior hemiblock pattern. Not uncommonly, the aberrantly conducted beats may reveal a combination of RBBB pattern and left anterior or posterior hemiblock pattern. At times, the QRS complexes may show 2 or more different configurations, such as a combination of LBBB pattern and RBBB pattern (Fig. 11–1) or a combination of LBBB pattern and left anterior or posterior hemiblock pattern on the same ECG tracing.

Aberrant ventricular conduction also may occur in sinus beats when there is marked variation of the ventricular cycle, such as is seen in marked sinus arrhythmia or in complete AV dissociation. Extremely rarely, aberrant ventricular conduction may be observed in the ventricular impulses, such as in ventricular premature beats, ventricular parasystolic beats, or artificial pacemaker-induced ventricular beats. In other words, the bizarre QRS complex of the ventricular impulse may become more bizarre because of either Ashman's phenomenon or a very short coupling interval. Because of varying coupling intervals in ventricular parasystole (Chapter 22), aberrant ventricular conduction is not uncommonly observed when the coupling interval becomes very short (Fig. 5–4). For a similar reason, aberrant ventricular conduction can be recognized when the supraventricular impulses with preexisting true LBBB or RBBB exhibit alteration of the QRS configuration, such as is seen in marked sinus arrhythmia, atrial flutter, or AT with varying AV response and in sinus tachycardia with Mobitz type I or II AV block. Under these circumstances, Ashman's phenomenon is almost always responsible for the development of aberrant ventricular conduction.

When the ventricular rate is extremely rapid in AF or atrial flutter with anomalous AV conduction in the WPW syndrome (Chapter 13), aberrant ventricular conduction may lead to markedly bizarre QRS complexes. In other words, aberrant ventricular conduction plus anomalous AV conduction results in extremely bizarre QRS complexes (Fig. 10–3).

The term "AV junctional beats or rhythm with aberrant ventricular conduction" had been used to describe escape beats or rhythm with slightly bizarre QRS complexes. However, electrophysiologic studies have demonstrated recently that the so-called AV JEBs or JER actually represents escape beats or rhythm originating from a fascicle of the left bundle branch system. It should be noted that AV JEBs or JER may show actual aberrant ventricular conduction on rare occasions.

Recognition of aberrant ventricular conduc-

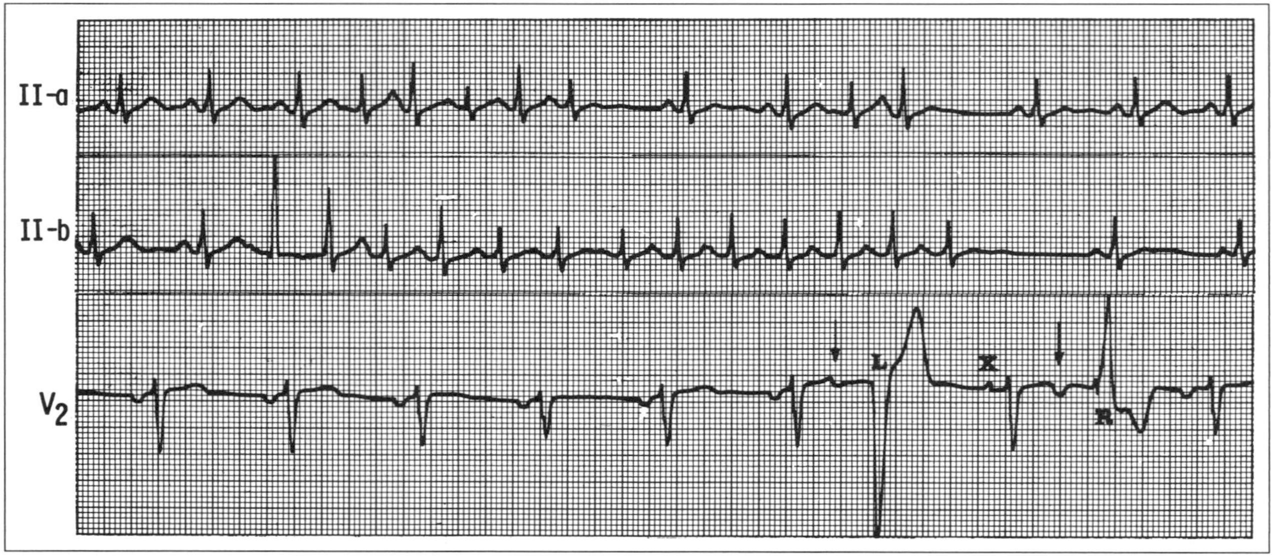


**Fig. 11–1.** Sinus rhythm and frequent APCs (indicated by arrows) with group beats and a short run of AT. Note that 1 APC shows aberrant ventricular conduction of LBBB pattern (L), whereas another APC exhibits aberrant ventricular conduction of RBBB pattern (R). In addition, 1 APC is followed by aberrant atrial conduction (Chung's phenomenon, marked X).

tion of supraventricular impulses is extremely important because it is commonly mistaken for ventricular ectopic beats or rhythm. As can be expected, aberrant ventricular conduction usually has little clinical significance, while ventricular arrhythmias may significantly influence the patient's morbidity and mortality.

Aberrant ventricular conduction is generally recognized with relative ease when the P wave precedes the QRS complex, as seen in APCs or AT. However, recognition of aberrant ventricular conduction is often difficult when it occurs in AF or atrial flutter with a very rapid ventricular response or when the P wave follows the QRS complex.

## DIAGNOSTIC CRITERIA

Aberrant ventricular conduction may occur in any supraventricular beat or rhythm when the impulses are conducted to the ventricles during the partial refractory phase. On rare occasions, the ventricular impulses may show aberrant ventricular conduction. The configuration of the QRS complex is commonly (about 80–85%) that of an RBBB pattern (Figs. 5–5, 5–16, and 10–5), and only 15–20% show an LBBB pattern (Fig. 11–2). In a small number of cases, the aberrantly conducted beats may show a combination of RBBB and left anterior or posterior hemiblock pattern. The aberrantly conducted beats with 2 or more different configurations in the same ECG tracing have been described previously (Fig. 11–1) in this chapter. In some cases, the QRS complexes of aberrantly conducted beats may be only slightly wide and bizarre in configuration and thus closely resemble a normally conducted beat (Fig. 5–7).

Regarding RBBB pattern in lead $V_1$, a triphasic pattern, such as rsR′, rSR′ or rsr′, is said to be the most common occurrence associated with a q wave and an R:S ratio greater than 1 in lead $V_6$. Less commonly, the QRS complex in lead $V_1$ may show a qRs, qR, R, or Rs pattern.

Although the initial force of the RBBB pattern during aberrant ventricular conduction is said to be often similar or even identical to that of the normally conducted beat, this finding is

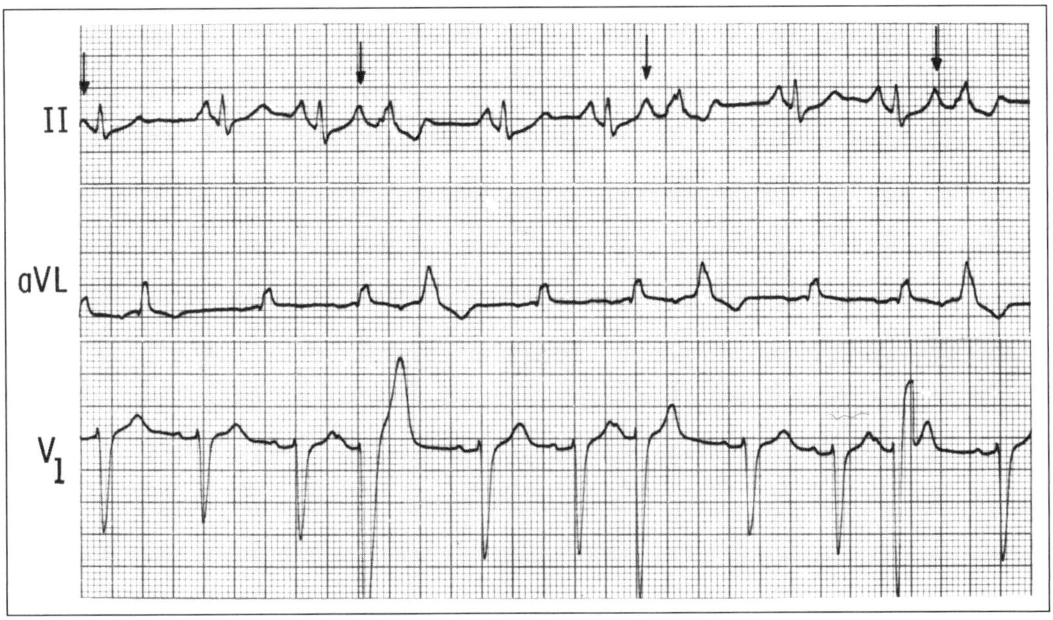


Fig. 11–2. Sinus rhythm and frequent APCs (indicated by arrows) with aberrant ventricular conduction of LBBB pattern.

not a reliable criterion for the diagnosis. In fact, more than 50% of the cases with aberrant ventricular conduction show the initial vector to be different from that of a normally conducted beat. In other words, the initial vector of the aberrant ventricular conduction may have various directions.

The T wave configuration, as expected, is also altered in aberrantly conducted beats, and this is a form of secondary T wave change. The degree of the T wave aberration usually parallels the degree of QRS aberration.

Aberrant ventricular conduction is diagnosed in various supraventricular beats or rhythm as follows.

## Aberrant Ventricular Conduction in Atrial Premature Contractions

Atrial premature contractions (APCs) may be followed by aberrant ventricular conduction when the coupling interval is very short (Fig. 5–4). The degree of aberrant conduction depends upon the degree of prematurity and the presence of Ashman's phenomenon. The longer the R-R interval immediately preceding the coupling interval, the greater is the degree of ventricular aberration. For this reason, aberrant ventricular conduction frequently occurs in atrial bigeminy (Fig. 5–5). Another factor that may influence the production of aberrant ventricular conduction is the status of the intraventricular conduction system. Thus, aberrant ventricular conduction may occur in a markedly impaired intraventricular conduction system even when the coupling interval is not too short. The pattern of the ventricular aberration may vary, particularly when APCs occur at different periods of the basic rhythm. For a similar reason, the QRS complex following an APC may show a true LBBB or RBBB pattern when the left or right bundle branch has impaired conduction. This is a form of rate-dependent BBB. On rare occasions, APCs may show aberrant ventricular conduction with RBBB pattern as well as LBBB pattern on the same ECG tracing (Fig. 11–1). Not uncommonly, APCs with aberrant ventricular conduction may demonstrate a combination of RBBB pattern and left anterior or posterior hemiblock pattern. Aberrant ventricular conduction in APCs closely resembles VPCs, but a prematurely appearing P wave preceding the QRS complex is a diagnostic clue for the former.

## Aberrant Ventricular Conduction in Atrial Tachycardia

Just as is seen in APCs, the QRS complex in AT may have a wide and bizarre configuration if there is an extremely rapid ventricular rate (Fig. 5–7). In addition, aberrant ventricular conduction is often observed in AT as a result of Ashman's phenomenon. Two or more forms of aberrant ventricular conduction may occur in AT with or without changing the ventricular rate (Fig. 5–7). The aberrant ventricular conduction, of course, occurs because the intraventricular conduction system is partially refractory as a result of the consecutive rapid impulses. For similar reasons, AT may be associated with LBBB or RBBB that was concealed during sinus rhythm. This occurs when 1 bundle branch is diseased and is thus unable to conduct rapid impulses beyond a critical rate. This is a form of rate-dependent BBB. When AT is associated with a wide QRS complex due to aberrant ventricular conduction, BBB, or the WPW syndrome, it certainly resembles VT, particularly if the P wave is not clearly discernible.

## Aberrant Ventricular Conduction in Atrial Flutter

A wide and bizarre QRS complex may occur in atrial flutter when the ventricular rate is extremely rapid, particularly during 1:1 AV conduction because of aberrant ventricular conduction. This occurs when rapid atrial impulses reach the ventricles during the relative refractory period of the intraventricular conduction system. On the other hand, wide QRS complexes may be observed in atrial flutter when preexisting RBBB or LBBB is present or rate-dependent RBBB or LBBB appears because of a rapid ventricular rate. In addition, the QRS complex may be wide in atrial flutter because of the WPW syndrome. Atrial flutter with a wide QRS complex often resembles VT.

## Aberrant Ventricular Conduction in Atrial Fibrillation

When the ventricular rate is rapid in AF, the QRS complex has a varying configuration because of aberrant ventricular conduction of varying degrees. When the aberrant ventricular conduction is marked, it may resemble isolated or coupled ventricular premature beats or even VT (Fig. 5–16). Aberrant ventricular conduction is prone to develop when the ventricular rate is extremely rapid because the rapidly transmitted atrial impulses find the ventricles in the relative refractory state. The degree of the ventricular aberration is extremely marked when the ventricular rates approach 250 beats/min. In addition, aberrant ventricular conduction tends to occur and the degree of the aberration is more pronounced in ventricular complexes following a longer R-R interval just before the appearance of a short R-R interval. In other words, the R-R interval immediately preceding a bout of rapid ventricular rhythm with aberrant ventricular conduction in AF is often long (Fig. 5–16). This occurs because the variability depends upon the irregularity of the cycle length. It can be said that the longer the ventricular pause (R-R interval), the longer is the refractory period following it; the shorter the pause, the shorter is the refractory period. Because of this, if 2 atrial impulses are conducted to the ventricles at the identical critically short time interval after the preceding beat, 1 may be conducted in a normal fashion following the short preceding R-R interval, and the other beat may show aberrant ventricular conduction following the preceding long R-R interval (Fig. 5–16). This finding is termed "Ashman's phenomenon." Aberrant ventricular conduction in AF is not followed by a long pause (Fig. 5–16). In contrast to this, paroxysmal tachycardia, either atrial, AV junctional, or ventricular, is almost always followed by a long pause because of the postdrive inhibition phenomenon.

It should be noted that the QRS complex in AF may be wide because of preexisting LBBB or RBBB (Fig. 5–17) or rate-dependent LBBB or RBBB or anomalous conduction because of the WPW syndrome (Fig. 10–3).

## Aberrant Ventricular Conduction in Atrioventricular Junctional Premature Contractions

It is not uncommon to observe a wide and bizarre QRS complex due to aberrant ventricular conduction. In general, the degree of aberrant ventricular conduction depends upon the degree of prematurity, the presence of Ashman's phenomenon, and the status of the intraventricular conduction system. Thus, aberrant ventricular conduction is prone to develop when the QRS complex of the AV junctional premature beat appears early in the cycle (short coupling interval) or following a long ventricular cycle preceding the coupling interval, because the ectopic impulse traverses the ventricles during their relative refractory period. Therefore, aberrant ventricular conduction is frequently observed after AV junctional bigeminy is established. Similarly, aberrant ventricular conduction often occurs only in the first of the 2 consecutively appearing AV JPCs.

Aberrant ventricular conduction in AV JPC may resemble VPC, but the former usually shows some resemblance to the QRS complex of the basic rhythm, or its configuration frequently exhibits RBBB pattern.

Rarely, the QRS complex of the basic rhythm immediately following an interpolated AV JPC may show aberrant ventricular conduction. This is observed because the sinus impulse reaches the ventricles during a relative refractory period because of an extremely short postectopic interval.

The QRS complex of the AV JPC may be

wide because of a preexisting or rate-dependent LBBB or RBBB or anomalous conduction due to the WPW syndrome.

## Aberrant Ventricular Conduction in Atrioventricular Junctional Tachycardia

The configuration of the QRS complex in AV JT is often normal, but it may be bizarre and wide when there is aberrant ventricular conduction. Aberrant ventricular conduction may occur because of a rapid ventricular rate. This is due to the fact that the rapid AV junctional impulses traverse the ventricles during the partially refractory period.

Until recently, the diagnosis of nonparoxysmal AV JT was made when regular tachycardia (rate: 60 to 150 beats/min) exhibited slightly bizarre QRS complexes. However, electrophysiologic studies have demonstrated that tachycardia with slightly bizarre QRS complexes originates from a fascicle of the left bundle branch system (fascicular tachycardia). When the configuration of the QRS complexes during regular tachycardia reveals incomplete RBBB pattern, the tachycardia is said to represent a left posterior fascicular tachycardia (Fig. 7–14). When there is preexisting or rate-dependent LBBB or RBBB, the QRS complex in AV JT will naturally be wide (Fig. 10–1).

## Aberrant Ventricular Conduction in Atrioventricular Junctional Escape Beats or Rhythm

It has been considered that AV JEBs or JER frequently produces aberrant ventricular conduction leading to slightly bizarre QRS complexes. The production of aberrant ventricular conduction under this circumstance was thought to be due to the fact that the AV junctional escape impulses are conducted to the ventricles via a preferential pathway, such as an accessory pathway demonstrated by Mahaim and by Lev and Lerner. However, electrophysiologic studies have demonstrated recently that so-called AV JEBs or JER with aberrant ventricular conduction represent fascicular escape beats or rhythm. A true aberrant ventricular conduction in AV JEBs or JER is observed only rarely.

## Aberrant Ventricular Conduction in Atrial or Atrioventricular Junctional Parasystole

Aberrant ventricular conduction may be observed when the ectopic atrial or AV junctional rhythm is generated by a parasystolic mechanism. It should be noted that so-called AV junctional parasystole with aberrant ventricular conduction in many cases has proven to be ventricular parasystole.

## Aberrant Ventricular Conduction in Reciprocal Beats or Rhythm

Aberrant ventricular conduction is occasionally observed in reciprocal beats or rhythm when the coupling interval is short, when Ashman's phenomenon is present, or when the ventricular rate is rapid. The mechanism responsible for the production of aberrant ventricular conduction in reciprocal beats or rhythm is essentially the same as seen in atrial or AV JPCs or tachyarrhythmias.

## Aberrant Ventricular Conduction in Sinus Beats

Occasionally, the configuration of the QRS complex of the sinus beat following an ectopic beat may be altered because of aberrant ventricular conduction. This is called "postectopic aberrant ventricular conduction" and is prone to occur following a very short postectopic pause, as seen in interpolated premature contractions (either atrial, AV junctional, or ventricular) because the sinus impulse traverses the ventricles during the partial refractory period. For a similar reason, aberrant ventricular conduction may be observed in the sinus beat (ventricular captured beat) in the presence of incomplete AV dissociation when the ventricular captured beat occurs very early in the cardiac cycle or when there is Ashman's phenomenon (Fig. 11–3).

### Aberrant Ventricular Conduction in Ventricular Beats

When the ventricular ectopic impulses, such as in VPCs, ventricular parasystolic beats, or artificial pacemaker-induced ventricular beats, are conducted to the ventricles during their partial refractory period, aberrant ventricular conduction is expected to occur. However, in most situations, aberrant ventricular conduction is not obvious because the configuration of the ventricular ectopic beats is bizarre without aberrant ventricular conduction. On the other hand, aberrant ventricular conduction can be recognized when the configuration of the ventricular ectopic beats is more bizarre than expected when compared with other ventricular ectopic beats in the same ECG tracing. In other words, aberrant ventricular conduction in the ventricular ectopic beats is manifested by a bizarre QRS complex in addition to the preexisting bizarre configuration (bizarre-plus).

Aberrant ventricular conduction is expected to occur when there is a very short coupling interval or Ashman's phenomenon. Ashman's phenomenon tends to occur when the ventricular cycle of the basic rhythm is extremely irregular, as seen in marked sinus arrhythmia, AT or atrial flutter with varying AV response, or varying degree Mobitz type I or II AV block. For the same reason, aberrant ventricular conduction tends to occur in ventricular parasystole because of varying coupling intervals (Chapter 22).

## DIFFERENTIAL DIAGNOSIS

Aberrant ventricular conduction in supraventricular arrhythmias often resembles ventricular arrhythmias. The differential diagnosis of these 2 entities is important because aberrant ventricular conduction is usually insignificant clinically, whereas ventricular arrhythmias often have serious clinical implications.

Preexisting LBBB or RBBB naturally produces wide QRS complexes in supraventricular arrhythmias (Figs. 5–17 and 10–1), but this is not aberrant ventricular conduction. Similarly, a wide QRS complex due to anomalous AV conduction in various supraventricular tachyarrhythmias associated with the WPW syndrome is not true aberrant ventricular conduction (Fig. 10–3). It should be noted that VT may coexist with atrial flutter or AF and can be easily misdiagnosed as aberrant ventricular conduction. Occasionally, VPCs occurring later in the cycle may resemble APCs with aberrant ventricular conduction because the sinus P wave immediately precedes the VPCs.

The following statements can be useful in differentiating aberrant ventricular conduction of supraventricular beats or rhythm from ventricular beats or rhythm, although they are not applicable in every instance.

1. Right bundle branch block pattern favors aberrant ventricular conduction.
2. An ectopic P wave preceding a wide QRS complex excludes ventricular arrhythmias.
3. Absence of the postectopic pause following consecutively appearing wide QRS complexes favors aberrant ventricular conduction.
4. In AF, fixed coupling intervals favor VPCs, whereas varying coupling intervals favor aberrant ventricular conduction, provided that ventricular parasystole is excluded.
5. An initial vector that is similar to or identical with that of a normally conducted beat favors aberrant ventricular conduction.
6. The presence of similar or identical bi-

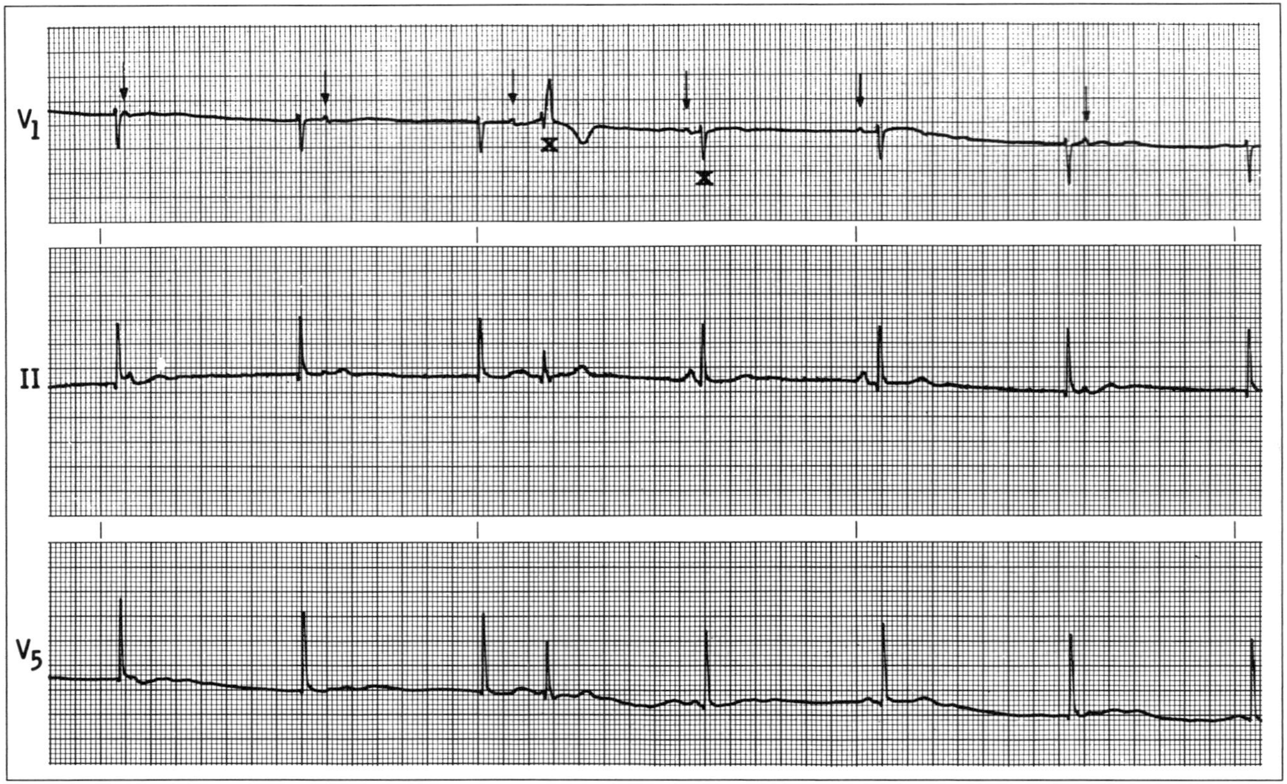


**Fig. 11–3.** Arrows indicate sinus P waves. The rhythm is marked sinus bradycardia (atrial rate: 38–40 beats/min) producing incomplete AV dissociation. Note that there are 2 ventricular captured beats (X), and 1 of them exhibits aberrant ventricular conduction (the fourth QRS complex).

zarre beats in a previous ECG during sinus rhythm can be the deciding factor for the diagnosis of VPCs in AF.

7. A long cardiac cycle preceding the coupling interval favors aberrant ventricular conduction (Ashman's phenomenon), whereas a short preceding cycle favors ventricular ectopic beats.
8. The presence of ventricular fusion beats favors ventricular ectopic beats.

## MECHANISM

The fundamental mechanisms responsible for the production of aberrant ventricular conduction in atrial or AV JPCs or reciprocal beats and in supraventricular tachyarrhythmias are essentially the same. The supraventricular impulse traverses the ventricles during the partial refractory phase because of a short coupling interval, Ashman's phenomenon, or a very rapid ventricular rate. The exact same underlying mechanisms as described above for the production of aberrant ventricular conduction in supraventricular impulses may produce aberrant ventricular conduction in ventricular ectopic impulses.

A pure RBBB or LBBB pattern of aberrantly conducted beats is considered to be due to a functional block within the corresponding bundle branch. The common occurrence of an RBBB pattern in aberrant ventricular conduction is thought to be due to the fact that the right bundle branch is more susceptible than the left bundle branch to a sudden variation of conductivity. In experimental animal studies, aberrant ventricular conduction has been shown, by sophisticated recording systems, to be the result of a functional block within the right bundle branch or left bundle branch. It has also been suggested that aberrant ventricular conduction showing left axis deviation results from a functional block within the anterior division of the left bundle branch and that a pattern of inferior (rightward) axis deviation results from a functional block within the posterior division of the left bundle branch. Grant initially proposed that a block of the left anterior division produced delayed activation of the anterolateral myocardium, leading to left axis deviation, whereas a block of the left posterior division caused inferior axis deviation. Experimental animal studies have substantiated this proposal.

Recently, Rosenbaum et al. have proposed that the escape impulses may arise at the ventricular level, from proximal segments of the main intraventricular conduction fascicles. These investigators further analyzed the origin of the escape beats according to the pattern of the QRS complex. In incomplete LBBB pattern, the ectopic beats arise from the main right bundle branch; in incomplete RBBB with left anterior hemiblock, the ectopic beats arise from the posterior division of the left bundle branch; in incomplete RBBB with left posterior hemiblock, the ectopic beats arise from the anterior division of the left bundle branch; in pure left posterior hemiblock, the ectopic beats arise from the pseudobifurcation.

## ASHMAN'S PHENOMENON

The most important factor for the production of aberrant ventricular conduction is Ashman's phenomenon (Figs. 5–5, 5–16, and 10–5), which is described in detail in Chapter 10.

## CLINICAL SIGNIFICANCE

There is no uniform agreement regarding the clinical significance of aberrant ventricular conduction. Some investigators believe that aberrant ventricular conduction indicates a pathologic conduction system, whereas others consider that it may be a physiologic phenomenon. From this author's experience, the occurrence of aberrant ventricular conduction is a physiologic phenomenon as long as 1 of the 3 major factors (very short coupling interval, Ashman's phenomenon, very rapid ventricular rate) is present. On the other hand, the unexpected occurrence of aberrant ventricular conduction without the above-mentioned factors may indicate abnormal intraventricular conduction.

Needless to say, aberrant ventricular conduction per se does not produce any clinical symptoms or signs.

# Chapter 12

# Carotid Sinus Stimulation

It has been known for many years that carotid sinus stimulation (CSS) is very useful in differentiating various tachyarrhythmias because the response to this procedure varies depending upon the origin and the nature of the arrhythmia. This is particularly true when dealing with regular ectopic tachycardia and wide QRS complex, where the differential diagnosis is often urgently needed. In addition, CSS is extremely valuable in terminating supraventricular (atrial or AV junctional) tachycardia. On the other hand, the danger of applying CSS to patients with suspected DI is well known. The reason for this is that VF may be induced during or after CSS in this circumstance. In addition, CSS should be avoided when sick sinus syndrome (SSS) is suspected.

## INDICATIONS FOR CAROTID SINUS STIMULATION

Carotid sinus stimulation is indicated for 2 major purposes, therapeutic and diagnostic.

### Therapeutic

1. Carotid sinus stimulation is extremely valuable in terminating paroxysmal atrial tachycardia (PAT) as well as AV JT.
2. In addition, regular and rapid tachycardia (rate: 160–250 beats/min) is often terminated by CSS even if the exact location of the ectopic focus and its mechanism are uncertain.
3. Carotid sinus stimulation may be effective whether the QRS complex is normal or wide.
4. Carotid sinus stimulation is often effective in terminating reciprocating tachycardia in WPW syndrome.

### Diagnostic Criteria

It has been known for many years that CSS is extremely useful in differentiating various tachyarrhythmias. This is particularly true when dealing with regular ectopic tachycardia and wide QRS complex. Various responses to CSS are described in Table 10–3. It should be emphasized that applying CSS to patients with DI or SSS is dangerous and may induce VF or ventricular standstill and even sudden death.

## RESPONSES OF VARIOUS ARRHYTHMIAS TO CAROTID SINUS STIMULATION

### Sinus Tachycardia

In general, it is not necessary to apply CSS either diagnostically or therapeutically in cases of sinus tachycardia. However, the procedure is occasionally useful when the rate of sinus tachycardia is very rapid (around 150–160 beats/min) and differentiation from AT is needed.

1. Sinus tachycardia slows only transiently in response to CSS.
2. Less commonly, CSS may produce varying degree (usually first degree or Wenckebach) AV block transiently.

### Atrial Tachycardia

Carotid sinus stimulation is extremely valuable in terminating PAT (Fig. 5–9). The patient with AT may respond to CSS in 1 of 4 ways:

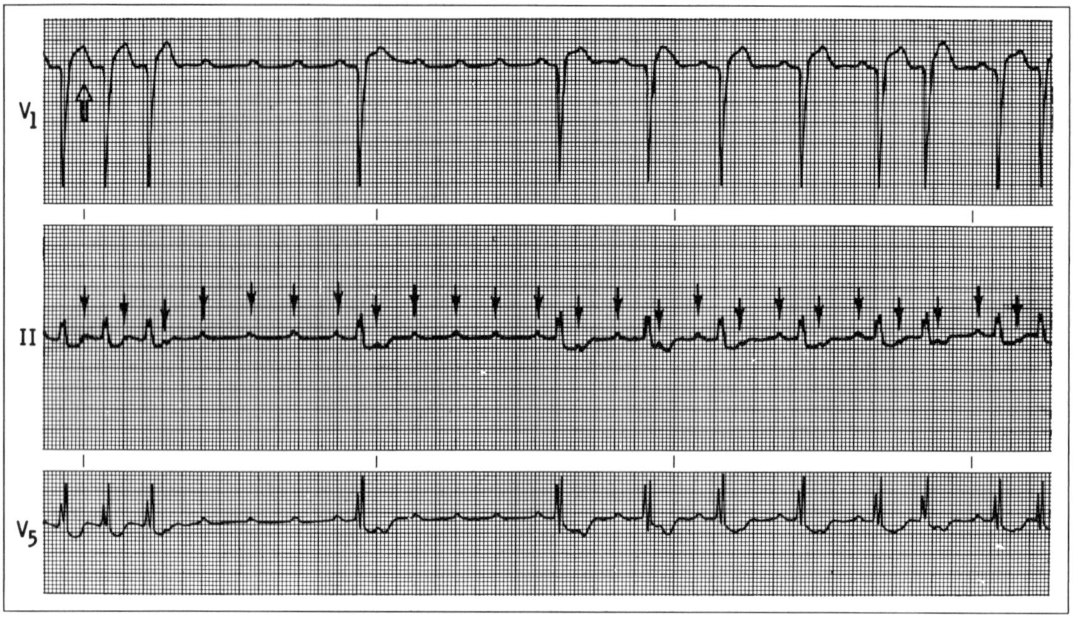


**Fig. 12–1.** Slowing of the ventricular rate in AT (rate: 155 beats/min) as a result of advanced AV block induced by CSS (indicated by upward arrow). Downward arrows indicate ectopic P waves.

1. Termination
2. No response
3. Slowing of ventricular rate due to increased AV block (Fig. 12–1)
4. Increased atrial rate

When slowing of the ventricular rate occurs in AT because of increased AV block, the underlying cause is usually DI (Chapter 17).

## Atrial Fibrillation or Flutter

1. When carotid sinus pressure is applied to patients with AF or atrial flutter, the ventricular rate invariably slows because of the increased AV block (Fig. 12–2).
2. Occasionally a long ventricular standstill may result when carotid sinus pressure is applied to an elderly patient with AF or atrial flutter or any patient with SSS.

## Atrioventricular Junctional Tachycardia

It is often difficult, and at times impossible, to distinguish between PAT and paroxysmal AV JT when only conventional ECGs are available. The P wave may be superimposed on the ST segment, T wave, or QRS complex of the preceding or succeeding beat. Therefore, the term "supraventricular tachycardia" is often used in this circumstance. Reciprocating tachycardia also belongs in this category. Nevertheless, it is believed that the response to CSS is similar in paroxysmal AV JT and PAT.

1. Paroxysmal AV JT may convert to sinus rhythm or may not respond to the procedure.
2. Nonparoxysmal AV JT, on the other hand, is usually unresponsive to CSS.
3. On rare occasions, the ventricular rate may be reduced by CSS in nonparoxysmal AV JT by inducing exit block.
4. Ventricular fibrillation may ensue if the

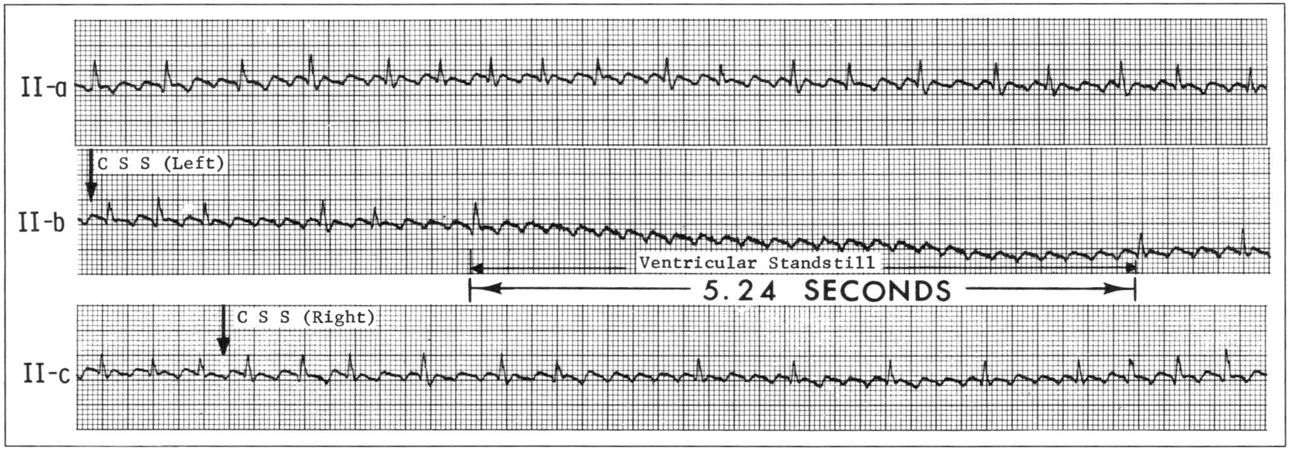


Fig. 12–2. Slowing of the ventricular rate with an area of a long ventricular standstill (5.24 seconds) in atrial flutter induced by CSS. Leads II-a and II-b are continuous.

underlying cause is DI. Thus, CSS is not recommended in the presence of nonparoxysmal AV JT, which is the most common sign of DI.

## Ventricular Tachyarrhythmias

Carotid sinus stimulation is often used to differentiate VT from supraventricular tachycardia, especially when the QRS complex is wide and bizarre.

1. In contrast to supraventricular tachyarrhythmias, as a rule, VT does not respond to CSS.
2. Therefore, any response to the procedure rules out VT in most cases.
3. It should be noted, however, that in VT, because of a parasystolic mechanism, CSS may slow or at times provoke a recurrence of the arrhythmia.
4. On extremely rare occasions, VT may be terminated by CSS. This unusual phenomenon is considered to occur on the basis of a parasympathetic action in the ventricles.

## Wolff–Parkinson–White Syndrome

1. Carotid sinus pressure can abolish the ventricular preexcitation.
2. In occasional instances, the procedure may cause ventricular preexcitation to appear.
3. When carotid sinus pressure is applied in the presence of WPW syndrome it can produce an AV junctional rhythm with a normal QRS complex, since the vagal stimulation tends to prolong AV conduction time or temporarily block the normal pathway and displace the pacemaker from the sinus node to the AV junction.
4. Carotid sinus pressure is often effective in terminating supraventricular (reciprocating) tachycardia associated with WPW syndrome (Fig. 12–3).

## Parasystole

1. The atrial or AV junctional parasystolic rate may be decreased by the application

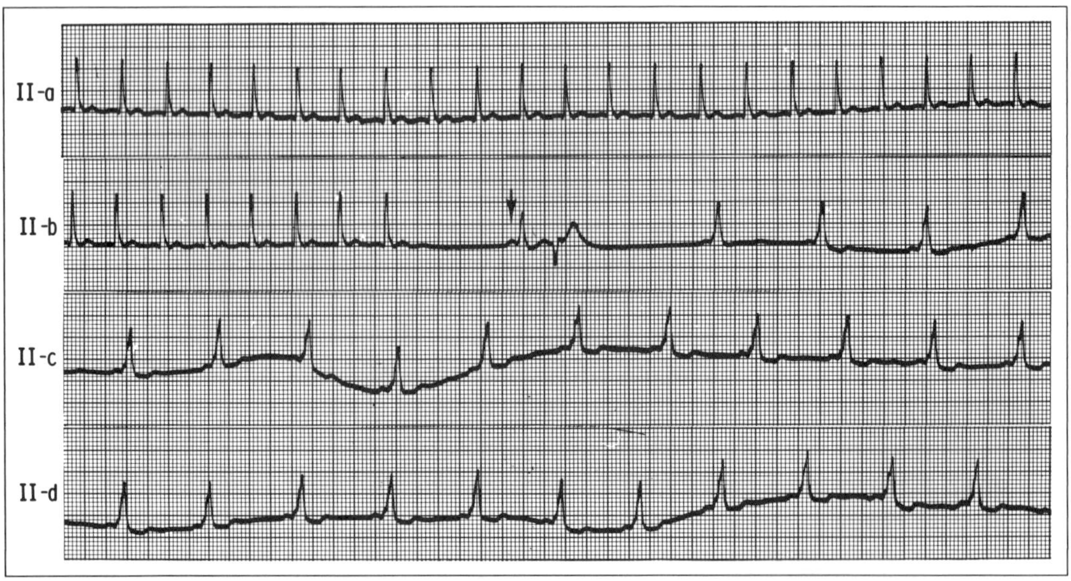


**Fig. 12–3.** Leads II-a, II-b, II-c, and II-d are continuous. Supraventricular (reciprocating) tachycardia (rate: 148 beats/min) is converted to sinus rhythm (indicated by arrow) by CSS. It is obvious that the underlying problem for the tachycardia is the WPW syndrome. Note a ventricular premature beat in lead II-b.

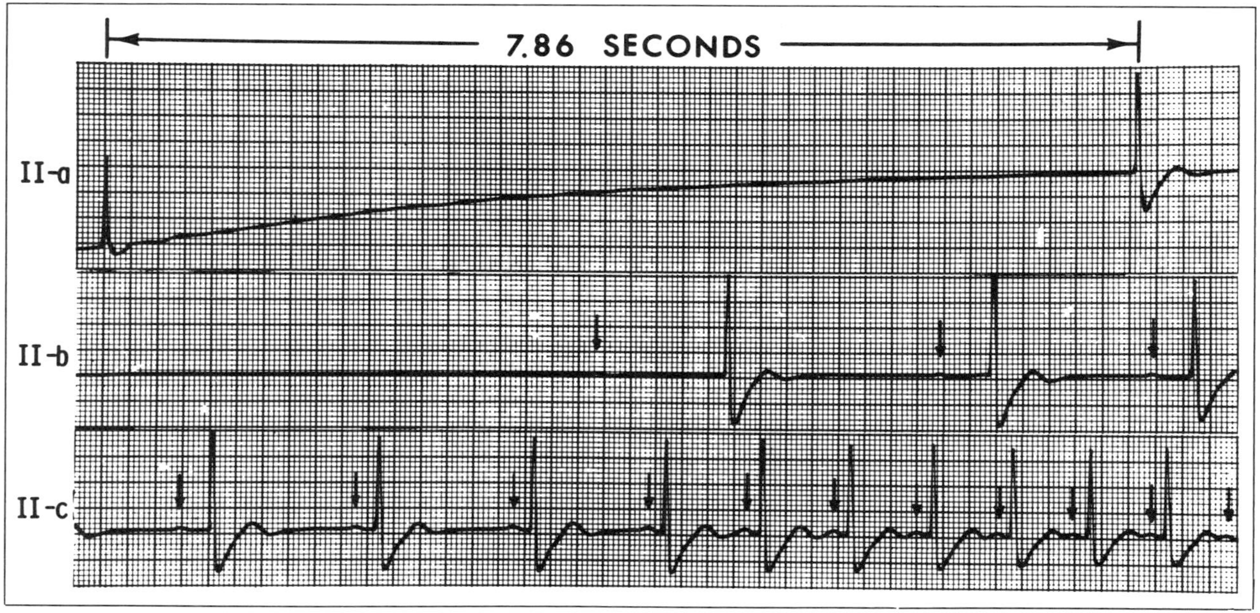


**Fig. 12–4.** Leads II-a, II-b, and II-c are continuous. Hypersensitive reaction to CSS is manifested by a long sinus arrest and occasional AV JEBs with a long escape interval (7.86 seconds). Note progressive acceleration of sinus cycle with progressive normalization of the P-R intervals following a long sinus arrest. Arrows indicate sinus P waves. Sick sinus syndrome is considered to be responsible for the production of a hypersensitive reaction to CSS.

of CSS. This phenomenon usually does not occur in other forms of atrial or AV junctional arrhythmias if the parasystolic mechanism is not present.
2. In ventricular parasystole, CSS may slow or even provoke the recurrence of the arrhythmia.
3. The disappearance of ventricular parasystole due either to the appearance of exit block or the disappearance of the protection block due to the same mechanism has been reported.
4. The disappearance of atrial parasystole by CSS has also been reported.
5. In certain cases, on the other hand, CSS may not influence the arrhythmia.

## Digitalis Intoxication (Chapter 17)

1. Some investigators observed that CSS frequently halts PAT with AV block not due to DI and is ineffective when digitalis is the etiologic factor.
2. On the other hand, a slowing of ventricular rate may result from increased AV block by the procedure when the underlying cause is DI (Fig. 12–1).
3. However, the author would like to emphasize the danger of applying CSS to patients with suspected DI because the patient may develop VF or ventricular standstill during or after CSS, which may result in a fatal outcome. Based on these observations, CSS should be avoided as much as possible on patients who are taking even small amounts of digitalis.

## Hypersensitive Patients and Sick Sinus Syndrome

1. Certain patients may be extremely sensitive to any pressure on the neck, including CSS.
2. These hypersensitive patients may develop long ventricular standstill and/or fainting episodes simply by turning the head, a tight collar, or light CSS (Fig. 12–4).
3. In general, SSS is the underlying disease process in patients with a hypersensitive reaction to CSS.
4. Obviously, CSS should be avoided in these patients, and most patients require permanent artificial pacemakers (Chapter 19).

## Artificial Pacemaker-induced Rhythm

1. Carotid sinus stimulation is a simple procedure to assess the function of a demand ventricular pacemaker when there is only the patient's own rhythm (either sinus or ectopic) without any artificial pacemaker activity.
2. This is observed when the patient's natural rhythm is faster than the preset demand pacing rate.
3. When a slowing of the sinus rate is produced by CSS in this case, the rhythm of the demand pacemaker will appear to control the ventricular activity as the pacing rate exceeds the sinus rate.

# Chapter 13

# Wolff-Parkinson-White Syndrome

The primary reason why every physician should be fully familiar with the Wolff-Parkinson-White (WPW) syndrome is the frequent occurrence of various ectopic tachyarrhythmias. In addition, the ECG findings in the WPW syndrome may closely resemble many other ECG abnormalities that are frequently misinterpreted in our daily practice. The WPW syndrome was first recognized as a clinical entity by 3 physicians, Wolff, Parkinson, and White, in 1930. The ECG findings that were later to be characteristic of this syndrome were described by Wilson in 1915, and again by Wedd in 1921.

The WPW syndrome has been known as a benign syndrome, and there are no subjective manifestations or hemodynamic alterations as long as there are no ectopic tachyarrhythmias. The tachyarrhythmias may occur at any time and may begin at birth or during infancy, childhood, or adult life. Sixty to seventy percent of the cases of WPW syndrome have been encountered in healthy individuals without organic heart disease.

The true incidence of the WPW syndrome is difficult to assess, but it has been estimated to be between 0.15 and 0.2% in the general population. The syndrome occurs more frequently in men than in women, with an incidence of between 54 and 70% in males.

## DIAGNOSTIC CRITERIA

Wolff-Parkinson-White syndrome can be diagnosed by 12-lead ECG, the His bundle ECG, or vectorcardiogram (VCG).

### Electrocardiographic Findings

1. The typical ECG findings include a short P-R interval and prolonged QRS interval due to a delta wave (initial slurring of the QRS complex) (Fig. 13–1).
2. A recognition of the delta wave is a key point in diagnosing the syndrome. In some cases with the WPW syndrome, however, the delta wave may not be obvious.
3. In addition, the P-R interval may be longer than 0.12 second, whereas the QRS interval may be narrower than 0.10 second in the proven WPW syndrome.
4. The acutal values of the P-R and the QRS intervals in the WPW syndrome are greatly influenced by the preexisting values of these intervals.
5. The term "Lown-Ganong-Levine (LGL) syndrome" has been used when the ECG shows a short P-R interval and narrow QRS complex without a clear-cut delta wave associated with recurrent tachyarrhythmias. In reality, the LGL syndrome is considered to be a variant of the WPW syndrome.
6. On the other hand, it should be emphasized that many normal individuals may have a short P-R interval, particularly during stressful situations. Obviously, this isolated ECG finding is usually meaningless.

### Vectorcardiographic (VCG) Findings

A unique finding in the WPW syndrome is the initial conduction delay of the QRS $s\hat{E}$ loop, which can be readily recognized by any physician who is familiar with VCG.

### His Bundle Electrocardiographic Findings

In equivocal cases of WPW syndrome, His bundle ECG may be necessary to confirm the

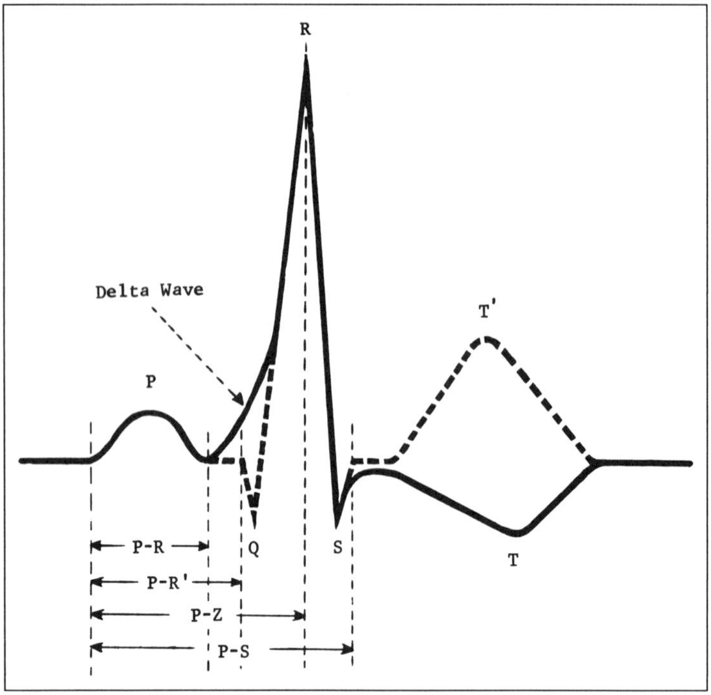


**Fig. 13–1.** The uninterrupted line indicates an anomalous conduction in WPW syndrome, whereas the dotted line indicates a normal conduction. P-R and P-R′ intervals are AV conduction times in WPW syndrome and normal conduction, respectively. The P-R interval is shorter than the P-R′ interval because of a delta wave. Note that the P-Z and P-S intervals are constant during anomalous and normal conduction. The T wave in WPW syndrome is inverted because of secondary T wave change.

diagnosis. In the His bundle ECG of the WPW syndrome, the H-V interval is shorter than normal; the His bundle potential may occur simultaneously with the ventricular deflection, or the His bundle potential may occur even later than the onset of the ventricular deflection. These findings are considered to occur because of a premature activation of a portion of the ventricles via anomalous conduction.

## CLASSIFICATION

The WPW syndrome has been traditionally classified into 2 types, types A and B, depending upon the direction of the delta wave. However, this classification is an oversimplification because many cases of WPW syndrome do not belong to either type A or B. The direction of the delta wave is primarily influenced by the location of the accessory pathway.

Nevertheless, the WPW syndrome is classified as follows:

### Type A Wolff-Parkinson-White Syndrome

1. In type A, the delta wave is directed anteriorly (commonly to the right and less commonly to the left).
2. In general, lead $V_1$ shows R, RS, Rs, RSr′, and Rsr′ patterns, whereas leads $V_5$ and $V_6$ show Rs or R deflection (Fig. 10–4).
3. Superficially, type A WPW syndrome resembles RBBB, RVH, and posterior MI.
4. When the QRS complexes in all precordial leads are upright, a type A WPW syndrome should be considered as the first diagnostic possibility.

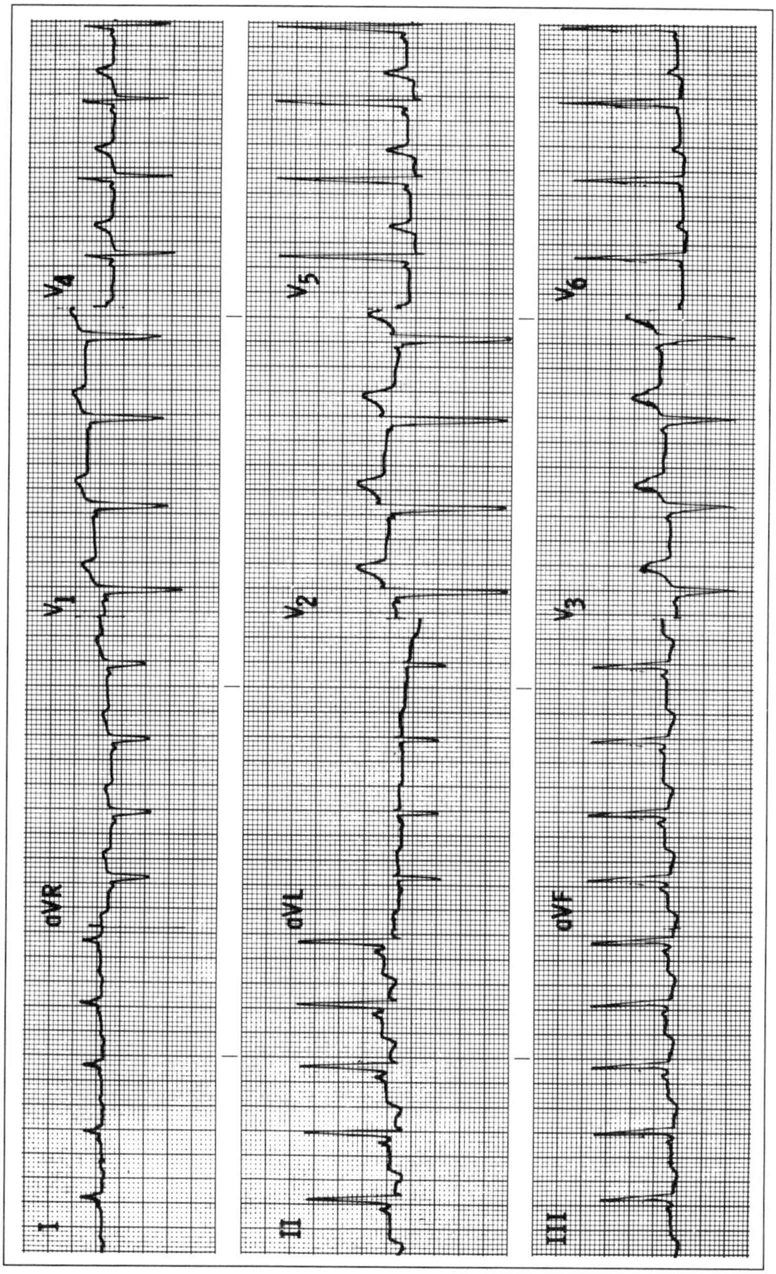


**Fig. 13–2.** Sinus arrhythmia with WPW syndrome, type B in an 11-year-old girl. Note pseudoanteroseptal MI with pseudo-LVH.

5. In type A, a premature activation occurs in the left ventricle.

### Type B Wolff-Parkinson-White Syndrome

1. In type B, the delta wave is directed posteriorly (commonly to the left and less commonly to the right).
2. Thus, the left precordial leads (leads I, aVL, and $V_{4-6}$) show tall R waves with delta waves, whereas leads $V_{1-2}$ show negative QRS complexes (QS waves) with delta waves (Fig. 13–2).
3. The ECG findings in type B WPW syndrome may closely resemble LBBB and LVH.
4. At times, a pseudoanteroseptal MI is produced in WPW syndrome, type B (Fig. 13–2)
5. In type B, a premature activation takes place in the right ventricle.

In both types A and B WPW syndrome, the delta wave is often directed superiorly. This ECG finding commonly produces QS or Q waves in leads II, III, and aVF that closely simulate diaphragmatic (inferior) MI (Fig. 10–4).

## TACHYARRHYTHMIAS

The most important clinical significance of the WPW syndrome is, of course, the frequent occurrence of supraventricular tachyarrhythmias. The incidence of tachyarrhythmias in WPW syndrome has been reported to be between 40 and 80%

### Reciprocating Tachycardia

1. Reciprocating tachycardia (the usual rate: 140–250 beats/min), is found in the majority of cases (75–80% of all tachyarrhythmias) (Fig. 12–3).
2. This type of tachycardia had been called "paroxysmal atrial tachycardia" until recently.
3. At present, the terms "reciprocating" or "reentrant" tachycardia are more commonly used because the tachycardia is considered to be due to a reentry phenomenon (Figs. 13–3 and 13–4). On the other hand, the term "circus movement tachycardia" has been frequently used in European literature to designate the same finding.
4. In reciprocating tachycardia, the QRS complex is usually normal (Fig. 12–3), and the broad QRS complex due to anomalous conduction is much less common.

### Atrial Flutter or Fibrillation

1. Atrial flutter or AF is rather uncommon in the WPW syndrome, and their incidence constitutes only 20–25% of all tachyarrhythmias.
2. Among these 2 rhythm disorders, atrial flutter is extremely rare.
3. The QRS complexes during AF or atrial flutter in the WPW syndrome are extremely bizarre and broad in most cases (Fig. 10–3).
4. The broad and bizarre QRS complexes are observed under this circumstance because of anomalous AV conduction due to the nature of the WPW syndrome itself plus aberrant ventricular conduction due to very rapid ventricular rate (ventricular rate: 250–300 beats/min).
5. Ventricular tachycardia or even VF is closely simulated when atrial flutter or AF with anomalous AV conduction occurs (Fig. 10–3).
6. In WPW syndrome, atrial flutter often exhibits 1:1 AV conduction, which results in extremely rapid ventricular rate.
7. It should be remembered that atrial flutter or AF in the WPW syndrome may terminate catastrophically.

### Ventricular Tachyarrhythmias

1. Although the occurrence of VT had been reported in the WPW syndrome previously, in most if not all instances, AF or

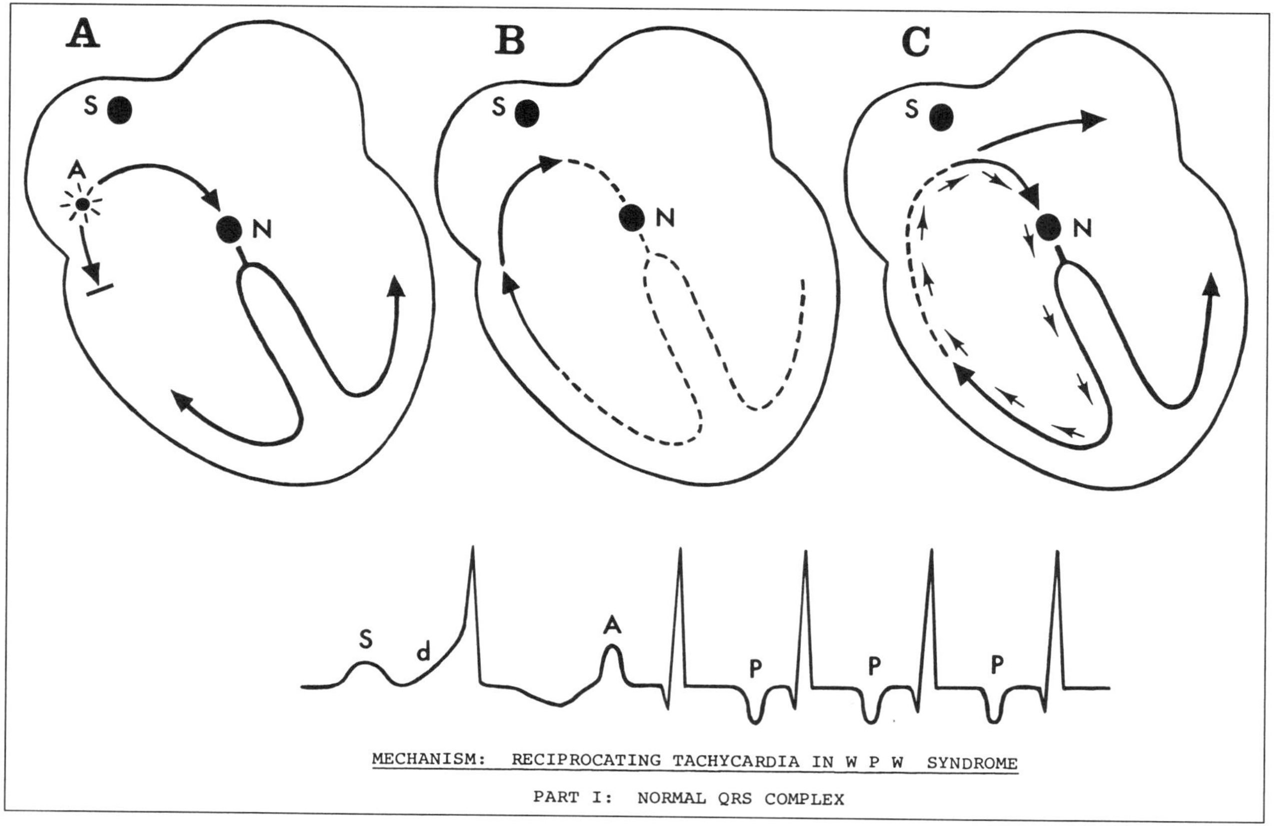


**Fig. 13–3.** Diagram illustrating the mechanism of a reciprocating tachycardia with normal QRS complex in the WPW syndrome. **A.** An atrial premature impulse (A) is conducted to the AV node (N), but the atrial premature impulse is blocked in the anomalous pathway. The atrial premature impulse is then conducted to both ventricles via the bundle branch system. **B.** The atrial impulse is conducted to the atria in retrograde fashion to produce an inverted P wave. **C.** The impulse is conducted in a clockwise fashion, producing reciprocating (reentry) cycle, and the same cycle may repeat indefinitely. Note that the QRS complex during the tachycardia is normal. d = delta wave; P = inverted P wave; S = sinus node.

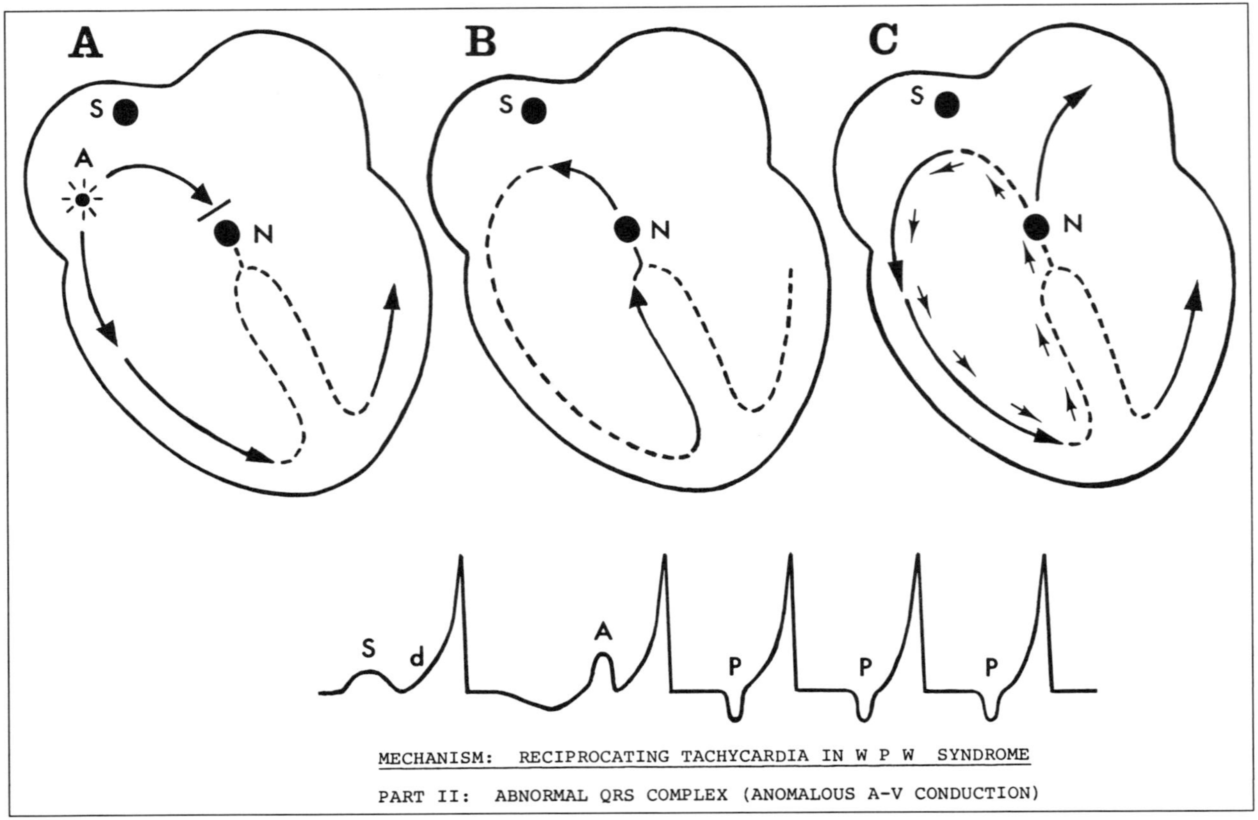


**Fig. 13–4.** Diagram illustrating a reciprocating tachycardia with anomalous conduction in the WPW syndrome. The reentry cycle is counterclockwise, which is exactly the reverse direction to that shown in Fig. 13–3.

atrial flutter with anomalous AV conduction had been simply misinterpreted.
2. On the other hand, a true incidence of VF has been reported in the WPW syndrome recently.
3. The sudden death in the WPW syndrome is most likely due to VF following atrial flutter or AF with extremely rapid ventricular response.

### Other Arrhythmias

Besides the above-mentioned tachyarrhythmias, various other arrhythmias, such as VPCs, AV dissociation, and ventricular or atrial parasystole, may simply coexist with the WPW syndrome.

## OTHER CLINICAL SIGNIFICANCE

In addition to the frequent association of various supraventricular tachyarrhythmias, recognition of the WPW syndrome is extremely important because the QRS complex in WPW syndrome often resembles various other ECG findings.

1. The diagnosis of diaphragmatic (inferior) MI is frequently made erroneously in the WPW syndrome (either type A or B), because of Q or QS waves in leads II, III, and aVF (Fig. 10–4). This ECG finding is observed when the delta wave is directed superiorly.
2. Type B WPW syndrome may closely resemble anterior or anteroseptal MI (Fig. 13–2).
3. Because of the broad QRS complexes due to the delta waves in the WPW syndrome, LBBB or RBBB is closely simulated.
4. Type A WPW syndrome may also be misdiagnosed as true posterior MI or RVH because of the tall R waves in leads $V_{1-3}$.
5. At times, a pseudolateral MI is produced in WPW syndrome.
6. It is also common to observe tall R waves in leads I, aVL, and $V_{4-6}$ with the secondary ST, T wave changes in the WPW syndrome, type B. This ECG finding closely mimics LVH.
7. When the WPW syndrome is observed intermittently (Fig. 13–5), the ECG finding resembles VPCs or even short runs of VT.
8. Recently, it has been demonstrated that a false positive exercise ECG test is common in the WPW syndrome (Fig. 13–6), especially in type B. Therefore, there is no significant diagnostic value to the exercise ECG test when the patient is known to have WPW syndrome.

## DISORDERS COMMONLY ASSOCIATED WITH WPW SYNDROME

1. It has been demonstrated that patients with WPW syndrome often suffer from some form of psychoneurotic disorders and hyperthyroidism. A direct relationship between these disorders and the WPW syndrome is not certain, however.
2. Some patients with AF in WPW syndrome not uncommonly suffer from RHD.
3. Congenital cardiac anomalies frequently associated with the WPW syndrome include Ebstein's anomaly, atrial septal defect, idiopathic hypertrophic subaortic stenosis (IHSS) and MVP syndrome.

## MECHANISMS—ELECTROPHYSIOLOGIC STUDIES

### Reciprocating Tachycardia

1. Electrophysiologic and pathologic studies suggest that the WPW syndrome occurs because of a premature activation of a portion of the ventricles as a result of an anomalous AV conduction via an accessory pathway directly from the atrium to the ventricles.
2. The remaining portion of the ventricular activation results from varying degrees

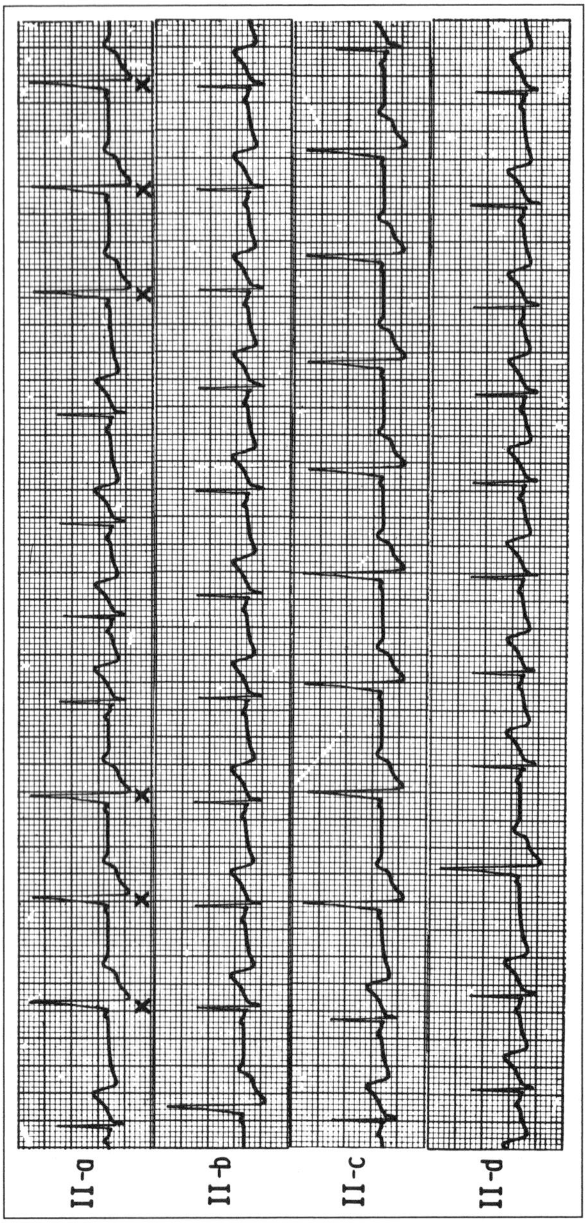


Fig. 13–5. Leads II-a, II-b, II-c, and II-d are continuous. The rhythm is sinus arrhythmia (rate: 74–98 beats/min). The tracing exhibits intermittent WPW syndrome (X), which closely resembles VPCs and nonparoxysmal VT.

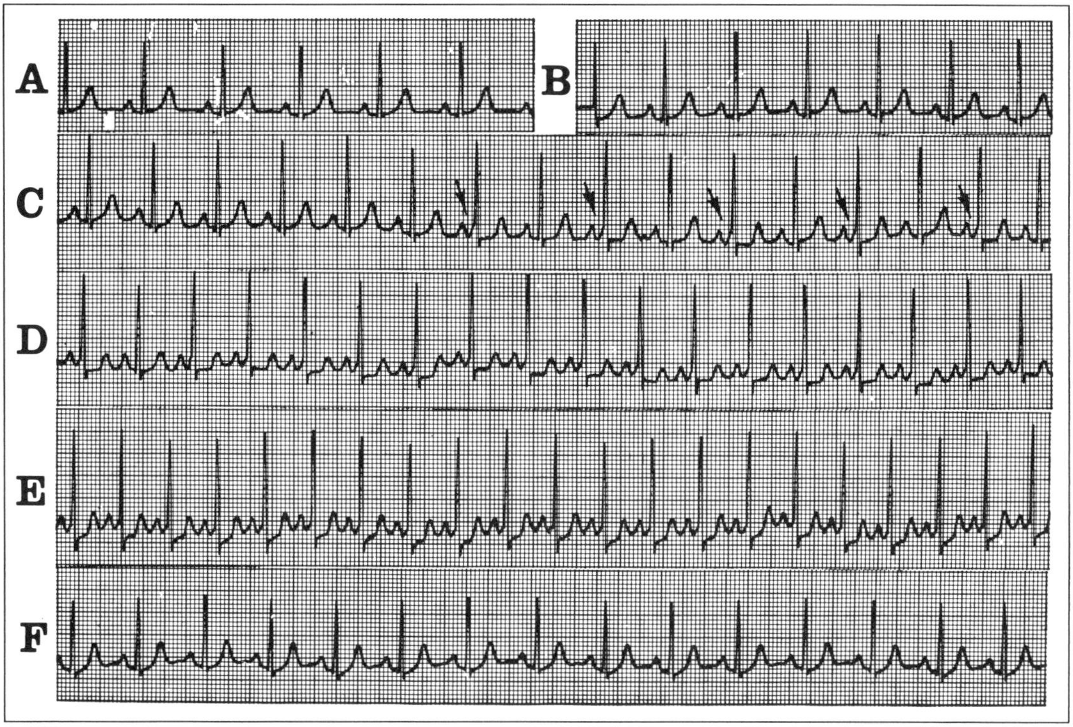


**Fig. 13–6.** Exercise (treadmill) ECG tracings in a 23-year-old man with intermittent WPW syndrome (indicated by arrows). During exercise (strips D and E), the tracing shows WPW syndrome. At rest (strips A and B) and after exercise (strip F), normal AV conduction is present. A false positive exercise ECG test is observed.

of fusion of transmissions via both the normal AV conduction system and the accessory pathway. In the majority of cases with WPW syndrome, the anomalous AV conduction is considered to occur through Kent bundle.

3. On the other hand, a normal P-R interval with delta wave may result from the slow conduction via Kent bundle or conduction via Mahaim tract.
4. Conduction through the James bundle, which is an AV nodal bypass tract, has been considered to be responsible for the LGL syndrome.
5. One of the important roles of the His bundle ECG is to diagnose WPW syndrome with accuracy and to understand the exact mechanisms of tachyarrhythmias associated with the syndrome.
6. In equivocal cases, the His bundle ECG can confirm the diagnosis of WPW syndrome by recognizing a shorter than normal H-V interval, simultaneous occurrence of His bundle deflection and ventricular deflection, or even the occurrence of ventricular deflection preceding the His bundle potential.
7. Electrophysiologic properties of both normal and anomalous AV pathways in patients with WPW syndrome can be examined by the His bundle recordings and atrial stimulation.
8. The P-delta interval is a duration of anomalous pathway conduction time, whereas the A-H interval (simultaneously recorded) indicates normal AV conduction time.
9. The configuration of the QRS complex in WPW syndrome depends upon the degree of fusion in ventricular activation between the impulse conducted via the anomalous conduction and the normal

AV conduction. The QRS complex is relatively narrow when the P-delta and A-H intervals are similar in duration, whereas the QRS contour is markedly bizarre when the A-H interval is long and the P-delta interval is short.

10. Refractory periods of both normal and anomalous pathways can be determined with the extrastimulus technique. It has been demonstrated recently that supraventricular tachycardia in WPW syndrome represents reciprocating tachycardia due to a reentry phenomenon.
11. The reason for the reentry is that marked discrepancy between the refractory periods in the normal and anomalous pathways predisposes to the initiation of reciprocating tachycardia. Diagrammatic illustrations of the mechanisms of reciprocating tachycardia in this syndrome are found in Figures 13–3 and 13–4.
12. Once the reentry is established, the impulse may be conducted antegradely to the ventricles via normal pathway and retrogradely to the atria via anomalous pathway (Figs. 12–3 and 13–3). In this case, the QRS configuration during the tachycardia is normal.
13. On the other hand, the reentry impulse may be conducted antegradely to the ventricles via anomalous pathway and retrogradely to the atria via normal pathway. Under this circumstance, the QRS complex during the tachycardia is bizarre (Fig. 13–4).
14. Clinically, the majority of cases with reciprocating tachycardia in WPW syndrome shows normal QRS complexes because the reentry cycle is carried out via antegrade normal AV conduction with retrograde anomalous conduction (Figs. 12–3 and 13–3).
15. The direction of the reentry cycles depends upon the availability of either normal or anomalous pathway, whichever is in a nonrefractory period. A premature impulse (commonly atrial and less commonly AV junctional or ventricular) will be blocked in a pathway that is refractory, whereas it will be conducted antegradely in another pathway that is nonrefractory. The reentry impulse, then, will be conducted to the atria in retrograde fashion via the pathway that was previously refractory (Figs. 13–3 and 13–4).
16. The reentry cycles may repeat once, twice, or even indefinitely. The reciprocating tachycardia is often terminated by a properly timed atrial premature beat (either spontaneous or induced).
17. Multiple accessory pathways in WPW syndrome have been reported by this author previously, and the His bundle ECG analysis on double accessory pathways has been described recently.

### Atrial Fibrillation and Flutter

1. The exact mechanism responsible for the initiation of AF in the WPW syndrome is not clearly understood.
2. It is considered that AF is triggered by the reentry impulse, which stimulates the atria during the atrial vulnerable period.
3. In AF or atrial flutter in the WPW syndrome, the rapid atrial impulses may be conducted to the ventricles via normal or accessory pathways, whichever is nonrefractory.
4. The QRS complexes during AF or atrial flutter in this syndrome are frequently bizarre and wide because of anomalous conduction plus the common occurrence of aberrant ventricular conduction due to an extremely rapid ventricular rate (Fig. 10–3).

## PREVENTION AND TREATMENT OF TACHYARRHYTHMIAS

No treatment is indicated when the WPW syndrome is not associated with tachyarrhythmias. Similarly, a transient arrhythmia with a short duration also requires no therapy. Paroxysmal reciprocating tachycardia in WPW syndrome is often terminated by vagal maneuvers, such as CSS or Valsalva maneuver (Fig. 12–3). On the other hand, many patients with tachyar-

**TABLE 13–1. Drugs on refractory period in normal and anomalous pathways**

| Drugs | AV Node | Accessory Pathway |
|---|---|---|
| Propranolol | ↑ | ○ |
| Digitalis | ↑ | ↓ |
| Lidocaine | ○ | ↑ |
| Quinidine | ↓ | ↑ |
| Procainamide | ○ | ↑ |
| Diphenylhydantoin | ↓ | Variable |
| Amiodarone | ↑ | ↑ |
| Ajmaline | ○ | ↑ |
| Verapamil | ↑ | Variable |

rhythmias in WPW syndrome require various antiarrhythmic agents (Table 13–1) either acutely or as long-term maintenance therapy. In urgent situations, especially in AF or atrial flutter with extremely rapid ventricular response, DC shock may be needed. When tachyarrhythmias become refractory, artificial pacemaker and even surgical therapy should be considered.

## Principles of Therapy

Therapy should be directed toward changing the conduction times in the normal AV and accessory pathways so that the reentry cycle becomes impossible. This can be accomplished in the following ways:

1. Equalizing the conduction times via the 2 pathways, either by accelerating the normal AV conduction or by slowing the conduction in the anomalous pathway
2. Inducing a functional or organic block in one or both pathways

The equalization of the conduction times can be achieved by atropine or isoproterenol (Isuprel) intravenously, by accelerating the normal AV conduction, but these methods provide only a transient effect. Thus, slowing the conduction in the accessory pathway seems to be a more physiologic approach. Various drugs can produce the slowing of the accessory pathway conduction (Table 13–1).

## Drug Therapy

The His bundle ECG has provided significant contributions to drug therapy for various tachyarrhythmias in the WPW syndrome. The drug of choice can be determined specifically according to the electrophysiologic properties of various antiarrhythmic agents for a given tachyarrhythmia in the WPW syndrome (Table 13–1). For example, it has been shown that lidocaine (Xylocaine) is extremely valuable in terminating supraventricular tachyarrhythmias, especially atrial flutter or AT, with anomalous conduction (Fig. 10–3) because the drug depresses the anomalous pathway. Procainamide and quinidine also are found to be very effective in this circumstance because these agents primarily produce the lengthening of the effective refractory period in the accessory pathway. In addition, quinidine is considered to be very effective because the drug is capable of suppressing atrial (less commonly AV junctional or ventricular) premature beats, which commonly initiate the paroxysmal reciprocating tachycardia in WPW syndrome.

On the other hand, propranolol (Inderal) is considered to be the drug of choice in the treatment of reciprocating tachycardia with normal QRS complexes in WPW syndrome (Fig. 12–3), because the drug depresses the normal AV pathway. In addition, it has been demonstrated that digitalis depresses normal AV conduction, but the drug may accelerate the anomalous conduction in WPW syndrome. Therefore, digitalis is very effective in the treatment of reciprocating tachycardia with normal QRS complex but is contraindicated in the treatment of tachyarrhythmias, particularly AF or atrial flutter, with anomalous AV conduction (Fig. 10–3).

There are several new drugs, such as amiodarone, ajmaline, and verapamil, which are found to be very effective in the treatment of various supraventricular tachyarrhythmias in the WPW syndrome (Table 13–1). Unfortunately, some of these agents are not available in the United States for clinical use.

In addition, various other agents, including phenytoin (Dilantin), acetycholine, neostigmine, atropine, amyl nitrate, and potassium salts, have been used in the past, but these drugs are not always effective in the treatment of rapid heart actions in the WPW syndrome.

To summarize:

1. Propranolol (Inderal) is the drug of choice in the treatment of reciprocating tachycar-

dia with normal QRS complexes in WPW syndrome. Digitalis is equally effective in this situation, but Inderal is considered to be superior to digitalis.

2. Lidocaine (intravenous injection) is considered to be the drug of choice for tachyarrhythmias, particularly AF or atrial flutter, with anomalous conduction. Procainamide or quinidine has been found to be effective in this circumstance. Digitalis is contraindicated in this case because it may accelerate the conduction via the accessory pathway.
3. For the prevention of arrhythmias, as maintenance doses, propranolol (10–30 mg 3–4 times daily by mouth) is the most useful agent, particularly for reciprocating tachycardia with normal QRS complexes. In the prevention of AF or atrial flutter, quinidine (0.3–0.4 g 4 times daily by mouth) is the drug of choice. In some malignant cases, a combined drug therapy (e.g., propranolol and quinidine) may be required.
4. New agents, such as amiodarone, ajmaline, and verapamil, are found to be very effective in certain cases, but some of these agents are not available for clinical use in the United States.

## Direct Current Shock

1. Direct current shock is the most effective treatment for any type of tachyarrhythmias associated with WPW syndrome.
2. In urgent situations, such as in supraventricular tachyarrhythmias with extremely rapid ventricular response, especially in AF or atrial flutter with anomalous conduction, DC shock is the treatment of choice.
3. In addition, any drug-resistant refractory tachyarrhythmias should be treated with DC shock under the usual precautions.
4. When the patient is taking digitalis, DC shock should be applied with extreme care because serious postcardioversion arrhythmias, such as VF, may be provoked. In order to prevent the postcardioversion arrhythmias under this circumstance, phenytoin 125–250 mg may be given intravenously a few minutes before the application of DC shock. In general, DC shock should be avoided if possible when the patient is taking digitalis.
5. For atrial flutter, only low energy (5–50 watt seconds) may be sufficient for its termination.
6. On the other hand, AF or other tachyarrhythmias usually require higher energy (above 100 watt seconds).
7. Needless to say, immediate application of defibrillator is the only life-saving measure if the patient suffers from VF.
8. Direct current shock is effective whether the configurations of the QRS complexes during tachyarrhythmias are normal or wide (either due to anomalous conduction or due to aberrant ventricular conduction).
9. However, DC shock is not indicated when the paroxysmal tachyarrhythmia is of short duration or is easily converted to sinus rhythm spontaneously or by a simple procedure, such as CSS (Fig. 12–3).
10. It should be noted that most patients with the WPW syndrome require various drugs (e.g., propranolol or quinidine) as outlined above following termination of the tachyarrhythmia in order to prevent its recurrence.

## Artificial Pacemakers

1. In the treatment of drug-resistant or DC shock-resistant tachyarrhythmias associated with WPW syndrome, the use of an artificial pacemaker should be considered. This is particularly true when the surgical approach is contraindicated or the procedure is declined by the patient.
2. The fundamental mechanism responsible for the termination of various tachyarrhythmias by artificial pacing is that the reenty cycle of the tachycardia can be considered to be interrupted by the pacing stimuli.

3. An appropriately timed pacing-induced atrial or ventricular impulse may block the reentry cycle either in the AV node or anomalous pathway so that the atria or ventricles become refractory to the reentry (reciprocating) impulse.
4. Artificial pacing is found to be most effective when the pacing electrodes are close to the anomalous pathway.
5. The pacing can be carried out by the transvenous approach to the right ventricle or coronary sinus (near the left atrium and left ventricle) or by transthoracic approach to the epicardium of any of the cardiac chambers.
6. As soon as the patient feels the tachycardia, artificial pacing can be initiated as the fixed-rate unit by means of a magnet placed over the implanted battery-powered demand pacemaker.
7. Artificial pacing by a radiofrequency device is found to be equally effective in terminating the reciprocating tachycardia in WPW syndrome. By this method, the development of AF is reported to be a potential risk when the rate of discharge is sufficiently high. It has been recommended that radiofrequency pacemakers should only be used when the refractory properties of the anomalous pathway are known. There has been no reported risk of the development of VF associated with the use of artificial pacemakers in the treatment of various tachyarrhythmias in the WPW syndrome.

## Surgical Approach

1. The surgical approach is considered only in selected patients who suffer from recurrent supraventricular tachyarrhythmias that cause significant disturbances in their lives in any way (socially, physically, or mentally) or life-threatening arrhythmias refractory to the usual drug therapy, as outlined above.
2. The rationale for surgical therapy is, obviously, to interrupt the reentry cycle, which is considered to be responsible for the tachyarrhythmias in WPW syndrome.
3. Electrophysiologically, the surgical approach will be the definitive way of therapy for tachyarrhythmias in the WPW syndrome. However, a successful surgical result is not always possible in every case.
4. Surgical treatment has been carried out in a relatively small number of patients, and the most data have been accumulated at Duke University Medical Center.
5. It has been shown that surgical results have been more favorable in patients with an anomalous pathway in the LV or RV free wall AV connections than in those with septal connections. In addition, there is a potential risk of damaging the normal AV conduction system in patients with septal connections.
6. In general, AF or atrial flutter in WPW syndrome is difficult to control by various drugs, and the surgical result is also not favorable.
7. It should be emphasized that the surgical approach is attempted only at medical institutions where multichannel, high-fidelity equipment for recording with facilities for cardiopulmonary bypass are available in the operating room. Needless to say, it requires a skillful electrophysiologist and surgical team who are fully familiar with the procedure.
8. The activation sequence of the human heart is measured by epicardial mapping for an accurate demonstration of the area of preexcitation. The epicardial mapping is performed by measuring local activation times at approximately 55 epicardial sites, and a point of the earliest epicardial preexcitation is identified. The incision is made through the atrial wall at its attachment to the mitral or tricuspid valve annulus.
9. The alternative surgical treatment for refractory tachyarrhythmias in WPW syndrome is the His bundle section. In this case, implantation of the permanent pacemaker is necessary. This method can prevent reciprocating tachycardia, but AF via the anomalous pathway cannot be prevented.

# Chapter 14

# Sick Sinus Syndrome

There has been an increasing awareness of the clinical entity, the sick sinus syndrome (SSS), in the past decade because the syndrome is found to be relatively common in our practice, particularly among elderly individuals, and it can be successfully treated with artificial cardiac pacing in most cases. Sick sinus syndrome has been used to describe a broad spectrum of clinical manifestations (e.g., syncope or near-syncope, dizziness, increased CHF, and/or angina and palpitations) as a result of a dysfunctioning sinus node. Electrocardiographic manifestations in the SSS may include (1) persistent and marked sinus bradycardia, (2) SA block, (3) sinus arrest, (4) long pause following an APC, (5) chronic AF or atrial flutter with slow ventricular rate, (6) carotid sinus hypersensitivity, (7) no stable sinus rhythm after cardioversion, (8) AV JER with or without slow and unstable sinus activity, and (9) BTS. These ECG findings in SSS are not drug induced.

Various terms have been used to describe these phenomena, including "sick sinus syndrome," "sinoatrial syncope," "sluggish sinus node syndrome," "inadequate sinus mechanism," "sick sinus node," and "lazy sinus node." When tachyarrhythmia components are present intermittently or periodically during slow rhythm, various terms, such as "bradytachyarrhythmia syndrome," "bradytachy syndrome," and "tachycardia-bradycardia syndrome," have been used. Although some investigators use the terms "SSS" and "BTS" interchangeably, BTS is one of the common manifestations of SSS in most cases.

As can be expected, the degree of sinus node dysfunction may be so minimal that the SSS may be manifested only by slight sinus bradycardia. In this case, the patient is usually asymptomatic. On the other hand, the sinus node may be severely diseased, leading to complete generator failure, that is, prolonged sinus arrest or AF with slow ventricular rate. Advanced SSS is nearly always symptomatic. Various symptoms in the SSS are usually related to either cardiac or cerebral dysfunction. The perfusion deficit in these organs is responsible for the production of various symptoms in the SSS. Syncope or near-syncope is the most common clinical manifestation of the SSS.

## ANATOMY AND ELECTROPHYSIOLOGY

The sinus node has both sympathetic and parasympathetic (vagal) innervation, but the latter is richer in the AV node. The electrophysiologic event, spontaneous phase 4 depolarization, is the determining factor to distinguish between the pacemaker cells and all cells in the body. The sinus node is the dominant pacemaker because the sinus node cells possess the fastest spontaneous depolarization. The spontaneous sinus node depolarization can be altered by parasympathetic and sympathetic influences. Vagal stimulation or acetylcholine can slow automaticity of the sinus node by reducing the slope of phase 4 depolarization as well as hyperpolarizing the cells. On the other hand, sympathetic stimulation or catecholamine infusion enhances the spontaneous sinus node discharge rate, primarily as a result of an increase in the rate of phase 4 depolarization

Various investigative studies confirmed that the sinus node is the primary pacemaker in the heart. Since the sinus node possesses the fastest inherent rate of any cardiac pacemakers, sinus rhythm is present in the majority of healthy individuals. In SSS, when the sinus node produces the cardiac impulses slower than usual (sinus bradycardia), fails to produce any impulse (sinus arrest), or the sinus impulse is not conducted to the atria due to SA block, the subsidiary pacemaker (commonly AV junction) will take over the ventricular activity as an escape mechanism. On the other hand, the chronic generator failure (sinus arrest) not uncommonly leads to the establishment of chronic AF (often with slow ventricular rate).

The size of the sinus node is approximately 15 mm in length, 5–7 mm in width, and 1.5–2.0 mm in thickness. The shape of the sinus node varies, but, by and large, it resembles an extended snail with its shell, which misleads one to think of the node as having a head, body, and tail. Since the sinus node is situated at a position that is less than 1 mm beneath the epicardial surface, the sinus node is vulnerable to many disease processes, including trauma or pericarditis. The superficial anatomic location of the sinus node may be responsible for the development of the SSS in many cases, directly or indirectly.

The sinus node artery in the human heart is commonly located near the center of the sinus node, but it may be eccentric. In approximately 55–60% of human hearts, the sinus node artery arises from the proximal 2–3 cm of the right coronary artery, whereas, in 40–45% of cases, it arises from the proximal 1 cm of the left circumflex coronary artery. Other origins of the sinus node artery are rare and account for about 2% of the total. At times, there are 2 branches of the sinus node artery of equal size. The sinus node artery, regardless of whether it arises from the right or left coronary artery, courses along the anteromedial atrial wall of the base of the superior vena cava, which it encircles. This artery anastomoses with other atrial arteries of both ipsilateral and contralateral origin. Generally, the primary arterial supply of the sinus node is practically always unilateral in origin. Smaller branches of the artery are distributed throughout the sinus node. Small veins are commonly found throughout the sinus node, whereas large veins are present infrequently.

Microscopically, the sinus node is composed of 3 types of cells, including P cells, transitional cells, and working cells. The term "P cells" has been used because of their pale appearance, which resembles primitive myocardial cells. The P cells are thought to be responsible for sinus node pacemaker function.

The Purkinjelike fibers, the internodal pathways that connect from the sinus node to the specialized atrial conduction tissue, have been described: the anterior, middle, and posterior internodal tracts. By electrophysiologic studies, it has been demonstrated that the cardiac impulse from the sinus node reaches the AV node more rapidly than it would if it were conducted through the ordinary myocardium. Although any 1 of 3 internodal pathways may be responsible for intraatrial conduction, the conduction is thought to be carried out preferentially via the anterior tract in most normal hearts. This view is not uniformly accepted, however.

## UNDERLYING CAUSES

Although such various drugs as digitalis, propranolol, and quinidine frequently cause dysfunction of the sinus node, these functionally reversible effects on the sinus node are not considered part of the SSS. The basic underlying causes of the SSS are anatomic, with physiologic consequences that produce a long-standing and often irreversible process in the sinus node.

### Coronary Artery Disease

1. Coronary artery disease (CAD), particularly MI, has been reported to be the most common underlying disease to produce the SSS.
2. Dysfunction of the sinus node was reported to occur in approximately 5% of acute MI. In addition, the sinus node dysfunction can be expected to be present in half of the patients with diaphragmatic MI.
3. Dysfunction of the sinus node is usually observed during the first 4 days of MI under this circumstance.
4. Commonly, sinus node dysfunction is manifested by a progressive sinus bradycardia followed by various supraventricu-

lar arrhythmias including AF or atrial flutter, and AV JER with a periodic restoration of sinus bradycardia and intermittent sinus arrest or SA block.

5. Atrial MI may cause sinus node dysfunction on rare occasions. Atrial damage including sinus node dysfunction is very common as a result of main right coronary artery occlusions (causing diaphragmatic MI) and left circumflex artery occlusions (causing anterolateral MI).

### Sclerotic-Degenerative Process

1. When one eliminates CAD as a cause of the SSS, most of the remaining cases show no clear evidence of clinical heart disease that is responsible for the production of the SSS. Under this circumstance, a sclerotic-degenerative process involving the sinus node is considered to be responsible for the SSS in most cases.
2. Pathologic studies revealed that severe fibrosis involving the sinus node and sinoatrial junction was the main feature of the SSS.
3. In some cases of the SSS, amyloid infiltration involving the sinus node was demonstrated.

### Other Disorders

In addition, many other underlying causes may be responsible for the SSS.

1. They may include RHD, cardiomyopathies, congenital heart disease, surgical trauma, hypertension, pericarditis, myocarditis, amyloidosis systemic lupus erythematosus, muscular dystrophy, Friedreich's ataxia, malignancy, hemochromatosis, and diphtheria.
2. Familial incidence of the SSS has been reported.
3. Its association with long Q-T syndrome also has been described.
4. Recently, the SSS associated with systemic embolism and MVP syndrome has been reported.

## ELECTROCARDIOGRAPHIC MANIFESTATIONS

Depending upon the degree of the sinus node dysfunction, various ECG abnormalities may be produced in SSS (Table 14–1). Persisting and severe sinus bradycardia (not due to drugs) is the most common (75–80% of all patients with SSS) and the earliest manifestation of SSS, and it is followed by various other ECG abnormalities as the syndrome progresses further. In a long-standing SSS, AF is the most common underlying rhythm. When the SSS is far advanced, it will be manifested by BTS in which a variety of cardiac rhythms will be observed in many cases. In addition, AV conduction disturbances and intraventricular block often coexist in many cases with advanced SSS

**TABLE 14–1. Sick sinus syndrome: ECG manifestations**

A. Marked and persisting sinus bradycardia
B. Sinus arrest and/or SA block
C. Drug (e.g., atropine, Isuprel)-resistant sinus bradyarrhythmias
D. Long pause following an atrial premature contraction
E. Prolonged sinus node recovery time determined by atrial pacing
F. Chronic atrial fibrillation or repetitive occurrence of atrial fibrillation (less commonly atrial flutter)
   1. With slow ventricular rate
   2. Preceded or followed by sinus bradycardia, sinus arrest, or SA block
G. AV junctional escape rhythm (with or without slow and unstable sinus activity)
H. Carotid sinus syncope
I. Failure of restoration of sinus rhythm following cardioversion
J. Bradytachyarrhythmia syndrome
K. Common coexisting AV block and/or intraventricular block
L. Any combination of the above

## Sinus Bradycardia

Although some degree of sinus bradycardia is very common in many healthy individuals, especially in athletes, a persisting and marked sinus bradycardia (not due to various drugs) deserves medical investigation.

1. Sick sinus syndrome should be strongly suspected when chronic sinus bradycardia shows a rate slower than 40–45 beats/min with or without symptoms.
2. Marked sinus bradycardia may produce symptoms, such as lightheadedness, near-syncope, or syncope.
3. It should be certain that sinus bradycardia is not due to drugs, such as propranolol (Inderal), digitalis, reserpine (Serpasil), guanethidine (Ismelin), and methyldopa (Aldomet).
4. On the other hand, SSS may be unmasked by small amounts of drugs, particularly digitalis or propranolol. In other words, marked sinus bradycardia following administration of a small amount of these drugs strongly suggests the SSS, especially in elderly individuals.
5. When sinus bradycardia is marked, one or more AV JEBs may occur and incomplete AV dissociation is often produced. At times, marked sinus bradycardia may lead to AV junctional escape-bigeminy, in which sinus beats and AV JEBs occur on every other beat. When the AV node is dis-

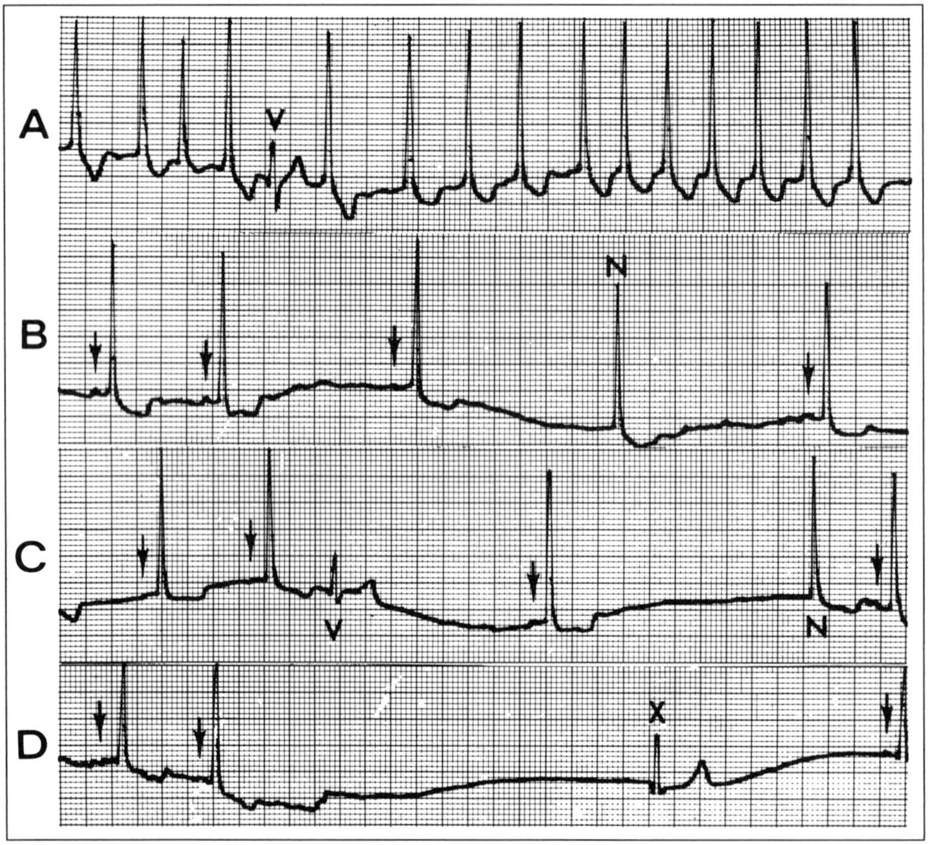


**Fig. 14–1.** The Holter monitor ECG rhythm strips A, B, C, and D are *not* continuous. Bradytachyarrhythmia as a manifestation of advanced SSS is shown in this Holter monitor ECG tracing. The ECG abnormalities include marked sinus bradycardia (indicated by arrows) and occasional AV junctional as well as ventricular escape beats (N and X) following sinus arrest, AF with rapid ventricular response, and VPCs (V).

eased together with sinus node—a common occurrence—the AV JER also produces a markedly slow rate.

6. At times, VEBs may appear to control the ventricular activity in severe sinus bradycardia when the AV node is unable to produce the expected escape impulses as a result of permanent disease of the AV node.
7. Marked sinus bradycardia is often irregular, and it may be followed by atrial or ventricular tachyarrhythmias leading to BTS (Figs. 14–1, 14–2, and 14–3).
8. First degree AV block (the P-R interval: 0.24 second or more) also commonly coexists.

## Sinus Arrest and/or Sinoatrial Block

1. When SSS further progresses, the sinus node fails to produce any cardiac impulse leading to sinus arrest (Fig. 14–1). The long P-P interval due to sinus arrest has no relationship to the basic P-P cycle.
2. During the sinus arrest, it is common to observe 1 or more AV JEBs (less commonly VEBs) to control the ventricular activity (Fig. 14–1).
3. In some other cases with SSS, SA block may be observed. In SA block, the sinus impulse is unable to conduct to the atria as a result of a block at the SA junction (Fig. 4–4).
4. Sinoatrial block has 2 forms, Mobitz type I and II. Mobitz type II SA block is characterized by intermittent absence of the expected P wave(s) in which the long P-P interval is a multiple of the basic P-P cycle. On the other hand, Mobitz type I (Wenckebach) SA block produces a progressive shortening of the P-P cycles until a pause occurs. Mobitz type I (Wenckebach) SA block is analogous to Mobitz type I (Wenckebach) AV block, and Mobitz type II SA block is analogous to Mobitz type II AV block.
5. In cases of far-advanced SA block or sinus arrest, the sinus activity is almost completely or, at times, entirely absent, leading to atrial standstill.
6. When the basic sinus cycle is irregular, it is impossible to distinguish between sinus arrest and SA block.

## Drug-resistant Sinus Bradyarrhythmias

1. When the sinus bradyarrhythmias fail to respond to atropine or isoproterenol (Isuprel), the diagnosis of the SSS is almost certain.
2. Diagnosis of the SSS is usually entertained if the sinus rate is not accelerated beyond 90 beats/min by intravenous injection of atropine sulfate (1–2 mg).
3. For a similar reason, the SSS can be diagnosed when intravenous Isuprel (1–2 mg/min) fails to enhance the sinus rate beyond 90–100 beats/min in sinus bradycardia.
4. It should be noted that Isuprel administration may provoke ventricular tachyarrhythmias.

## Long Pause Following an Atrial Premature Contraction

In general, an APC is not followed by a full compensatory pause because the sinus node is passively activated by the ectopic atrial impulse. Thus, the automaticity of the sinus node is momentarily disturbed by the ectopic atrial impulse. Occasionally, an APC is followed by a full compensatory pause when an APC occurs during late cardiac cycle so that the sinus node impulse formation is not disturbed. In this case, the interference (collision) between the sinus impulse and ectopic atrial impulse occurs at the SA junction, in the atria, or at the AV junction.

1. Although a postectopic pause following an APC is not fully compensatory, the returning cycle (the interval from the ectopic P wave to the first sinus P wave) is usually longer than the basic sinus P-P cycle because of a transient suppression of the

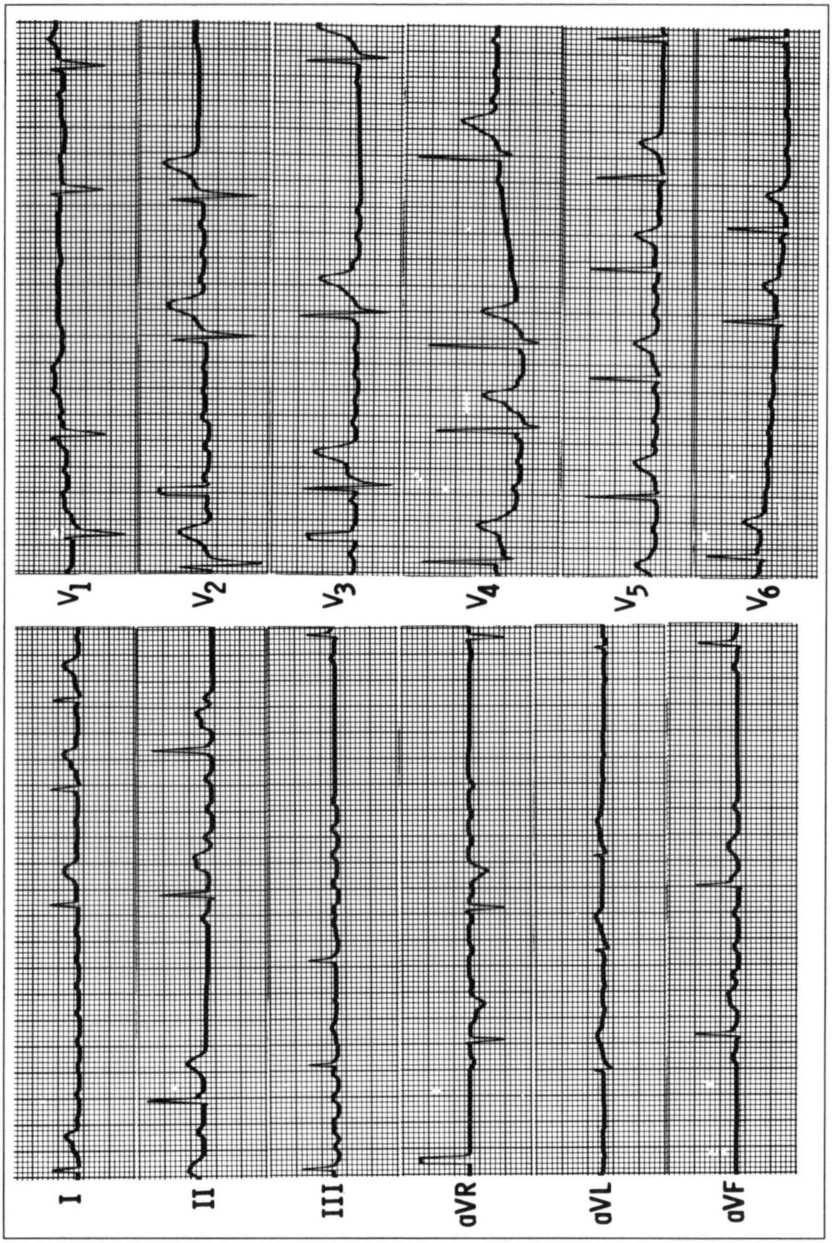


**Fig. 14–2.** Sick sinus syndrome is manifested by marked sinus bradycardia and intermittent atrial flutter with advanced AV block.

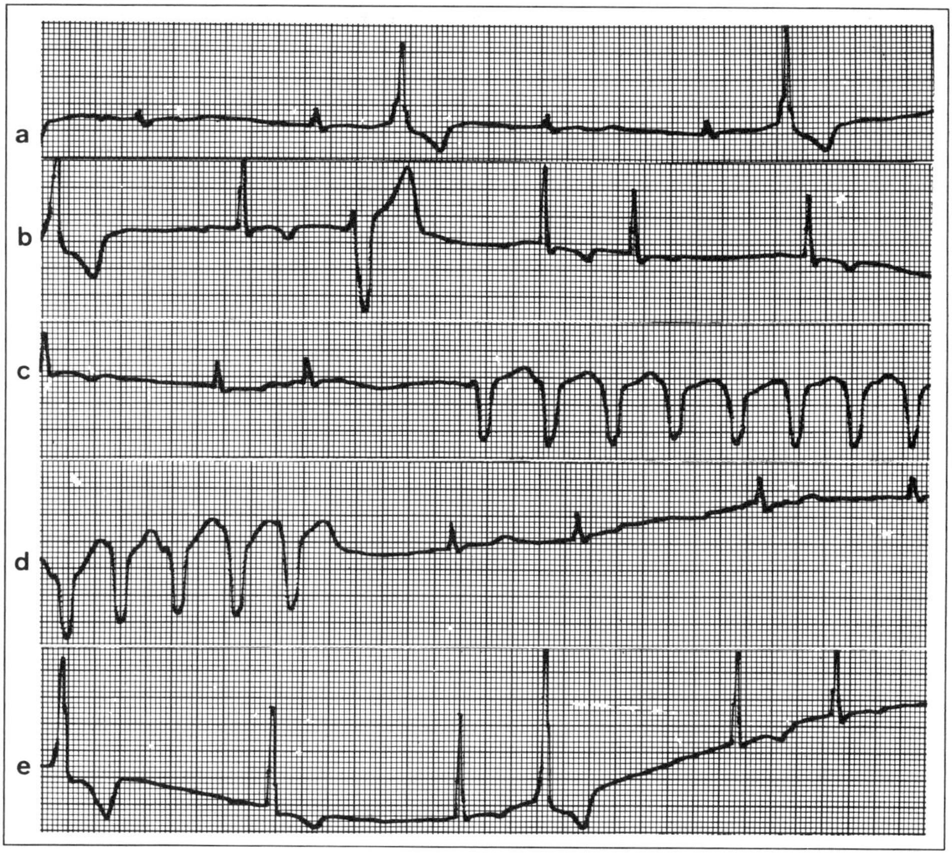


**Fig. 14–3.** The Holter monitor ECG rhythm strips a, b, c, d, and e are not continuous. Bradytachyarrhythmia as a manifestation of SSS is demonstrated in this Holter monitor ECG tracing. The ECG abnormalities include unstable sinus bradycardia (P waves are not clearly evident) with first degree AV block, frequent multifocal VPCs, and a short run of VT.

sinus node by the ectopic atrial impulse—a physiologic phenomenon.

2. When the returning cycle is longer than usual, however, an abnormally prolonged refractory period of the sinus node is suspected.
3. In cases of markedly prolonged sinus node recovery time due to SSS, a single APC may be sufficient to produce sinus arrest, leading to absence of the sinus P waves for a long period of time.
4. Atrioventricular JER or VER frequently appears to activate the ventricles under this circumstance.

## Prolonged Sinus Node Recovery Time Determined by Atrial Pacing

The prolonged sinus node recovery time determined by a rapid atrial pacing (rate: 120–150 beats/min) is a reliable indicator of the SSS. The rapid atrial pacing is particularly valuable when the ECG manifestations of the SSS are not obvious and when the clinical symptoms of the syndrome are vague. Detailed descriptions regarding the determination of the sinus node recovery time and its usefulness are given under Diagnostic Approach.

## Chronic Atrial Fibrillation or Repetitive Occurrence of Atrial Fibrillation (Less Commonly, Atrial Flutter)

1. Chronic AF is the most common underlying rhythm in patients with far-advanced SSS, in which the sinus node is no longer capable of producing the cardiac impulse.
2. In this case, AF is often associated with slow ventricular rate (rate: 30–50 beats/min) as a result of advanced AV block, and 1 or more AV JEBs (less commonly VEBs) may occur.
3. Until AF is well established as a chronic form, it is often preceded by or followed by marked sinus bradycardia, sinus arrest, or SA block, with or without first degree AV block (Fig. 14–1).
4. Less commonly, atrial flutter is the underlying rhythm in advanced SSS, and again the ventricular rate is often slow due to advanced AV block (Fig. 14–2).
5. Until atrial flutter is well established, it is often preceded by or followed by marked sinus bradycardia, sinus arrest, or SA block in SSS.
6. In some cases with the SSS, however, the ventricular rate is relatively fast in AF or atrial flutter, leading to BTS (Fig. 14–1).

## Atrioventricular Junctional Escape Rhythm (with or without Slow and Unstable Sinus Activity)

1. When marked sinus bradycardia is further deteriorated, it is often followed by sinus arrest, and AV JER may become the underlying rhythm with or without any unstable sinus activity (Fig. 6–2).
2. The AV JER is commonly irregular until it becomes well established as a chronic form.
3. In chronic AV JER, its cycle is usually regular.
4. Under this circumstance, retrograde P waves may be preceded by or followed by the QRS complexes, and at times, no P wave is discernible (Fig. 6–2).

## Carotid Sinus Syncope

It has been reported that sudden development of sinus arrest by CSS lasting more than 3 seconds is highly suggestive of inappropriate sinus node responsiveness—the SSS (Fig. 12–4). Similarly, the appearance of a long ventricular standstill in chronic AF or atrial flutter induced by CSS probably represents the same clinical significance.

## Failure of Restoration of Sinus Rhythm Following Cardioversion

The SSS is strongly suspected when there is an inability of the heart to restore stable sinus rhythm for a long period of time following termination of any ectopic tachyarrhythmias by DC shock. This is particularly true following the termination of AF or atrial flutter. Under this circumstance, AV JER becomes the dominant rhythm in many cases with or without unstable sinus P waves. In far-advanced SSS, AF may persist with unstable AV JER or VER following the termination of ventricular tachyarrhythmias by DC shock.

## Bradytachyarrhythmia Syndrome

Although some investigators use the terms "BTS" and "SSS" interchangeably, they are by no means identical. It should be reemphasized that BTS is often 1 of the common manifestations of advanced SSS.

1. In the BTS, the bradyarrhythmia component is commonly marked sinus bradycardia and less commonly chronic AF with slow ventricular rate.

2. The most common tachyarrhythmia component in BTS is AF with rapid ventricular response and less commonly atrial flutter with rapid (often 2:1) ventricular response (Figs. 14–1 and 14–2).
3. Paroxysmal atrial tachycardia or AV JT as a tachyarrhythmia component in BTS is not very common.
4. The occurrence of ventricular tachyarrhythmia in BTS has been reported to be 8–10% by different authors (Fig. 14–3).

### Common Coexisting Atrioventricular Block and/or Intraventricular Block

Although AV block or intraventricular block per se is not a part of the SSS, they often coexist because the same underlying disease process—degenerative-sclerotic change—may involve diffusely the entire conduction system. This is the reason that advanced or even complete AV block often occurs in chronic AF or atrial flutter, leading to a very slow ventricular rate in advanced SSS. In addition, first degree AV block (P-R interval greater than 0.24 second) is extremely common in BTS, and it is often preceded by or followed by AF with slow ventricular rate. Furthermore, various forms of intraventricular block frequently coexist with the SSS.

### Any Combination of Above Findings

As can be expected, various ECG manifestations of the SSS itself may be present, or common coexisting ECG abnormalities (e.g., AV block, intraventricular block, AV JER or VER) may occur together with the SSS. For example, 1 ECG tracing with advanced SSS may consist of marked sinus bradycardia, sinus arrest, AV JER and VER, paroxysmal AF, and VPCs. Another example of the SSS may be manifested by sinus bradycardia, intermittent SA block, LBBB, and VEBs.

## CLINICAL CONSIDERATIONS

Laslett described syncopal attacks associated with bradycardia for the first time in 1909. There have been increasing interest and awareness of the therapeutic problems regarding the SSS and the BTS among physicians since Short described the therapeutic dilemma in patients presenting sinus bradycardia and tachyarrhythmia associated with syncope.

The clinical manifestations in patients with the SSS are fundamentally due to hypoperfusion of the vital organs, particularly the brain, heart, and kidney as a result of markedly slow ventricular rate that may or may not be associated with tachyarrhythmias.

### Sex and Age

There is no particular sexual preponderance in SSS, but the syndrome has been reported more frequently among elderly females than males.

1. Sick sinus syndrome may involve any age group, although the syndrome is primarily a disease of elderly individuals.
2. The peak incidence of the SSS has been reported to be in the sixth and seventh decades of life.
3. It has been suggested that the SSS may be the cause of sudden death in some young athletes.
4. A recent report described 8 Africans with SSS, and all of them were age 32 or younger.
5. Recent literature indicates that SSS is not uncommon in young people in some parts of the world. The life expectancy in the different parts of the world seems to influence greatly the peak incidence of the SSS.

### Underlying Heart Diseases

1. As described previously in this chapter, the most common underlying heart disease in SSS has been reported to be CAD (about 50% incidence).

2. The next common underlying disease process seems to be idiopathic, i.e., sclerotic-degenerative change in the sinus node and other conduction system (about 30–35% incidence).
3. Of course, many patients with SSS may have more than 1 underlying cardiac disease.
4. Less common underlying diseases of SSS may include RHD, congenital heart disease, hypertension, cardiomyopathy, amyloidosis, hemochromatosis, surgical injury, myocarditis, pericarditis, Friedreich's ataxia, progressive muscular dystrophy, collagen disease, and metastatic disease.

## Clinical Manifestations

Clinical manifestations of the SSS may be multifaceted, and they may occur only intermittently. The most common manifestations of advanced SSS are lightheadedness, near-syncope, or actual syncope, but in mild cases, the patient may be totally asymptomatic, or SSS may be extremely difficult to recognize or evaluate in the early stage.

**Cerebral Manifestations:**

1. In mild cases or early stages of SSS, diminished cerebral arterial blood flow may be manifested by generalized fatigue, muscle ache, or slight personality changes, including irritability, intermittent memory loss, and insomnia.
2. When SSS progresses further, cerebral manifestations may include slurred speech, pareses, erroneous judgment, lightheadedness, and near-syncope followed by actual fainting episodes.
3. Severe cerebral manifestations, such as syncope or near-syncope, are almost always due to marked slowing of the heart rate or cardiac arrest, and the tachycardia component seldom produces significant cerebral symptoms.
4. Since the SSS is primarily the disease of elderly individuals, the various cerebral manifestations are frequently misinterpreted as cerebrovascular accidents or simply as "senility."
5. Syncope or near-syncope has been reported to occur in 40–70% of patients with the SSS. The incidence of dizziness was reported to be 6–7% of patients with the SSS.

**Cardiac Manifestations:** As can be expected, various cardiac manifestations are the second most common finding in SSS.

1. In the early stage of mild SSS, cardiac manifestations, other than a slow heart rate or mixture of slow and rapid cardiac rhythms may be completely absent.
2. The 3 most common cardiac manifestations in SSS include palpitations, increased signs of CHF, and increased angina.
3. In some instances, a sudden occurrence of or episodic acute pulmonary edema may be the first sign of the SSS because the patient may not seek medical attention during the mild stage of the syndrome.
4. Feelings of palpitations may be due to extremely slow rhythm itself (e.g., sinus bradycardia or AF with advanced AV block), irregular rhythm, or a mixture of slow and rapid rhythms (BTS).
5. Most patients experience palpitations when the cardiac rhythm suddenly changes from slow rhythm to rapid rhythm, or vice versa.
6. The occurrence of the 3 common cardiac manifestations (palpitations, angina, and CHF) of the SSS is closely interrelated, and 1 symptom frequently aggravates the others.
7. In far-advanced cases of the SSS, patients may develop prolonged cardiac arrest or VF leading to death.

**Other Manifestations:** Various nonspecific manifestations, such as oliguria, gastrointestinal distress, and so on are not uncommon in the SSS, but these findings are usually secondary due to hypoperfusion to the heart itself.

**TABLE 14–2. Sick sinus syndrome: Diagnostic approach**

A. Clinical manifestations
B. Routine 12-lead ECG
C. Ambulatory (Holter monitor) ECG
D. Carotid sinus stimulation and Valsalva maneuver
E. Cardioversion
F. Exercise (stress) ECG test
G. Drugs (e.g., atropine, isoproterenol)
H. Electrophysiologic studies
   1. Determination of sinus node recovery time by atrial pacing
   2. Determination of SA conduction time by atrial extrastimulus technique
   3. His bundle ECG

# DIAGNOSTIC APPROACH

In mild cases of the SSS, it is not always easy to diagnose with certainty (Table 14–2). A high index of suspicion is often necessary in many cases to reach a correct diagnosis during the early stage of SSS. Marked and persisting sinus bradycardia (not due to drugs) should always raise the possibility of the SSS even in totally asymptomatic young individuals including athletes.

## Clinical Manifestations

Diagnosis of the SSS cannot be made with certainty by recognizing clinical findings alone. However, the SSS must be included among differential diagnosis when dealing with any patient with a history of syncope or near-syncope. Similarly, SSS should be suspected as a possible underlying disorder in any individual with unexplained pulmonary edema, palpitations, or angina, particularly when these findings (singly or together) are associated with slow heart rate not due to drugs (e.g., digitalis, propranolol).

## Routine 12-lead Electrocardiogram

Diagnosis of advanced SSS can be confirmed by the typical ECG findings shown on a routine 12-lead ECG or long rhythm strips.

## Ambulatory (Holter Monitor) Electrocardiogram

When the typical ECG findings of SSS are not documented on the routine 12-lead ECG because the finding is intermittent, the Holter monitor ECG is the best diagnostic tool.

## Carotid Sinus Stimulation and Valsalva Maneuver

Sinus arrest lasting more than 3 seconds with CSS is strongly suggestive of inappropriate sinus node responsiveness (Fig. 12–4), the SSS. As with CSS, the response to the Valsalva maneuver may be useful to demonstrate sinus node dysfunction. The Valsalva maneuver produces the expected changes in aortic pulse pressure but causes little or no change in pulse rate. In contrast, physiologic bradycardia of the elderly demonstrates the expected acceleration of the heart rate during the strain phase (phase II) and the subsequent slowing of the heart rate during the BP overshoot (phase IV). However, it should be noted that these procedures provide no direct diagnostic evidence of sinus node disease but give a clue to the functional status of the sinus node. Further investigation is often indicated in many cases.

## Cardioversion

Needless to say, cardioversion is not a diagnostic method for SSS. However, a failure of restoration of sinus rhythm following the termination of any ectopic tachyarrhythmia by the procedure is strongly diagnostic of SSS.

## Exercise Electrocardiography

When the sinus rate does not increase significantly by the standard exercise ECG (e.g., treadmill) protocol, the SSS may be suspected providing that inappropriate sinus rate change is not influenced by drugs (e.g., propranolol).

Of course, healthy individuals in good physical condition (e.g., daily runners, athletes) may not show significant increment of the heart rate by the exercise ECG protocol simply because of insufficient workload rather than sinus node dysfunction.

## Drugs

1. The SSS is often suspected when any individual, particularly an elderly person, develops marked sinus bradycardia following administration of a small amount of digitalis or propranolol (Inderal). However, this finding is not always reliable in the diagnosis of SSS.
2. Recently, atropine has been used frequently to evaluate the response of the sinus node. Physiologic sinus bradycardia responds to the intravenous administration of atropine by a normal or exaggerated acceleration of the sinus rate.
3. On the other hand, no significant increment of the sinus rate is observed in SSS following atropine administration.
4. It has been suggested that when intravenous atropine sulfate (1–2 mg) fails to increase the sinus rate beyond 90 beats/min in sinus bradycardia and when the sinus node recovery time remains prolonged by rapid (pacing rate: 120–140 beats/min for 2–4 minutes) atrial pacing after atropine injection, the diagnosis of SSS can be made.
5. Similarly, the diagnosis of the SSS may be entertained when the sinus rate does not increase beyond 90–100 beats/min in sinus bradycardia following intravenous administration of isoproterenol (1–2 mg/min).

## Electrophysiologic Studies

**Determination of Sinus Node Recovery Time:**

1. Among various electrophysiologic studies, determination of the sinus node recovery time (postpacing pause) by rapid atrial pacing is the most reliable provocative test to detect indirect evidence of SSS.
2. It can be obtained by the use of a pervenous right atrial pacing catheter and conventional ECG recordings.
3. Artificial pacing can be performed by placing the catheter either within the coronary sinus or at the junction of the superior vena cava and right atrium, whichever location provides the most effective and consecutive atrial capture.
4. The initial pacing rate is usually 90 beats/min, and it is progressively increased thereafter by 10 beats every 2–4 minutes up to 150 beats/min.
5. The pacing is terminated suddenly at the end of each period, and the post-pacing pause (the interval from the last pacing spike to the onset of the next sinus P wave) is measured.
6. When there is complete absence of sinus P wave (atrial standstill) following the termination of pacing, the first AV junctional escape interval is measured.
7. Atrial pacing must be restarted immediately, however, when there is complete cardiac arrest for 4 seconds in order to avoid a syncopal episode.
8. The postpacing pause is expected to occur in individuals with normal as well as diseased sinus node, and this electrophysiologic phenomenon is comparable to the posttachyarrhythmia pause. However, the diseased sinus node requires an abnormally long recovery time until the automaticity as a primary pacemaker is reestablished. Thus, it has been documented that there is a clear distinction between normal and abnormal responses.
9. It has been reported that the actual sinus node recovery time following the termination of atrial pacing is closely related to the resting sinus rate—the slower the resting sinus rates, the longer the maximum postpacing pause.
10. When the resting sinus rate is between 75 and 85 beats/min, the maximum

postpacing pause is estimated to be 115 and 128% of the resting cycle length (postpacing pause: 800–900 msec).

11. In sinus bradycardia (rate: 45–60 beats/min), the maximum postpacing pause is expected to be much longer, and the abnormally prolonged sinus node suppression can be easily recognized.
12. In sinus rhythm with a rate of 60 beats/min (cycle length: 1,000 msec) the postpacing pause showing 125% of the resting value (1,250 msec) is strongly suggestive of SSS. The diagnosis of SSS is almost certain when the postpacing pause is longer than 1,250 msec under this circumstance.
13. When the resting sinus rate is 45 beats/min (cycle length: 1,420 msec), the postpacing pause of 1,700 msec or greater is diagnostic of the SSS, although the percentage increase is only 120%. In severe SSS, the postpacing pause may reach between 2,000 and 6,000 msec.

**Determination of Corrected Sinus Node Recovery Time:** Narula et al. proposed the corrected sinus node recovery time (CSRT)—the difference between the postpacing pause and the resting sinus P-P cycle. Normal maximum CSRT is calculated to be 525 msec or less, whereas the abnormal CSRT is calculated to be 1,880 ± 1,079 msec.

**Determination of Sinoatrial Conduction Time:** By other methods of electrophysiologic study, the SA conduction times (SACT) were measured indirectly by atrial extrastimulus technique. In 1 study, prolonged (more than 152 msec) calculated SACT was associated with a high incidence of sinus node and/or atrial disease. On the other hand, SACT was not significantly different between the control group and patients with SSS who were studied by others.

**His Bundle Electrocardiography:** Since SSS is often associated with various abnormalities in impulse formation and conduction elsewhere in the heart, the His bundle ECG can provide useful information. For example, abnormal electrophysiologic properties within the AV junction may indirectly support the diagnosis of the SSS. By recognizing the coexisting conduction disturbance, a specific type of artificial pacing may be selected for a given patient with SSS.

## THERAPEUTIC APPROACH

The fact that antiarrhythmic drug therapy alone has been unsatisfactory in the treatment of SSS has been repeatedly emphasized. At present, the use of a permanent artificial pacemaker is the treatment of choice for all patients with SSS. Drug therapy alone for SSS is unsuccessful for the following reasons:

1. The agent for treatment of the tachyarrhythmia component is harmful to or aggravates the bradyarrhythmia component, and vice versa.
2. The lack of therapeutic effects of pharmacologic agents (e.g., atropine sulfate or isoproterenol) for bradyarrhythmias.
3. Significant and intolerable side effects of all pharmacologic agents in many instances.

Currently, it is generally agreed that artificial pacemaker therapy is mandatory in almost every case of advanced SSS even if the patient is asymptomatic. In fact, the most common indication for artificial pacemaker at the present time is considered to be SSS.

### Artificial Pacemaker Therapy

1. The most ideal pacing mode for the majority of patients with SSS is a bifocal (AV sequential) demand pacing because many patients have coexisting AV block.
2. The multiprogrammable pacemaker, which is a new artificial pacing design, is the most suitable for most patients with SSS because various pacemaker parameters (functions), such as the pacing rate and the energy output, can be easily adjusted at any time after implantation so that pacemaker functions most appropriate to a given patient's clinical circumstance can be provided.
3. On the other hand, the ordinary ventricu-

lar pacemaker is satisfactory for many elderly patients with SSS.

4. When the atria are paced, the chance of suppressing various atrial tachyarrhythmias is much greater than when the ventricles are paced in patients with BTS.
5. However, 1 or more antiarrhythmic agents may be indicated when the tachyarrhythmia component persists even after artificial pacing in BTS.

## Antiarrhythmic Drug Therapy

1. As indicated earlier in this chapter, antiarrhythmic drug therapy alone is unsatisfactory and often hazardous for SSS. However, antiarrhythmic drug therapy can be instituted with relative safety following implantation of a permanent pacemaker.
2. Antiarrhythmic agents are often required for SSS because the tachyarrhythmia component is usually not suppressed by the pacing alone, although atrial pacing may be capable of eliminating atrial tachyarrhythmias.
3. Indications for specific antiarrhythmic agents are similar to the general recommendations for various tachyarrhythmias not associated with SSS.
4. Digitalis is the drug of choice for AF, atrial flutter, or AT with rapid ventricular response.
5. Digitalis and diuretics may improve myocardial function and indirectly suppress atrial tachyarrhythmias in patients with SSS associated with CHF.
6. At times, propranolol or verapamil may be added when atrial tachyarrhythmia with rapid ventricular response is not well controlled by digitalis alone.
7. Quinidine is very useful for the prevention of atrial tachyarrhythmias.
8. When ventricular tachyarrhythmia is not controlled by artificial pacing, various drugs, such as procainamide (Pronestyl), quinidine, phenytoin (Dilantin), disopyramide (Norpace), or propranolol (Inderal), may be tried as a single agent or combined drug therapy.

## PROGNOSIS

1. The natural course of disease of the sinus node seems to be chronic, progressive, and long standing, but it is difficult to determine the long-term prognosis with certainty.
2. To present knowledge, the diseased sinus node cannot be cured, and, in most cases, only symptomatic treatment with hemodynamic improvement, i.e., artificial pacing to replace the natural pacemaker, can provide a productive life for the patient with SSS.
3. The exact duration from the onset of the first manifestation of SSS until death is unknown, but it seems to take many months to 5–10 years in most cases.
4. It will be more difficult to evaluate the natural course of SSS at the present time because of the ready availability of artificial pacemakers in the early stage of SSS.
5. The danger of sudden death is always possible in untreated patients with SSS.
6. The initial stage of SSS is marked and chronic sinus bradycardia, and it is progressively followed by development of sinus arrest and/or SA block.
7. Advanced SSS is manifested by chronic AF or atrial flutter with slow ventricular rate due to advanced AV block and/or BTS.
8. Although chronic AF is considered to be the end stage of SSS, it is difficult to predict its appearance in every individual with SSS.
9. In addition, it is also difficult to predict the life expectancy of individuals with SSS after the development of chronic AF.

# Chapter 15

# Therapeutic Approach to Cardiac Arrhythmias

Since DC cardioverters and artificial pacemakers have become readily available (Chapters 19 and 20), the therapeutic results of the management of various arrhythmias have improved markedly in the past decade. The best therapeutic results can be obtained when a precise diagnosis of the arrhythmia is determined because some drugs are more effective or even almost specific for certain arrhythmias. For instance, digitalis is usually the drug of choice for AF with rapid ventricular response. Conversely, digitalis is ineffective or even contraindicated in the treatment of ventricular tachyarrhythmias (Chapter 16).

It is essential to eliminate the cause if it is still present. For example, the most important and the first step in treating digitalis-induced arrhythmias is immediate discontinuation of digitalis (Chapter 17), and the first therapeutic approach to quinidine-induced polymorphous VT (torsade de pointes) is to discontinue quinidine immediately. Underlying etiologic factors also significantly influence the therapeutic result. For example, VT associated with acute MI is best treated with lidocaine (Xylocaine), whereas digitalis-induced VT responds best to phenytoin (Dilantin) or potassium (Chapter 17).

For alcohol-induced cardiac arrhythmias, immediate discontinuation of alcohol consumption is the most important therapeutic aspect. The term "holiday heart syndrome" has been used to describe sudden occurrence of various tachyarrhythmias following consumption of large amounts of alcohol because these episodes are commonly observed following holidays or weekends.

Prevention of the recurrence of tachyarrhythmia is another important aspect of management. For this reason, maintenance therapy with digitalis and many antiarrhythmic drugs (Chapters 16 and 18) is often necessary for long periods of time or even indefinitely. Quinidine is known to be the best agent, for the prevention of recurrence of AF or atrial flutter, whereas procainamide (Pronestyl) is known to be the best agent for the prevention of ventricular tachyarrhythmias for long-term therapy. Propranolol (Inderal) is shown to be the most effective agent in the treatment of catecholamine-induced arrhythmias and arrhythmias related to WPW syndrome. Many new antiarrhythmic agents have been introduced in clinical medicine recently, and some of them are still under investigation. These new antiarrhythmic agents are discussed in Chapter 18. Various antiarrhythmic agents have been classified into 4 major categories according to their electrophysiologic properties and pharmacologic actions (Chapter 18).

Antibradyarrhythmic agents (Chapter 18) are used much less frequently because of the ready availability of artificial pacemakers (Chapter 19). Commonly used antibradyarrhythmic agents include atropine and isoproterenol (Isuprel), especially during acute MI (Chapter 18).

It is not uncommon to use various antiarrhythmic drugs in conjunction with DC cardioverters and artificial pacemakers when dealing with refractory cardiac arrhythmias (Chapters 19 and 20).

Since electrophysiologic studies have been carried out extensively, it is now possible to use a specific antiarrhythmic agent for a specific cardiac arrhythmia. For example, reciprocating tachycardia with normal QRS complexes in WPW syndrome is best treated with either propranolol (Inderal) or digitalis because these drugs block the normal AV conduction (Chapters 13 and 18). On the other hand, lidocaine (Xylocaine) is found to be extremely effective in terminating AF with anomalous AV conduction in WPW syndrome (Chapters 13 and 18).

Recently electrophysiologic investigative studies using an extrastimulation technique have shown that the best antiarrhythmic agent for a specific tachyarrhythmia can be chosen according to its efficacy. For example, when VT under a given clinical circumstance cannot be induced by an extrastimulation (arrhythmic induction) technique following administration of a certain antiarrhythmic agent (e.g., quinidine) in an electrophysiologic laboratory, that particular drug will be the agent of choice for that clinical circumstance. This extrastimulation technique is very useful when dealing with refractory VT, and the technique is also extremely beneficial for a long-term prophylactic antiarrhythmic therapy.

## GUIDE TO ANTIARRHYTHMIC THERAPY

1. The purpose of drug therapy for cardiac arrhythmias is the prevention of various untoward sequelae of the arrhythmias.
2. The common untoward sequelae of arrhythmias include CHF, angina pectoris, fainting, dizziness, weakness, palpitations, skipped heartbeats, convulsion, feeling of impending death, cerebral ischemia, and even death.
3. Correct diagnosis of a given arrhythmia is essential. There are 3 major categories (Chapter 1):
   a. Tachyarrhythmias, including premature contractions (extrasystoles) of various origins
   b. Bradyarrhythmias
   c. Bradytachyarrhythmias
4. Careful consideration of indications and contraindications for various agents by electrophysiologic approaches (Chapter 18) is essential.
5. All physicians should be familiar with the recommended dosages of various antiarrhythmic agents (Chapter 18).
6. Prevention of side effects and toxicity of various agents is essential.
7. Eliminate the direct or indirect cause of a given arrhythmia if possible, before any antiarrhythmic agent is used.
8. When dealing with any unexplainable tachyarrhythmia, especially in young individuals, common underlying problems should be considered before initiating any antiarrhythmic agent. Common underlying factors or disorders that frequently cause various cardiac arrhythmias include:
   a. Excessive usage of coffee, tea, or cola drinks, cigarette smoking, and emotional stress
   b. Hyperthyroidism (thyrotoxicosis)
   c. Mitral valve prolapse syndrome
   d. Wolff-Parkinson-White syndrome (Chapter 13).
9. Various antiarrhythmic agents may show synergistic or antagonistic actions. For example, the serum digoxin level often rises excessively when digoxin and quinidine are administered together, so that the incidence of digoxin toxicity increases significantly. Digitoxin and quinidine do not seem to show any synergistic action.
10. Prevention of recurrent cardiac arrhythmia is another important aspect of antiarrhythmic therapy.
11. Refractory arrhythmias often require a combination of 2 or more antiarrhythmic agents.
12. Not uncommonly, some patients require DC shock and artificial pacemaker in addition to the antiarrhythmic agents.
13. Antiarrhythmic drug therapy alone is unsatisfactory in the treatment of SSS in the majority of cases. Thus, the use of an artificial pacemaker is the treatment of choice for SSS. In some cases with BTS (commonly a manifestation of advanced SSS), 1 or more antiarrhythmic agents are indicated even after pacing (Chapter 14).

14. For torsade de pointes (polymorphous VT), not only are the conventional antiarrhythmic agents ineffective, but also more serious arrhythmias may be produced. Intravenous infusion of isoproterenol is shown to be the most effective agent under this circumstance. Artificial pacing with overdriving rate (80–120 beats/min) is often a more effective and safer treatment for this VT. Of course, a causative agent (commonly quinidine) should be discontinued immediately.

## ELECTROPHYSIOLOGIC STUDY

It has been well documented that various antiarrhythmic agents may alter the response of patients with VT to programmed ventricular stimuli or ventricular pacing. Many commonly used antiarrhythmic drugs occasionally enhance the response to the stimuli. At times, the characteristics of the VT itself may be altered by certain agents. Most antiarrhythmic agents are given intravenously or, less commonly, by mouth during the acute phase of the electrophysiologic evaluation. In addition, long-term oral antiarrhythmic drug therapy can be guided by the results of the electrophysiologic study. When an effective antiarrhythmic agent is selected for a given patient based on the electrophysiologic test results, VT can be effectively treated and prevented.

Since it is almost impossible to predict which antiarrhythmic agent will be effective to suppress VT in a given patient, various commonly used drugs are usually evaluated consecutively. In general, refractory VT requires in-depth electrophysiologic study. During the electrophysiologic study, even when an effective antiarrhythmic agent is selected, all other effective drugs are usually tested, so that an alternative effective drug can be quickly given if the patient develops serious untoward effects from the first drug chosen.

As a rule, it will take at least several days to complete the electrophysiologic evaluation of common antiarrhythmic agents because only 1 drug can be evaluated each day, except for lidocaine, which has a short half-life. It is essential to wait until the effects of each antiarrhythmic agent are completely dissipated before the next drug is evaluated. For example, lidocaine and procainamide may be evaluated during the initial complete electrophysiologic study, and it may be followed by the evaluation of other drugs, including quinidine, propranolol, phenytoin, and disopyramide on consecutive days. When any new antiarrhythmic agents under investigation are also to be tested, additional days will be necessary. During the electrophysiologic study, a pervenous RV electrode is often left in place, and continuous ECG monitoring is usually carried out for close observation of the patient.

The usual electrophysiologic study on various antiarrhythmic drugs is conducted in the following manner. Before any antiarrhythmic agent is tested, VT has been induced and terminated by ventricular pacing in a given patient. When procainamide is to be evaluated, a loading dose of the drug (1–2.5 g) is administered by intravenous infusion at a rate of about 50 mg/min. Then, the programmed ventricular stimulation will be repeated. When the VT cannot be provoked by the stimulation, blood is drawn to determine the concentration of procainamide, and oral therapy is initiated. The oral dosage of the drug is estimated by the intravenous doses required for suppression of the VT. By and large, the effective doses and the therapeutic blood concentrations are reported to be greater than those conventionally acceptable values. In 1 study, the effective doses of procainamide (Pronestyl) ranged from 6 to 12 g/day, with the therapeutic blood concentrations ranging from 4.3 to 32.3 mg/liter (average: 13.6 mg/liter). The efficacy of procainamide has been repeatedly documented on follow-up electrophysiologic evaluation during oral drug therapy.

The usual intravenous doses for the electrophysiologic evaluation of other antiarrhythmic agents are as follows. Lidocaine (Xylocaine) is given at a dosage of 300 mg at a rate of 20–30 mg/min, and the usual dosage of phenytoin (Dilantin) is 1000 mg at 20 mg/min. When propranolol (Inderal) is to be tested, 0.1–0.2 mg/kg of body weight is administered at 1 mg/min. The usual dosage of quinidine gluconate is 400–1600 mg at 20 mg/min. Disopyramide (Norpace) is administered orally for the study. The drug is given by mouth before the initiation of the electrophysiologic study in a loading dosage of 200–400 mg, followed by 100–300 mg every 6 hours for 36 hours. As a rule, relatively large amounts of each agent are given in order to obtain the therapeutic effect, providing no significant untoward effect is produced.

During short-term electrophysiologic evaluation of various antiarrhythmic agents, the study is terminated when VT is suppressed or significant side effects are observed. By and large, the evaluation should be discontinued immediately when the QRS duration or the Q-T interval is increased to more than 25–50% of the preexisting values or when serious adverse effects, such as hypotension, are produced.

There is a good correlation between the results of the electrophysiologic study using various antiarrhythmic agents and the efficacy of a given drug in suppressing VT in clinical settings. In some patients, VT may be well controlled by a given drug even when the tachycardia is still inducible by programmed stimulation. It can be said from the above observation that programmed stimulation may be more potent in provoking VT than spontaneous VT during antiarrhythmic drug therapy.

When dealing with patients who have recovered from cardiac arrest, cardiac arrhythmias (usually ventricular in origin) that were responsible for the production of the cardiac arrest can be reproduced, in many cases, by the electrophysiologic study. Thus, an effective antiarrhythmic drug program to prevent VT or VF can be established.

It has been demonstrated that the rate of VT is often decreased by various antiarrhythmic drugs regardless of whether or not a given drug is capable of reducing the ease of provoking the tachycardia by programmed stimulation. Occasionally, however, certain drugs may accelerate the rate of VT. In general, the rate of VT is nearly always reduced by quinidine, procainamide, and disopyramide when sufficient amounts are administered because the conduction velocity of the reentry cycle is slowed as a result of prolonged refractoriness in the involved ventricular myocardium by the drug.

It has been shown that the effect of procainamide on the tachycardia zone varies considerably. The drug may cause narrowing or widening of the tachycardia zone, and at times, there may be no change. Although quinidine and disopyramide possess similar antiarrhythmic effects on spontaneous or induced VT, it is not possible to predict with certainty the true efficacy of these drugs in every case. Propranolol and verapamil show little effect on the rate of VT or the tachycardia zone.

One of the serious side effects of some antiarrhythmic agents is the ability of these drugs to accelerate the rate of VT in certain cases. This side effect has been observed occasionally during administration of lidocaine and phenytoin.

## MANAGEMENT OF PREMATURE CONTRACTIONS (EXTRASYSTOLES)

1. The first step in management is to remove any possible cause of premature contractions regardless of the origin of the ectopic impulses. For example, digitalis-induced premature contractions, particularly ventricular in origin, are treated best by discontinuation of digitalis (Chapter 17).
2. Sedation is another important method in eliminating premature beats, especially when dealing with high-strung or nervous individuals.
3. Premature contractions are often eliminated by stopping heavy smoking or excessive ingestion of coffee.
4. If the VPCs are frequent (30 beats or more per hour), particularly in a diseased heart, such as in acute MI, various antiarrhythmic agents may be required.
5. Supraventricular (atrial or AV junctional) premature contractions are best treated with quinidine if symptomatic (e.g., palpitations). Propranolol (Inderal) is almost equally effective in this situation. By and large, supraventricular pre-

mature beats are self-limited, and no active treatment is necessary as long as the arrhythmia does not cause any symptoms.

6. Digitalis is particularly effective when premature contractions are associated with CHF.
7. Lidocaine (Xylocaine) is the drug of choice for the treatment of VPCs associated with acute MI or during catheterization and cardiac surgery.
8. In the following situations, treatment of VPCs is considered to be indicated:
   a. Frequent VPCs (30 or more beats/hour)
   b. R-on-T phenomenon (VPC superimposed on top of T wave of the preceding beat—vulnerable period)
   c. Multifocal VPCs
   d. Grouped or paired VPCs
   e. VPCs after the termination of VT or VF
9. For long-term therapy of VPCs, procainamide (Pronestyl) or quinidine is the drug of choice. Alternatively, disopyramide (Norpace) or phenytoin (Dilantin) may be used.
10. Phenytoin (Dilantin) is probably the best agent for the treatment of digitalis-induced premature beats (Chapter 17).
11. Beta-blocking agents (e.g., propranolol) are shown to be most effective in the treatment of various cardiac arrhythmias, particularly premature contractions associated with MVP syndrome.
12. Likewise, catecholamine-induced premature contractions are best treated with beta-blocking agents.
13. Calcium antagonists (e.g., verapamil or nifedipine) are the agents of choice for the treatment of VPCs associated with coronary artery spasm.

## MANAGEMENT OF SUPRAVENTRICULAR TACHYARRHYTHMIAS

1. The first step in management is elimination of the cause if it is present. For example, AF associated with thyrotoxicosis cannot be treated satisfactorily unless the thyroid function returns to euthyroid level.
2. Carotid sinus stimulation is often very effective in terminating PAT or AV JT (Chapter 12).
3. Digitalis is usually the drug of choice in the treatment of AF with rapid ventricular response (Fig. 5–14).
4. In digitalis-induced supraventricular tachyarrhythmias, digitalis must be discontinued immediately. In addition, phenytoin (Dilantin) or potassium is found to be very effective in terminating digitalis-induced supraventricular tachyarrhythmias (Chapter 17).
5. Quinidine is the best agent to prevent the recurrence of AF or atrial flutter.
6. Propranolol (Inderal) is shown to be the most effective agent in the treatment of arrhythmias precipitated by exercise, emotional distress, or excessive sympathetic stimulation and WPW syndrome or supraventricular tachyarrhythmias related to MVP syndrome.
7. Procainamide (Pronestyl) is less commonly used for the treatment of supraventricular tachyarrhythmias, and lidocaine (Xylocaine) is rarely used in this situation except in the WPW syndrome.
8. Verapamil is a very useful drug in the treatment of various supraventricular tachyarrhythmias including those associated with WPW syndrome.
9. Direct current shock is often very effective in terminating various acute supraventricular tachyarrhythmias. In addition, elective cardioversion is another important therapy for terminating chronic AF or atrial flutter (Chapter 20).
10. In holiday heart syndrome, various tachyarrhythmias may be observed, but paroxysmal AF is the most common arrhythmia in this entity. Immediate discontinuation of alcohol consumption is the most important and the first therapeutic approach.
11. Artificial pacemakers (overdriving rate) are occasionally needed in the suppres-

sion of various supraventricular tachyarrhythmias that are refractory to antiarrhythmic agents and/or DC shock (Chapter 19).

12. Sedation is often beneficial for the treatment of supraventricular tachyarrhythmias in conjunction with other therapeutic measures.

## MANAGEMENT OF VENTRICULAR TACHYARRHYTHMIAS

1. It is essential to eliminate any possible cause of ventricular tachyarrhythmias if present. Digitalis should be stopped immediately when ventricular tachyarrhythmias are due to DI (Chapter 17).
2. Quinidine or any other causative agents (procainamide or disopyramide) must be discontinued immediately in the treatment of torsade de pointes (polymorphous or atypical VT). In addition, artificial pacing with slight overdriving rate (80–120 beats/min) or intravenous infusion of isoproterenol is often indicated. Quinidine syncope or sudden death during quinidine therapy is often attributed to torsade de pointes (Chapter 18).
3. Direct current shock is the most effective way of terminating VT, ventricular flutter, and VF (Chapter 20). Defibrillation should be carried out immediately for the treatment of VF or ventricular flutter, in addition to cardiopulmonary resuscitation (CPR) as needed. However, DC shock should be avoided insofar as possible if VT is induced by digitalis, since DC shock often produces new cardiac arrhythmias, particularly VF, in this situation.
4. Lidocaine (Xylocaine) is the drug of choice for the treatment of VT associated with acute MI or during anesthesia and cardiac catheterization. Procainamide (Pronestyl) and quinidine are the next commonly used drugs in this situation.
5. Bretylium (a new antiarrhythmic agent) is found to be a very effective drug for refractory ventricular tachyarrhythmias.
6. Disopyramide (Norpace) or propranolol (Inderal) is less commonly used for the treatment of ventricular tachyarrhythmias.
7. Phenytoin (Dilantin) is the best drug for the treatment of digitalis-induced VT (Chapter 16).
8. Ventricular tachyarrhythmias associated with coronary artery spasm are best treated with calcium antagonists (e.g., nifedipine).
9. When ventricular tachyarrhythmias are refractory to antiarrhythmic agents and/or DC shock, the use of an artificial pacemaker (overdriving pacing rate: 100–120 beats/min) is often a life-saving measure (Chapter 19).

## MANAGEMENT OF SINUS BRADYCARDIA, SINUS ARREST, AND SINOATRIAL BLOCK

1. The therapeutic approaches vary markedly, depending upon the fundamental mechanism responsible for the production of bradyarrhythmias, the ventricular rate, and the underlying cause and degree of symptoms.
2. Sinus bradycardia of mild degree (rate: 50–59 beats/min) is not uncommon in healthy individuals, especially in young athletes and elderly persons. When the sinus rate is between 40 and 50 beats/min, there may be some symptoms. Marked sinus bradycardia with a rate below 40 beats/min often produces significant hemodynamic alterations, especially when it is associated with acute MI.
3. The most common causes of sinus bradycardia include the therapeutic or toxic effects of various drugs—including digitalis, propranolol, reserpine, and guanethidine, methyldopa (Aldomet)—and acute diaphragmatic MI. Drug-induced sinus bradycardia, sinus arrest, or SA block is best treated by stopping that particular drug.
4. Active treatment is indicated when marked sinus bradycardia persists and

becomes symptomatic, especially when it is associated with acute MI. The treatment of choice in this case is atropine, and the next commonly used agent is isoproterenol (Isuprel).

5. Essentially the same therapeutic approach may be used in the treatment of symptomatic sinus arrest or SA block.
6. In drug-resistant sinus bradycardia, sinus arrest, or SA block, a temporary or even a permanent artificial pacemaker is the treatment of choice.
7. When dealing with persisting and drug-resistant sinus bradyarrhythmias, the underlying disorder is commonly SSS. For symptomatic or advanced SSS, permanent artificial pacemaker implantation is the treatment of choice (Chapter 14).

## MANAGEMENT OF ATRIOVENTRICULAR BLOCK

1. Atrioventricular block per se does not require treatment. Therapeutic indication for AV block depends primarily on the degree, site, and etiology of the AV block, the ventricular rate, and the presence or absence of symptoms.
2. First degree AV block usually requires no particular treatment, except that the direct cause, such as DI, should be eliminated. It has been reported that atropine is effective in abolishing digitalis-induced first and second degree AV block. Isoproterenol (Isuprel) may be effective in this circumstance, but the drug often produces untoward reactions, such as increasing ventricular irritability.
3. Wenckebach (Mobitz type I) AV block (Fig. 8–1) usually does not require active treatment unless significant symptoms are produced. Wenckebach AV block usually represents AV nodal block (Chapter 8).
4. On the other hand, Mobitz type II AV block (Fig. 8–3) requires an artificial pacemaker because Mobitz type II AV block is considered to be an advanced form of BBBB. Mobitz type II AV block represents infranodal block (Chapter 8).
5. In complete AV block, the therapeutic approach depends upon the ventricular rate, the exact site of the block, and the degree of symptoms. Active treatment is usually not indicated when the ventricular rate is relatively rapid (40–60 beats/min) in AV JER due to complete AV block, such as is seen in acute diaphragmatic MI, unless symptomatic. On the other hand, a permanent artificial pacemaker is indicated when the ventricular rate is slow (slower than 40 beats/min) in ventricular escape (idioventricular) rhythm due to complete AV block, such as is seen in acute anterior MI, or in elderly individuals with degenerative changes in the conduction system.
6. Complete AV block in acute diaphragmatic MI represents AV nodal block, whereas complete AV block in acute anterior MI usually represents infranodal block, complete TFB (Chapters 8 and 9).
7. In general, AV nodal block is relatively benign and self-limited, and thus, active treatment is not indicated. On the other hand, infranodal block is usually irreversible, and permanent pacemaker implantation is necessary in most cases (Chapters 8 and 9).
8. Bilateral bundle branch block (BFB and TFB) of varying degrees often requires a permanent artificial pacemaker, especially when symptomatic (Chapter 19).
9. In urgent situations, before the insertion of an artificial pacemaker, such agents as isoproterenol (Isuprel) or epinephrine (Adrenalin) may be tried.

*Chapter 16*

# Digitalization

Digitalis is one of the most important drugs in managing CHF and various cardiac arrhythmias, particularly those of supraventricular origin. From the time digitalis was introduced by a British physician, William Withering, into the practice of medicine in 1785, it has been probably the most valuable drug available for various cardiac and many noncardiac diseases. It has been shown that 1 of 5 patients receiving cardiac glycosides in general hospitals has some degree of DI. The incidence of DI has been relatively high because the margin between therapeutic and toxic doses is narrow. This narrow margin becomes further reduced in elderly and seriously ill patients. The therapeutic dose is estimated to be approximately 60% of the toxic dose. The incidence of DI increases markedly when there are various modifying factors, such as hypokalemia, myxedema, renal failure, and COPD.

Although digitalis is 1 of the essential drugs in the treatment of CHF, the drug may cause or aggravate CHF if the patient develops DI. Aggravation of CHF by DI may be the first recognizable evidence of DI without any other manifestation.

Although such gastrointestinal symptoms as anorexia, nausea, and vomiting have been said to be the most common early symptoms, cardiac arrhythmias are frequently the earliest signs and may be the only evidence of DI in the absence of such signs. Cardiac arrhythmias are particularly common when using the purified glycosides and, in fact, have been a more common manifestation than gastrointestinal symptoms. Since the most serious and life-threatening manifestations of DI are cardiac arrhythmias, they must be immediately treated, for preexisting CHF becomes rapidly worse under superimposed arrhythmias.

Levels of serum digoxin or digitoxin are determined at many institutions in order to assess the therapeutic and toxic doses of digitalis, but the clinical implications of these levels are not fully understood. This is so because there is a significant overlap between the therapeutic and toxic doses. Nevertheless, a markedly increased serum digitalis level certainly indicates DI, whereas a very small amount of digitalis in the serum usually indicates underdigitalization. Serum digitalis determination is extremely valuable when dealing with patients who suffer from intractable CHF and/or complex cardiac arrhythmias when little or no information regarding previous digitalization is available.

Patients may differ greatly in required dosage and tolerance to digitalis. Some may experience signs of toxicity with small amounts, while others may receive more than the usual quantity for digitalization without the development of toxicity. Toxic and therapeutic dosages may be almost the same in patients with severe CHF.

Other situations predisposing to toxicity, even with dosages usually nontoxic, include further deterioration of the underlying lesion, hypokalemia, myxedema, thyrotoxicosis, renal failure, hypoxia due to various causes, COPD, and advanced age. Therefore, any patients who are receiving a digitalis preparation may develop DI at any time during therapy. A search for DI should be a routine part of the management of patients with CHF, as an early recognition of DI simplifies therapy and minimizes morbidity and mortality. It is not uncommon to fail to recognize DI even when it is severe enough to cause death, for DI does not produce pathognomonic evidence. In retrospect, an inadequate explanation of the cause of death in patients with refractory CHF can be attributed to digitalis.

## FUNDAMENTAL PRINCIPLES OF DIGITALIZATION

Before a physician attempts to administer digitalis to a patient, the physician should be fully aware of the following information regarding the patient and the cardiac glycoside chosen for use.

### Indications and Contraindications for Digitalization

1. One should know whether or not digitalis is definitely indicated. One should know whether or not the patient is suffering from CHF and/or supraventricular tachyarrhythmias. Two major indications of digitalis include CHF and various supraventricular tachyarrhythmias, particularly AF or atrial flutter with rapid ventricular response, except those induced by digitalis.
2. In addition, one should be aware that there are some clinical situations in which digitalis is contraindicated (i.e., DI and possibly IHSS). The reason is that digitalis improves the contractile state of the LV myocardium, which further reduces the LV outflow tract. The clinical status of a patient with IHSS deteriorates during digitalization but usually improves upon discontinuation of digitalis administration.

### Information on Previous Digitalization

1. Physicians should try their best to obtain precise information about previous digitalization. In particular, full information regarding past digitalization up to 3–4 weeks prior to the present digitalization is important.
2. Not only the duration of digitalization but also exact information concerning the preparation, dosage, and route of administration are indispensable.
3. If the clinical symptoms are rather mild and a history of previous digitalization is equivocal, it is preferable not to give any more digitalis until a definite indication for digitalization is established.
4. Serum digitalis determination by radioimmunoassay is extremely valuable when a history of previous digitalization is unclear. It has been well documented that the serum digoxin level rises considerably when digoxin and quinidine are administered together. Thus, a possibility of DI will be greater under this circumstance. The serum digitoxin level, however, does not seem to be influenced by quinidine therapy.

### Electrocardiograms Before and During Digitalization

1. It is essential to take a control ECG immediately before digitalization regardless of the clinical situation except in the case of the unusually acute patient in a critical state. The most important reason for this is to confirm a fundamental mechanism of the cardiac rhythm, so that it will be clearly evident if any new cardiac arrhythmia develops after digitalization.
2. Any form of a new cardiac arrhythmia that develops during or after digitalization strongly suggests DI, since almost every known type of rhythm disturbance may be induced by digitalis.
3. Another reason for the necessity of a control ECG is to know if there are any unexpected ECG abnormalities, such as acute MI or hypokalemia, that directly influence the efficacy of digitalis and the incidence of DI.
4. In addition to the control ECG, frequent follow-up ECG tracings are needed until the patient becomes fully digitalized and the patient's condition becomes stable.
5. An ECG should be taken immediately, when there is any change in the cardiac rhythm detected by physical examination, or when DI is clinically suspected.

6. For the confirmation of the current cardiac mechanism, long rhythm strips of leads II and $V_1$ should be obtained.

## Choice of Preparation and Method

1. Choice of preparation and method of digitalization, directly and indirectly, influence the efficacy of digitalis and the development of DI.
2. For urgent situations, such as acute pulmonary edema, particularly associated with supraventricular tachyarrhythmias, a short-acting preparation, such as deslanoside (Cedilanid-D) or digoxin should be given intravenously.
3. If there are any modifying factors, short-acting preparations are always preferable.
4. If the clinical situation is not urgent, the slower method oral administration is advisable.
5. Every physician should be fully familiar with the preparation chosen. Precise oral and parenteral dosages as well as various advantages and disadvantages of the particular preparations should be clearly understood.
6. Every physician should be fully familiar with at least 1 preparation for intravenous use for very rapid digitalization and 1 preparation for oral use for slow digitalization.
7. Digoxin has proven to be the most useful preparation that can be given in most clinical situations.
8. There is no point in changing from 1 preparation to another unless there will be a definite advantage or allergy to the former preparation is discovered.

## Factors Modifying Efficacy of Digitalis

Various modifying factors, such as hypokalemia and various cardiac as well as noncardiac diseases, directly influence digitalis efficacy and the development of DI. Therefore, these factors should be carefully considered.

## Determination of Serum Digitalis Level

In the past 20 years, various methods have been developed to determine the serum digitalis level in order to assess an optimal therapeutic dosage and to diagnose DI with accuracy. Serum digitalis determination by the radioimmunoassay method is extremely valuable when the values of serum digitalis levels are interpreted in conjunction with the total clinical picture and ECG findings. The usual therapeutic range of serum digoxin level is 1–2 ng/ml. Remember that the therapeutic serum digoxin or digitoxin levels are significantly lower when there are various modifying factors (e.g., old age, myxedema, renal failure, hypokalemia, COPD).

## Evaluation of Refractory Congestive Heart Failure

1. Refractory CHF requires careful evaluation in order to determine whether the patient needs more digitalis or whether digitalis must be discontinued.
2. The presence of any modifying factors and the reevaluation of the initial diagnosis are to be considered in treating refractory CHF.
3. It should be reemphasized that DI is 1 of the important causes of refractory CHF.

## Evaluation of Complex Arrhythmias

At times, digitalis-induced arrhythmias may be so complex that experienced electrocardiographers argue about the mechanism of the cardiac rhythm. A given tracing may suggest a variety of mechanisms, and the cardiac rhythm may change quickly from 1 form to another every few seconds or minutes. It may be reasonable to state that an argument regarding the mechanism of the cardiac rhythm during digitalization is, in itself, often sufficient evidence to suspect DI.

### Digitalis Effect on Electrocardiogram

During digitalis therapy (particularly during long-term oral administration), many patients develop slight ST segment depression or ST segment sagging with biphasic to slightly inverted T waves involving many leads. This ECG change is termed the "digitalis effect" and is totally unrelated to DI.

## INDICATIONS FOR DIGITALIZATION

1. Congestive heart failure regardless of underlying heart disease (except when digitalis induced).
2. Most supraventricular tachyarrhythmias (except when digitalis induced).
   a. Atrial fibrillation
   b. Atrial flutter
   c. Atrial tachycardia
   d. Paroxysmal AV JT
   e. Reciprocating tachycardia
3. Digitalis is the drug of choice for AF with rapid ventricular response (Fig. 5–14) regardless of the clinical circumstances. In addition, digitalis is also very effective for atrial flutter with rapid ventricular response (most commonly 2:1 AV response) (Fig. 5–11).
4. When the supraventricular tachyarrhythmias occur only transiently and when these arrhythmias last only for a short duration, digitalis is not indicated.
5. It is also important to remember that the same tachyarrhythmia may be treated differently. Other antiarrhythmic agents can be used, or DC shock may be used depending upon the clinical circumstance (Chapters 18 and 20).

## CONTRAINDICATIONS TO DIGITALIZATION

### Absolute Contraindications

1. Digitalis intoxication
2. Idiosyncrasy to digitalis

### Relative Contraindications

**Idiopathic Hypertrophic Subaortic Stenosis:** Digitalis is relatively contraindicated in patients with IHSS because the drug improves the contractile state of the LV outflow tract, leading to increased obstruction of LV outflow, LV systolic pressure, LV-aortic pressure gradient, and a diminution of the effective orifice size of the LV outflow tract. Deterioration in the clinical status by digitalization of this entity improves when digitalis is discontinued. However, if patients with IHSS develop AF, digitalis may be required to reduce the heart rate.

**Ventricular Tachycardia:** There is disagreement as to whether cardiac glycosides are indicated or contraindicated for treatment of VT. If it is certain that VT is a result of CHF or CHF is a result of VT not due to digitalis, the drug may be indicated and often is effective. Digitalis should be given with caution under these circumstances, however.

**Complete Atrioventricular Block:** Although digitalis is not absolutely contraindicated in the presence of complete AV block, if CHF is present, the effect of the drug is often not striking. It is generally agreed that CHF with complete AV block is often improved by increasing the heart rate with an artificial pacemaker. Digitalis should be continued even after artificial pacemaker implantation if CHF persists. However, in such emergency situations as acute pulmonary edema in patients with complete AV block, a clinical trial of rapid digitalization may be necessary.

**Acute Myocardial Infarction:** During the first 72 hours of acute MI, digitalization should be avoided if possible because often digitalis not only is ineffective but also may induce various life-threatening cardiac arrhythmias. When digitalis is considered to be definitely indicated (e.g., AF with very rapid ventricular response) a smaller than usual dosage should be administered with caution.

**Sick Sinus Syndrome:** The same precautions and principles should be applied when treating cardiac patients with SSS (Chapter 14). As a rule, an artificial pacemaker is the treatment of choice for SSS. When CHF persists even after artificial pacing, digitalis may be indicated.

**Wolff-Parkinson-White Syndrome:** For any tachyarrhythmias, particularly AF with anomalous AV conduction in WPW syndrome (Chapter 13) (Fig. 10–3), digitalis should not be used. The reason for this is that digitalis enhances the conduction via the anomalous pathway, leading to an extremely rapid ventricular rate. In some cases, VF may be provoked under this circumstance, and sudden death may occur subsequently.

## METHODS OF DIGITALIZATION

Choice of the proper digitalis preparation and the method of digitalization directly influences the therapeutic effect of digitalis and the incidence of DI. By and large, there are 5 ways to digitalize in most clinical situations (Table 16–1).

1. Very rapid parenteral digitalization (within 12 hours)
2. Rapid oral digitalization (within 24 hours)
3. Moderately rapid oral digitalization (within 2–3 days)
4. Slow oral digitalization (within 5–8 days)
5. Digitalization with maintenance doses

These may be carried out depending upon the degree of urgency, the nature of the underlying heart disease, and/or the presence or absence of cardiac arrhythmias. Recently it has been shown that very slow digitalization can be carried out by giving a maintenance dosage for mild cases. In spite of the fact that there are marked variations in dosages in different individuals and even variations in the same individual, extensive clinical experience enables us to set guidelines concerning average doses and the usual ranges of dosages for full digitalization and maintenance use. Methods of digitalization in adults are shown in Table 16–1.

### Digitalization (Digoxin) in Children

**Intravenous Administration:**

1. Initial dosage is between one quarter and one half of the estimated total digitalizing dose based upon the age and weight of the child.
   a. Under 2 years: 0.02–0.03 mg/pound
   b. Over 2 years: 0.01–0.02 mg/pound
2. Full digitalization dosage follows the initial dosage with one quarter of the estimated total digitalizing dose every 8–12 hours until the patient is digitalized.

**Oral Administration:**

1. Initial dosage is between one quarter and one half of the estimated total digitalizing dose based upon the age and weight of the child.
   a. Under 2 years: 0.03–0.04 mg/pound
   b. Over 2 years: 0.02–0.03 mg/pound
2. Full digitalization dosage follows the initial dosage with one quarter of the estimated total digitalizing dose every 6–8 hours until the patient is digitalized.
3. Maintenance dosage is one quarter of the total digitalizing dosage.

## MAINTENANCE DOSAGES

The usual maintenance dosages of commonly used digitalis preparations are as follows:

1. Digoxin: 0.125–0.75 mg (average: 0.25 mg)
2. Digitoxin: 0.05–0.2 mg (average: 0.1 mg)
3. Digitalis leaf: 0.05–0.2 g (average: 0.1 g)

**TABLE 16–1. Methods of digitalization**

| | Very Rapid Digitalization (within 12 h) | Rapid Digitalization (within 24 h) | Moderately Rapid Digitalization (within 2–3 Days) | Slow Digitalization (within 5–8 Days) | Digitalization with Maintenance Dose |
|---|---|---|---|---|---|
| Digoxin | 0.5–1 mg IV injection initially, then 0.25–0.5 mg $\overline{q}$ 2–4 h as needed | 1–1.5 mg by mouth initially, then 0.5 mg $\overline{q}$ 6 h until digitalized | 0.5 mg tid by mouth for 2–3 days until digitalized | 0.25 mg tid by mouth for 5–8 days until digitalized | 0.125–0.75 mg (average: 0.25 mg) by mouth daily |
| Deslanoside | 0.8–1.6 mg IV injection initially, then 0.4 mg $\overline{q}$ 2–4 h as needed | — | — | — | — |
| Ouabain | 0.25–0.5 mg IV injection initially, then 0.1 mg $\overline{q}$ ½ h as needed | — | — | — | — |
| Digitoxin | — | 0.8 mg by mouth initially, then 0.2 mg $\overline{q}$ 6 h until digitalized | 0.2 mg tid by mouth for 2–3 days until digitalized | 0.1 mg tid by mouth for 5–8 days until digitalized | 0.05–0.2 mg (average: 0.1 mg) by mouth daily |
| Digitalis leaf | — | 0.8 g by mouth initially, then 0.2 g $\overline{q}$ 6 h until digitalized | 0.2 g tid by mouth for 2–3 days until digitalized | 0.1 g tid by mouth for 5–8 days until digitalized | 0.05–0.2 g (average: 0.1 g) by mouth daily |

IV, intravenous; $\overline{q}$, every; h, hours.
Reproduced with permission from Chung: Principles of Cardiac Arrhythmias, 3rd ed. Baltimore, Williams & Wilkins, 1983.

# Chapter 17

# Digitalis Intoxication

It is well documented that digitalis may produce almost every known type of cardiac arrhythmia via an alteration of impulse formation, conduction, or both. The diagnosis of DI is commonly made by recognizing a variety of cardiac arrhythmias rather than by evaluating various clinical manifestations (Table 17–1). The most common digitalis-induced arrhythmia is probably nonparoxysmal AV JT, especially in the presence of AF. Ventricular premature contractions, both multifocal and grouped, are probably equally common in DI. Various digitalis-induced arrhythmias are listed in order of frequency in Table 17–2. It is commonly observed that patients with DI demonstrate various combinations of cardiac arrhythmias. Arrhythmias may change from one to another in the same ECG tracing. In general, cardiac arrhythmias occur in 80–90% of patients presenting with DI.

It is interesting and important to note that certain cardiac arrhythmias are not produced by digitalis. Under this circumstance, the term "nondigitalis-induced arrhythmias" is used. Typically, parasystole and Mobitz type II AV block are not digitalis-induced arrhythmias. Various nondigitalis-induced arrhythmias are listed in Table 17–3. Various clinical manifestations of DI are discussed in Chapter 16.

## DISTURBANCES OF SINUS IMPULSE FORMATION AND CONDUCTION

1. Minor toxic effects of digitalis may induce sinus arrhythmia and/or sinus bradycardia, but these arrhythmias may lead to more serious arrhythmias, such as sinus arrest and SA block when digitalization continues.

**TABLE 17–1. Manifestations of digitalis toxicity**

| Common | Uncommon |
|---|---|
| *Gastrointestinal symptoms* | |
| Anorexia, nausea, vomiting | Abdominal pain, constipation, diarrhea, hemorrhage |
| *Cardiac symptoms* | |
| Worsening of congestive heart failure, ventricular premature contractions, atrial tachycardia with AV block, nonparoxysmal AV junctional tachycardia, AV block, sinus bradycardia | Atrial fibrillation, atrial flutter, ventricular tachycardia, ventricular fibrillation, sinus arrest, SA block, atrial premature contractions, junctional premature contractions |
| *Visual symptoms* | |
| Color vision (green or yellow) with halos | Blurring or shimmering vision, scotoma, micropsia, or macropsia, amblyopia |
| *Neurologic symptoms* | |
| Fatigue, headache, insomnia, malaise, confusion, vertigo, depression | Neuralgia, convulsions, paresthesia, delerium, psychosis |
| *Nonspecific symptoms* | |
| | Allergic reaction, idiosyncrasy, thrombocytopenia, gynecomastia |

Reproduced with permission from Chung: Principles of Cardiac Arrhythmias, 3rd ed. Baltimore, Williams & Wilkins, 1983.

**TABLE 17–2. Digitalis-induced arrhythmias (in order of frequency)**

1. Nonparoxysmal AV junctional tachycardia in the presence of atrial fibrillation
2. Nonparoxysmal AV junctional tachycardia (pure form)
3. Nonparoxysmal AV junctional tachycardia in the presence of other arrhythmias
4. Ventricular premature contractions (multifocal or grouped)
5. Wenckebach (Mobitz type I) AV block
6. Sinus bradycardia
7. First degree AV block
8. Atrial tachycardia with varying degree AV block (PAT with block)
9. Advanced or complete AV block (AV nodal block)
10. Atrial or AV junctional premature contractions
11. Sinus arrest or SA block
12. AV junctional escape rhythm
13. Reciprocal beats, rhythm, or tachycardia
14. Multifocal or bidirectional ectopic tachycardia
15. Atrial flutter or fibrillation

Reproduced with permission from Chung: Principles of Cardiac Arrhythmias, 3rd ed. Baltimore, Williams & Wilkins, 1983.

**TABLE 17–3. Nondigitalis-induced arrhythmias**

1. Sinus tachycardia
2. Paroxysmal AV junctional tachycardia
3. Mobitz type II AV block
4. Complete infranodal AV block
5. Parasystole or parasystolic tachycardia
6. Nonparoxysmal ventricular tachycardia (idioventricular tachycardia or accelerated ventricular rhythm)
7. Hemiblocks, bundle branch block, bifascicular block, and trifascicular block

Reproduced with permission from Chung: Principles of Cardiac Arrhythmias, 3rd ed. Baltimore, Williams & Wilkins, 1983.

2. Sinoatrial block with or without the Wenckebach phenomenon is not uncommon in DI, particularly in children.
3. In fact, digitalis may be the most common cause of SA block.

## Atrial Arrhythmias

1. Although digitalis is the drug of choice in the treatment of most atrial tachyarrhythmias, the drug is also capable of producing various atrial arrhythmias.
2. Atrial tachycardia with AV block was described by Sir Thomas Lewis in 1906 and was attributed to digitalis by Sir James MacKenzie in 1911.
3. Although the frequent occurrence of digitalis-induced AT with AV block of varying degree is emphasized by some investigators, its average incidence as reported by different authors is only 10% of the total digitalis-induced cardiac arrhythmias. In fact, many different series demonstrated a much lower incidence of this arrhythmia.
4. Digitalis-induced AT is commonly associated with varying degree Wenckebach AV block (Fig. 5–8).
5. In addition, AT often coexists with other digitalis-induced arrhythmias, such as nonparoxysmal AV JT and VPCs.
6. Regarding the mechanism responsible for the production of atrial tachyarrhythmias, the indirect vagal-stimulating action of digitalis results in a markedly shortened refractory period of the atrial musculature. Thus, increased conductivity within the atrial muscle can produce various rapid atrial arrhythmias. A combination of the depressive effect on the AV conduction and the shortening effect on the refractory period results in rapid atrial arrhythmias with varying degrees of AV block.
7. Besides AT, AF or atrial flutter may be induced by digitalis, but they occur very rarely.
8. Multifocal atrial tachycardia (MAT), likewise, is considered to be not digitalis-induced arrhythmia, although many patients may have MAT during digitalization because of underlying COPD.
9. Although APCs are not as common as VPCs, if the former occur, the ectopic atrial beats are frequently not conducted to the ventricles (nonconducted or blocked APCs). The combination of impaired AV conduction in the atrial ectopic beats plus the increased excitability in the atria results in frequent nonconducted APCs or APCs with markedly prolonged P-R interval.

## ATRIOVENTRICULAR JUNCTIONAL ARRHYTHMIAS

1. It is well documented that digitalis frequently induces various AV junctional arrhythmias because of passive impulse formation, resulting in AV JER, or enhancement of AV junctional impulse formation, resulting in nonparoxysmal AV JT.
2. Digitalis-induced AV junctional arrhythmias, especially nonparoxysmal AV JT, are very common in the presence of AF (Fig. 6–4), particularly in elderly individuals. It can be said that nonparoxysmal AV JT, particularly in the presence of AF, is probably the most common digitalis-induced arrhythmia.
3. In a rare form of AV dissociation, the atria and ventricles may be controlled by 2 different pacemakers in the AV junction. In this circumstance, the atria are activated in retrograde fashion. Each pacemaker at the AV junction may produce an AV JER or nonparoxysmal AV JT.
4. If there is further progression of the DI, exit block of various degrees may develop so that ventricular action may become slower or irregular. When the exit block is of the Wenckebach type, the cardiac rhythm will show regular irregularity.
5. On the other hand, digitalis may induce further acceleration of AV junctional impulse formation, resulting in bidirectional AV JT.
6. The incidence of digitalis-induced AV junctional arrhythmias is probably as high as the incidence of VPCs.
7. Digitalis-induced AV JPCs are occasionally observed.
8. Not uncommonly, nonparoxysmal AV JT coexists with AT, producing double supraventricular tachycardias in advanced DI.
9. It should be noted that the patient with an artificial pacemaker is not immune to DI. Thus, digitalis-induced AV JER or nonparoxysmal AV JT induced by DI is occasionally observed in the presence of artificial pacemaker-induced ventricular rhythm. Under these circumstances, regularly occurring independent retrograde P waves are observed in the presence of artificial pacemaker-induced ventricular rhythm (Fig. 17–1).

## VENTRICULAR ARRHYTHMIAS

1. Ventricular premature contractions (VPCs) are the most common and often

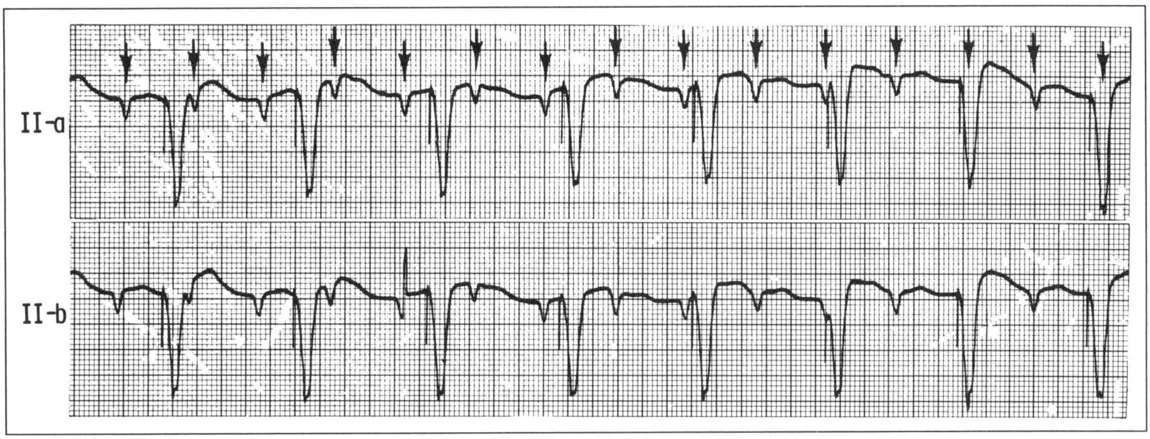


**Fig. 17–1.** Arrows indicate retrograde P waves. Leads II-a and II-b are not continuous. The rhythm is digitalis-induced nonparoxysmal AV JT (atrial rate: 107 beats/min) in the presence of artificial pacemaker-induced ventricular rhythm.

the earliest manifestation of DI in the adult population. Various investigators have reported that the incidence is approximately 50% of all digitalis-induced arrhythmias.

2. It has been known for many years that ventricular bigeminy is a specific arrhythmia in diagnosing DI during digitalis therapy (Fig. 7–5).
3. In children, supraventricular arrhythmias and AV conduction disturbances are a more common occurrence than VPCs.
4. Ventricular premature contractions may originate from a single focus or multiple foci, but multifocal VPCs are more pathognomonic for DI.
5. Ventricular premature contractions may appear as group beats or may lead to short runs of VT.
6. When VPCs become frequent, particularly when multifocal or bidirectional, a brief period of VT may develop, producing unidirectional or bidirectional tachycardia or even VF.
7. The average incidence of VT is approximately 10% of all digitalis-induced arrhythmias.
8. The mortality of patients with digitalis-induced VT is extremely high (68–100%).
9. Bidirectional VT is considered to be a more pathognomonic feature of DI than the unidirectional entity. This arrhythmia is more common in advanced heart disease, and frequently the basic atrial mechanism is AF, atrial flutter, or AT (Fig. 7–13).
10. In VT, either unidirectional or bidirectional, the average heart rate is between 150 and 180/min, the latter often having a faster rate.
11. Whenever an impulse from the sinus node or atria is unable to conduct to the ventricles because of SA block, sinus arrest, or complete AV block, idioventricular rhythm may appear, particularly when the AV junction is unable to produce AV JER. Idioventricular rhythm is usually slow (30–40 beats/min) with bizarre QRS complexes. Terminally, the idioventricular rhythm gradually slows, and finally ventricular standstill ensues.

## ATRIOVENTRICULAR CONDUCTION DISTURBANCES

1. Digitalis may produce various degrees of AV conduction disturbances due to both the direct and indirect actions of the drug. These actions are very important for the drug's therapeutic effect on various supraventricular tachyarrhythmias, particularly AF.
2. The degrees of AV block in DI depend on the dose of the drug, underlying heart disease, preexisting AV conduction disturbances, and the possible presence of electrolyte imbalance.
3. First degree AV block during digitalization definitely should be considered as a manifestation of DI.
4. Various studies indicate that the average incidence of second degree AV block is 11%, and Wenckebach AV block is the most common incomplete AV block in DI (Fig. 8–1).
5. Wenckebach AV block may be associated with 2:1 AV block, but in this case 2:1 AV block is a variant of Wenckebach AV block (Chapter 8).
6. This is in contrast to the Mobitz type II AV block, which has not been reported as a manifestation of DI.
7. It is important to remember that DI causes AV nodal block, and the drug never produces Mobitz type II AV block, which represents infranodal block (Chapter 8).
8. High degree (advanced) AV block is very common in DI when the underlying cardiac rhythm is AF.
9. If any form of second or high degree AV block progresses, it results in complete AV block.
10. It is reported that DI is the second most common cause of complete AV block.

Again, advanced or complete AV block in DI is always due to AV nodal block (Chapter 8).

## DETERMINATION OF SERUM DIGITALIS LEVEL BY RADIOIMMUNOASSAY METHODS

1. In the past 10–15 years, various methods for determining serum cardiac glycosides have been utilized in order to assess an optimal therapeutic dosage and to diagnose DI with accuracy.
2. The radioimmunoassay method is most commonly used at present.
3. The clinical implications of serum cardiac glycoside levels are based on the fact that there is a reasonably close correlation between the blood and tissue contents of digitalis, so that the blood levels reflect total body and myocardial concentrations.
4. It is generally agreed that patients with unequivocal DI have significantly higher serum or plasma levels of digoxin or digitoxin than nontoxic patients. Nevertheless, substantial overlap between toxic and nontoxic serum or plasma cardiac glycoside levels cannot be avoided.
5. The optimal dosage of digitalis not only varies from patient to patient but also may vary from time to time even in the same patient. Similarly, toxic and nontoxic serum or plasma digitalis levels may differ among patients, depending largely upon various modifying factors, including electrolyte imbalance, thyroid diseases, renal diseases, acute or chronic lung disease, and particularly the nature and severity of the underlying heart disease.
6. In general, serum digoxin levels of 2.0 ng/ml or below and serum digitoxin levels of 20 ng/ml or below are considered to be nontoxic, although toxic patients may have serum levels below these values. Many investigators feel that the therapeutic levels of digoxin and digitoxin are 0.5–2.5 ng/ml and 15–30 ng/ml, respectively.
7. Very low (digoxin levels below 0.4 ng/ml or digitoxin levels below 10 ng/ml) serum cardiac glycoside concentrations usually indicate underdigitalization.
8. Ventricular tachycardia, particularly when bidirectional, always represents a very advanced DI that is often irreversible.
9. A serum digoxin level above 10 ng/ml is, in general, incompatible with life.

### Methods and Procedures

The method of choice, at present, for the measurement of serum digoxin levels is radioimmunoassay for the following reasons:

1. Speed: Assay in 1–2 hours or less
2. Sensitivity: 0.2 ng/ml (approximately 5 times more sensitive than other tests)
3. Precision: Standard deviation 4% (standard error ±1.3% or less over 0.5–10 ng/ml range)
4. Specificity: No false positives (even from closely related steroids)
5. Extraction of glycoside: None needed

**Procedure for Serum Digoxin Determination (Fig. 17–2):**

1. One milliliter of the patient's blood is drawn, and the cells are separated from the liquid portion of the blood (either serum or plasma).
2. Samples of 0.2 ml of this liquid are added to tubes along with radioactive digoxin tritium ($^3$H-digoxin) and the antibody of a digoxin–albumin antigen.
3. The concentrations of antibody and digoxin tritium are fixed such that approximately 50% of the radioactivity of digoxin tritium binds to the antibody.
4. If there is nonradioactive digoxin (from the patient's blood), it will displace or compete with radioactive digoxin for binding to the antibody.
5. The amount of radioactive digoxin that is displaced or never bound can be related to a known amount of nonradioactive digoxin by a standard curve in which

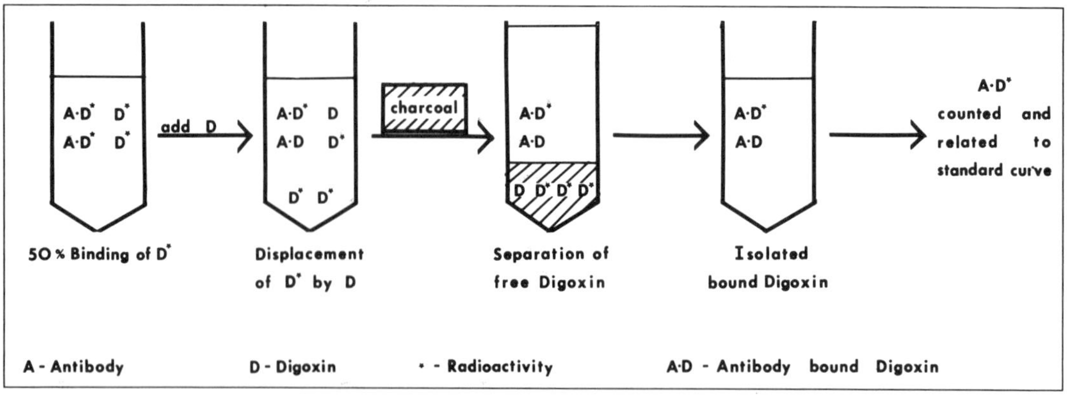


**Fig. 17–2.** The radioimmunoassay of digoxin. $^3$H-Digoxin (D*) is added to digoxin-specific antibodies (A) to give 50% of D* bound; A forming A-D*. Nonradioactive digoxin (D) from serum or standard solution added to A-D* displaces D* proportionate to its concentration. Dextranized charcoal added to the solution absorbs free D and D*. Measurement of radioactivity (i.e., D* still remaining bound to A) in the supernatant when related to the standard curve gives the concentration of D originally added. The standard curve is prepared by displacing D* from A-D* by known amounts of D.

amounts of nonradioactive digoxin (from 0 to 10 ng) have displaced radioactive digoxin from a standard amount of antibody.

6. As concentrations of nonradioactive digoxin increase, the digoxin tritium associated with the antibody will be bound to a lesser extent (less than 50%).
7. The system is established so that only digoxin tritium bound to the antibody is actually followed, and therefore as nonradioactive digoxin increases, the radioactivity associated with the antibody decreases.
8. The system is essentially linear from 1 to 4 ng of digoxin/ml. This is the critical area as far as the concentration of digoxin in human blood is concerned (refer to the nontoxic amounts).

The clinical usefulness of the serum digoxin or digitoxin levels determined by radioimmunoassay methods is still far from ideal, primarily because of the considerable overlap between toxic and nontoxic patients. However, these methods are extremely valuable when the values of serum cardiac glycoside levels are interpreted in conjunction with the total clinical picture and ECG findings. The determination of serum digitalis levels is very useful when little or no information about previous digitalization is available. Knowing the serum digitalis levels in a given patient under this circumstance permits much more accurate determination of additional digitalis dosage. On the other hand, the serum digitalis level may indicate DI. Serum digitalis levels are valuable when dealing with patients who have various modifying factors, where daily regulation of digitalis dosage is indicated. Another role of the serum digitalis level determination is to assess underdigitalization, which may be difficult or even impossible to ascertain clinically and/or electrocardiographically, especially in the presence of sinus rhythm.

## DETERMINATION OF SALIVA ELECTROLYTES

Recently, it has been shown that the electrolyte content in the saliva has a close relationship with DI. It has been demonstrated that patients with DI have disproportionately high concentrations of potassium and calcium. This test also shows some overlapping between toxic and nontoxic groups, although the mean values of saliva potassium and calcium were significantly higher in the group with DI. Further clinical evaluation will be needed to assess the value of the saliva test.

## NONDIGITALIS-INDUCED CARDIAC ARRHYTHMIAS

Although it is extremely important to recognize various digitalis-induced cardiac arrhythmias, a full understanding of cardiac rhythm disturbances that are not due to DI is equally essential. The term "nondigitalis-induced cardiac arrhythmias" is used for all cardiac rhythm disturbances that are totally unrelated to DI. The nondigitalis-induced cardiac arrhythmias include parasystole, nonparoxysmal VT (idioventricular tachycardia or accelerated ventricular rhythm), paroxysmal AV JT, various intraventricular conduction disturbances (hemiblocks, BFB, and TFB; Chapter 16), Mobitz type II AV block, and sinus tachycardia (Table 17–3).

It should be noted, however, that any of these nondigitalis-induced cardiac arrhythmias may be present in patients with DI, but digitalis is not responsible for the development of a given nondigitalis-induced arrhythmia.

### Parasystole

Parasystole is characterized by varying coupling intervals and constant shortest interectopic intervals with frequent occurrences of fusion beats (Chapter 22). In other words, a parasystolic rhythm produces an independent ectopic rhythm to the basic rhythm. When a long interectopic interval is present, it is usually a multiple of the shortest interectopic interval, usually due to exit block.

Ventricular parasystole closely simulates frequent VPCs. Although they resemble each other very closely on the ECG, clinically VPCs are commonly due to DI, whereas ventricular parasystole is unrelated to digitalis. Parasystolic VT is frequently misinterpreted as digitalis-induced ventricular arrhythmia.

A less common form of parasystole is AV junctional parasystole; atrial parasystole is rarely observed.

### Nonparoxysmal Ventricular Tachycardia (Idioventricular Tachycardia or Accelerated Ventricular Rhythm)

It has been known for many years that paroxysmal (ordinary) VT is not uncommon in advanced DI, but nonparoxysmal VT (Fig. 7–11) has not been reported in patients with DI. The usual rates of nonparoxysmal VT are between 70 and 130 beats/min, and the tachycardia often competes with the basic sinus rhythm with similar heart rates to produce incomplete AV dissociation. Nonparoxysmal VT is relatively common during the first 72 hours of acute MI, and it is usually self-limited (Chapter 7).

### Paroxysmal Atrioventricular Junctional Tachycardia

There are 2 forms of AV JT. Nonparoxysmal AV JT (usually a slower rate: 70–130 beats/min) is nearly always due to DI, whereas paroxysmal AV JT (usually a fast rate: 160–250 beats/min) has not been reported in DI. Paroxysmal AV JT has an abrupt onset and termination, as its name designates.

### Mobitz Type II AV Block

Mobitz type II AV block is characterized by constant P-R intervals in all conducted beats, with intermittent occurrences of blocked P waves (Fig. 8–3), and thus it does not have the Wenckebach phenomenon. Mobitz type II AV block has not been encountered in DI, but Wenckebach (Mobitz type I) AV block is commonly digitalis induced. Mobitz type II AV block is frequently associated with BBB and is considered to be a precursor of complete AV (infranodal) block. It should be pointed out that Mobitz type II AV block represents incomplete infranodal block, i.e., incomplete TFB (Chapter 8).

## TREATMENT OF DIGITALIS INTOXICATION

The most important treatment for DI is the immediate discontinuation of the drug, not reduction of the dosage. Most patients with mild DI, such as first degree AV block, sinus bradycardia, and occasional VPCs, can recover from DI by discontinuing the drug for several days. If DI is manifested by serious cardiac arrhythmias, more active therapeutic measures are required. Generally, in every patient with DI, emotional and physical activities should be restricted, and all factors that may aggravate the toxicity should be prevented and corrected.

Various agents, including potassium, phenytoin, beta-adrenergic receptor blocking agents, sodium ethylenediamine tetraacetate, have been used with varying success. Recently, reversal of advanced digoxin intoxication with Fab fragments of digoxin-specific antibodies has been reported.

### Potassium

1. Potassium is probably one of the most effective agents in abolishing various atrial tachyarrhythmias and ventricular arrhythmias in DI.
2. The amount of potassium administered depends upon the severity of the toxicity, the degree of suspected potassium deficiency in the myocardium, and the response to potassium therapy.
3. Potassium is definitely contraindicated in the presence of renal failure and hyperkalemia.
4. Potassium is relatively contraindicated in the presence of a second degree or complete AV block unless the serum potassium is very low, although occasionally digitalis-induced AV block may be abolished by potassium therapy.
5. Potassium in the form of potassium chloride may be administered orally in doses of 20–80 mEq/liter daily or by a slow intravenous infusion in doses of 40–60 mEq/liter over a 2–3-hour period initially.
6. Intravenous administration is preferred because the exact amount received by the patient can be controlled and the drug may be discontinued at any time indicated.
7. Oral administration is widely used for milder cases with DI when hypokalemia is suspected or present.
8. During intravenous administration of potassium, continuous ECG monitoring is essential in order to prevent or avoid toxic signs of hyperkalemia or any cardiac arrhythmia.
9. Frequent determinations of serum potassium are also indicated.

### Phenytoin (Dilantin)

1. Various clinical investigations have demonstrated that Dilantin is effective in treating digitalis-induced arrhythmias, including PAT, AV junctional rhythm, wandering atrial pacemaker, ventricular bigeminy, multifocal VPCs, and VT.
2. Most patients respond within 3 seconds to 5 minutes via intravenous administration. The duration of response varies from 5 minutes to 4–6 hours. Detailed descriptions of the usual dosage and toxic manifestations of Dilantin are given in Chapter 18.
3. Dilantin is not only effective therapeutically for various tachyarrhythmias but may also be effective in certain cases of mild digitalis-induced AV block. However, this drug is not recommended when there are second or third degree AV block and/or SA block.
4. It has been shown recently that Dilantin is of prophylactic value prior to DC shock in a digitalized patient, since the drug is capable of preventing arrhythmias induced by cardioversion by increasing the threshold of excitability of the heart by counteracting the electrophysiologic actions of digitalis.
5. Dilantin is probably the safest and most effective drug in the treatment of all types of digitalis-induced tachyarrhythmias.

## Beta-Adrenergic Blocking Agents

Various beta-adrenergic blocking agents are capable of abolishing various arrhythmias, including those induced by digitalis and those resistant to digitalis. In particular, propranolol (Inderal) is commonly used in treating digitalis-induced tachyarrhythmias, especially when potassium or Dilantin is found to be ineffective or contraindicated. The usual dosage and side effects of propranolol are fully discussed in Chapter 18.

## Procainamide (Pronestyl) and Quinidine

Procainamide and quinidine may be effective in abolishing supraventricular and ventricular tachyarrhythmias induced by digitalis. Procainamide or quinidine may be used if potassium, Dilantin, and propranolol are ineffective or contraindicated. However, it is important to remember that the serum digoxin level is often raised when quinidine is administered in digitalized patients. Thus, DI may be further aggravated by quinidine administration. Detailed descriptions of procainamide and quinidine are given in Chapter 18.

## Xylocaine (Lidocaine)

Xylocaine may be used in the treatment of digitalis-induced ventricular tachyarrhythmias or frequent VPCs when potassium and Dilantin are ineffective or contraindicated. The usual dosage and side effects of Xylocaine are discussed in Chapter 18.

## Chelating Agents

Sodium ethylenediamine tetraacetic acid (EDTA) is occasionally of value in the treatment of digitalis-induced ventricular arrhythmias and AV block. The chief advantage of this drug is its rapid onset of action, while its disadvantages include transient effect, occasional hypotension, and renal damage following large doses. Chelating agents may be used when potassium and Dilantin are contraindicated or ineffective.

## Magnesium

Recent clinical as well as experimental investigative studies have shown that hypomagnesemia predisposes to DI. Thus, the administration of magnesium sulfate should be tried when DI is associated with hypomagnesemia. The drug may be given by slow (1 $cm^3$/min) intravenous infusion (20 $cm^3$ of 20% solution) under continuous ECG monitoring.

## Direct Current Shock

Cardioversion should not be attempted on patients with suspected or proven digitalis-induced arrhythmias because the procedure frequently induces more serious and irreversible arrhythmias, such as VT or VF. If cardioversion is considered to be definitely needed, the prophylactic administration of Dilantin or potassium may prevent the occurrence of serious arrhythmias. It is essential to discontinue cardiac glycosides prior to the application of cardioversion. If a short-acting preparation has been given, the procedure should be postponed for at least 24–48 hours. If long-acting preparations have been used, the procedure should be delayed for at least 3–5 days.

In general, when treating the digitalis-induced tachyarrhythmias, cardioversion should be attempted only as a last resort after all other available measures have been exhausted.

## New Agents for Digitalis Intoxication

Recently, various new agents, including potassium canrenoate, diphenidol polarizing solution, and aprindine HCl, have been introduced in the treatment of DI with various degrees of success. These new agents are available primarily for investigative purposes in humans or for animal studies. In addition, Smith et al. have successfully reversed severe digoxin-induced advanced AV block with areas of ventricular standstill as a result of suicidal attempt by using Fab fragments of digoxin-specific antibodies in conjunction with the use of an artificial pacemaker. A 39-year-old man with rheumatic heart disease had ingested 22.5 mg (90 tablets of 0.25 mg) of digoxin with suicidal intent. The serum digoxin level before Fab infusion was 17.6 ng/ml. Sinus rhythm was restored 10 minutes after complete Fab infusion in this case.

## Artificial Pacemakers

The primary indications for artificial pacemakers are in treating AV block and advanced SSS. Although DI is reported to be the second most common cause of complete AV block, the Adams-Stokes syndrome as a manifestation of digitalis overdose has been found to be rare, since the ventricular rate in digitalis-induced complete AV block tends to be faster than that in complete AV block due to other causes. However, if the underlying rhythm is AF, the incidence of Adams-Stokes seizures increases. When the Adams-Stokes syndrome develops owing to DI, a temporary demand pacemaker is suitable because the AV block induced by digitalis is often transient and intermittent. Permanent pacemaker implantation for the treatment of digitalis-induced AV block is rarely called for unless other causes of AV block coexist. Artificial pacemakers are discussed in detail in Chapter 19.

## Lactones

There are 2 saturated lactones (tetrahydrofurfuryl alcohol and gammabutyrolacetone) that have in animals been effective in treating digitalis-induced cardiac arrhythmias. Further investigation of these compounds is needed in order to establish their value in clinical medicine.

## Intensive Care Unit

It is ideal to treat all patients with serious cardiac arrhythmias in an intensive care unit that is similar or identical to a CCU. As emphasized repeatedly, the mortality rate from DI is high and may reach 100% in patients with ventricular tachyarrhythmias unless recognized early and treated promptly. In addition, various cardiac arrhythmias may change from one type to another in a short period of time. Therefore, admittance of all patients with serious digitalis-induced arrhythmias to the CCU is highly recommended.

# Chapter 18

# Antiarrhythmic Drug Therapy

## ANTITACHYARRHYTHMIC AGENTS

As emphasized previously, the best therapeutic results can be obtained when a precise diagnosis of the arrhythmia is determined because some drugs are more effective or even almost specific for certain arrhythmias (Chapter 15). In addition, indications for various antitachyarrhythmic agents (Table 18–1) vary markedly, depending upon the underlying cause of the tachyarrhythmias. Proper selection of various antiarrhythmic agents using electrophysiologic study in the treatment of refractory ventricular tachyarrhythmias is discussed in detail in Chapter 15.

The most commonly used antitachyarrhythmic agents include cardiac glycosides, quinidine, lidocaine (Xylocaine), procainamide (Pronestyl), phenytoin (Dilantin), and propranolol (Inderal). The various antiarrhythmic agents are classified into 4 groups (some investigators classify them into 5 groups). New antitachyarrhythmic agents include bretylium, disopyramide (Norpace), verapamil, nifedipine, amiodarone, aprindine, tocainide, encainide, acecainide, mexiletine, metoprolol, and acebutolol. Many of these agents are still under investigation and are not available for routine clinical use. Various effects of commonly used drugs on conduction time are summarized in Table 18–2. Digitalis therapy and digitalis-induced cardiac arrhythmias are described in Chapters 16 and 17.

### Quinidine

Quinidine has been probably the most valuable antiarrhythmic agent available for more than 50 years. Quinidine has 2 major effects, direct and indirect. The direct effect of the drug is on the cell membrane, and the indirect effect is anticholinergic. As a result of the net clinical effect of combined anticholinergic and direct actions, a marked prolongation of the refractory period in the atria and a lesser degree of prolongation of the ventricles are produced. In addition, a shortening of the refractory period in the AV junction is induced by quinidine. When the refractory period in the atria is significantly prolonged during quinidine therapy, the atrial flutter cycle is often progressively reduced, and the atrial rate may become as slow as 120–180 beats/min (Fig. 5–12). Even though the atrial rate is extremely slow because of the quinidine effect, the characteristic features of atrial flutter waves are usually maintained under this circumstance (Chapter 5). It is very important to remember that the clinical situation may become extremely serious when quinidine is given to the patient with atrial flutter with 2:1 AV conduction (Fig. 5–11) without digitalis therapy, because the cardiac rhythm may become 1:1 AV conduction with atrial flutter as a result of the enhancement of AV conduction and slowing of the atrial flutter rate produced by quinidine, leading to a much faster ventricular rate.

It has been clearly documented that the serum digoxin level is frequently raised when quinidine is given together with digoxin, leading to a higher incidence of DI (Chapter 17). The serum digitoxin level is not shown to be influenced by concomitant quinidine therapy, however.

The sinus rate tends to be slowed by the direct effect of quinidine, but the indirect (vagolytic) effect tends to reverse this. As a result, the sinus rate may not be altered significantly by quinidine or it may even be accelerated.

It is a well-known fact that Q-T interval prolongation is most commonly produced by quin-

TABLE 18–1. Antitachyarrhythmic agents, including dosage,

| Drug | Full Dosage | Maintenance Dosage | Onset of Action | Maximum Effect |
|---|---|---|---|---|
| Digoxin (Lanoxin) | 0.5–1 mg IV initially, then 0.25–0.5 mg q̄ 2 h as needed (total: 1–2.5 mg) | 0.125–0.75 mg (average: 0.25 mg) daily (PO) | 10–30 min (IV route) | 2–3 h (IV route) |
| Deslanoside (Cedilanid-D) | 0.8–1.6 mg IV initially, then 0.4 mg q̄ 2 h as needed (total: 1.2–2 mg) | — | 10–30 min | 2–3 h |
| Ouabain (G-Strophantin) | 0.25–0.5 mg IV initially, then 0.1 mg q̄ ½ h as needed (total: 0.5–1.2 mg) | — | 3–10 min | ½–1 h |
| Lidocaine (Xylocaine) | 75–100 mg direct IV q̄ 10–20 min as needed (total: 750 mg) or 200–250 mg IM | 1–5 mg/min IV infusion | At once | At once |
| Procainamide (Pronestyl) | 1–2 g/200 ml 5% D/W IV drip 100 mg q̄ 2–4 min (1 g in ½–1 h) (total: 2 g) or 1 g PO initially, then 0.5 g q̄ 2–3 h (total: 3–5 g) | 0.25–0.5 g q̄ 3 h (PO) | At once (IV route)<br>Rapid | Minutes (IV route)<br>1–2 h |
| Quinidine gluconate | 0.8 g/200 ml 5% D/W IV drip 25 mg/min or 0.4–0.6 g IM initially, then 0.4 g q̄ 2–4 h (total: 2.6 g) | — | 10–15 min<br>10–15 min | Not immediate<br>30–90 min |
| Quinidine sulfate | Oral route (see text) | 0.3–0.4 g q̄ 6 h (PO) | — | 2–3 h |
| Phenytoin (Dilantin) | 125–250 mg IV q̄ 10–20 min as needed (total: 750 mg/h) | 100–200 mg q̄ 6 h (PO) | At once (IV route) | Minutes (IV route) |
| Propranolol (Inderal) | 1–3 mg IV initially, then second dose may be repeated after 2 min. Additional medication should not be given less than 4 h (total: 10 mg) | 10–40 mg q̄ 6 h (PO) | At once (IV route) | Minutes (IV route) |
| Disopyramide (Norpace) | 300 mg PO initially, followed by 100–200 mg q̄ 6 h | 100–200 mg q̄ 6 h (PO) | 1 h | 2–3 h |
| Bretylium | 5–10 mg/kg direct IV (slow) q̄ 15–20 min as needed (total: 30 mg/kg) | 5–10 mg/kg (slow) IV or IM q̄ 6–8 h or IV infusion at 1–2 mg/min | 5–10 min for antifibrillatory effect and 20 min–2 h for prevention of V arrhythmias | — |
| Verapamil | 0.075–0.15 mg/kg direct IV (slow) followed by 5–10 mg IV, repeated at 30 min or IV infusion at 0.005 mg/kg/min | IV infusion at 0.005 mg/kg/min or 40–80 mg PO q̄ 8 h (maximum: 720 mg/day) | 5 min (IV) 2 h (PO) | 2–5 h |

IV, intravenous injection; IM, intramuscular injection; q̄, every; D/W, dextrose in water; PO, orally; h, hours; IV block, intraventricular block; LE, lupus erythematosus; GI, gastrointestinal; AFI, atrial flutter; SV tachyarrhythmias, supraventricular tachyarrhythmias; V tachyarrhythmias, ventricular tachyarrhythmias; SB, sinus bradycardia.

Reproduced with permission from Chung: Principles of Cardiac Arrhythmias, 3rd ed. Baltimore, Williams & Wilkins, 1983.

action, indications, adverse effects, and toxicity

| Therapeutic Plasma Levels | Duration of Action | Indications | Adverse Effects and Toxicity |
|---|---|---|---|
| 0.5–2.5 ng/ml | 3–6 days | SV tachyarrhythmias (especially for AF and AFl) | Almost every known arrhythmia, aggravation of CHF, anorexia, nausea, vomiting, color vision, blurring vision, headache, dizziness, confusion, allergic manifestations (urticaria, eosinophilia), idiosyncrasy, thrombocytopenia, GI hemorrhage, and necrosis |
| — | 3–6 days | | |
| — | 12 h–3 days | | |
| 2–5 $\mu$g/ml | Minutes | Primary: V tachyarrhythmias<br>Secondary: SV tachyarrhythmias with anomalous conduction in WPW syndrome | Dizziness, drowsiness, confusion, muscle twitching, disorientation, euphoria, cardiac and respiratory depression, convulsion, hypotension, AV and IV block |
| 3–10 $\mu$g/ml | 6 h | Primary: V tachyarrhythmias<br>Secondary: SV tachyarrhythmias including those with anomalous conduction in WPW syndrome | AV and IV block, ventricular arrhythmias, LE, nausea, vomiting, lymphadenopathy, hypotension, convulsion, allergic manifestations (eosinophilia, urticaria), agranulocytosis |
| | 6–8 h | | |
| — | 6–8 h | Primary: SV tachyarrhythmias including those with anomalous conduction in WPW syndrome<br>Secondary: V tachyarrhythmias | AV, IV block, nausea, vomiting, photophobia, diplopia, headache, tinnitus, diarrhea, ventricular arrhythmias, respiratory depression, hypotension, convulsion, rashes (macular or papular), thrombocytopenic purpura, thrombocytopenia, hemolytic anemia |
| | 6–8 h | | |
| 2–6 mg/ml | 6–8 h | | |
| 5–20 $\mu$g/ml | 4–8 h | Primary: Digitalis-induced arrhythmias<br>Secondary: Nondigitalis-induced V tachyarrhythmias | Cardiac depression, hypotension AV, SA block, sinus bradycardia, ataxia, tremor, gingival hyperplasia, allergic manifestations (urticaria, purpura, and eosinophilia) |
| 50–100 ng/ml | 3–6 h | Various tachyarrhythmias (very effective for those in WPW syndrome and MVP syndrome) | Marked SB, SA, AV block, CHF, nausea, vomiting, diarrhea, asthma, hypotension, shock, erythematous rashes, paresthesias of hands and fever |
| 2–6 $\mu$g/ml | 6–9 h | Primary: V tachyarrhythmias<br>Secondary: SV tachyarrhythmias including those with anomalous conduction in WPW syndrome | Dry mouth, urinary hesitancy or retention, blurred vision, constipation, precipitation of glaucoma, prolonged Q-T interval, V tachycardia or fibrillation, syncope, CHF, hypotension, AV block, IV block, aggravation of SSS, skin rash, jaundice, psychosis, hypoglycemia, agranulocytosis |
| 1.33 $\mu$g/ml | 5–10 h | Life-threatening or recurrent refractory V tachycardia or VF | Hypotension (especially postural), dizziness, vertigo, syncope, nausea, vomiting, parotid pain, new V arrhythmias, worsening of preexisting V arrhythmias |
| — | 3–7 h | SV tachyarrhythmias (AF, AFl, AT, AV JT) including those in WPW syndrome | Nausea, headache, dizziness, rash, flushing, urinary retention, constipation, ankle edema, hypotension, AV block, SB, sinus arrest |

**TABLE 18–2. Effects of cardiac drugs on conduction time**

| Drugs | A-H Interval (AV Nodal Conduction Time) | H-V Interval (His-Purkinje Conduction Time) |
|---|---|---|
| Digitalis | Increase (slowing) | No change |
| Propranolol (Inderal) | Increase (slowing) | No change |
| Quinidine | Decrease (accelerating) | Increase (slowing) |
| Procainamide (Pronestyl) | No change or increase (slowing) | Increase (slowing) |
| Phenytoin (Dilantin) | Decrease (accelerating) or no change | No change |
| Lidocaine (Xylocaine) | No change | No change |
| Disopyramide (Norpace) | No change | Increase (slowing) |
| Verapamil | Increase (slowing) | No change |
| Atropine | Decrease (accelerating) | No change |
| Isoproterenol (Isuprel) | Decrease (accelerating) | No change or decrease (accelerating) |

Reproduced with permission from Chung: Principles of Cardiac Arrhythmias, 3rd ed. Baltimore, Williams & Wilkins, 1983.

idine. Although the prolonged Q-T interval per se during quinidine therapy is not harmful, torsade de pointes (atypical VT), VF, and even sudden death may easily be provoked by any stimulus (commonly a VPC) as a result of a markedly prolonged Q-T interval with very broad T wave leading to the R-on-T phenomenon (Fig. 7–5).

**Indications:**

1. Quinidine has been an indispensable drug primarily to convert AF or atrial flutter to sinus rhythm. Before DC cardioverters were available, large amounts of quinidine sulfate had to be used to restore sinus rhythm, but it is no longer necessary to do so except when a DC cardioverter is not available.
2. At present, the role of quinidine is primarily to prevent the recurrence of AF or atrial flutter following a restoration of sinus rhythm by either digitalization or DC shock (Chapters 16 and 20).
3. In addition, quinidine is useful in the treatment of various acute supraventricular as well as ventricular tachyarrhythmias. In acute tachyarrhythmias, quinidine is found to be more effective for the treatment of supraventricular than ventricular ones.
4. Quinidine is also useful in the suppression of premature beats of various origin, including VPCs.
5. Quinidine is very effective in the treatment of supraventricular tachyarrhythmias with anomalous conduction in the WPW syndrome (Chapter 13).

**Full Dosage:**

1. For the treatment of acute tachyarrhythmias, quinidine gluconate 0.8 g diluted in 200 ml of 5% dextrose in water may be given intravenously at a rate of about 25 mg/min, under continuous ECG monitoring.
2. Intramuscular administration of quinidine gluconate may be carried out by giving 0.4–0.6 g initially, followed by 0.4 g every 2–4 hours as needed. Total dosage by intramuscular route should not exceed 2–4 g.

**Maintenance Dosage:** The usual maintenance dosage of quinidine sulfate for the prevention of recurrence of various arrhythmias is 0.3–0.4 g every 6 hours.

**Side Effects and Toxicity:**

1. Side effects or mild toxic manifestations include nausea, vomiting, diarrhea, tinnitus, slight impairment of hearing and vision, and slight widening of the QRS complex and/or Q-T interval.
2. When quinidine toxicity is advanced, the above manifestations become more severe. Thus, the patient may develop blurring vision, disturbed color perception, photophobia, diplopia, abdominal pain, headache, confusion, and ventricular tachyarrhythmias.
3. When the patient has an unusual sensitivity or idiosyncrasy to quinidine, he may develop respiratory depression, hypotension, convulsion, urticaria, macular or

papular rashes, fever, thrombocytopenia, hemolytic anemia, and even sudden death.

4. The most serious side effect and toxicity of quinidine is the production of multiformed and irregular VT (torsade de pointes), which is usually initiated by VPCs with the R-on-T phenomenon as a result of a markedly prolonged Q-T interval with broad T wave induced by quinidine. Torsade de pointes (Fig. 7–5) is most commonly initiated by VPCs, and the coupling interval is usually very long (Fig. 7–5). Since digoxin toxicity is easily produced when quinidine and digoxin are given together (Chapter 16), torsade de pointes may be easily provoked under this circumstance (Fig. 7–5). This serious arrhythmia often transforms to VF, leading to death.
5. It has been shown that so-called quinidine syncope or sudden death from quinidine is attributed to VF as a result of R-on-T phenomenon initiated by the multiform VT (Fig. 7–5).

## Lidocaine (Xylocaine)

The discovery of the antiarrhythmic properties of lidocaine (Xylocaine) is probably the most important addition to the therapeutic approach to cardiac arrhythmias. Lidocaine has a similar structure to quinidine or procainamide, but its electrophysiologic properties are different. Since lidocaine has little effect on the atria, the drug is of little use in the treatment of atrial tachyarrhythmias except for those associated with WPW syndrome. Lidocaine depresses diastolic depolarization and automaticity in the ventricles. It is of interest that lidocaine, in standard doses, has no effect on conduction velocity and generally shortens both the action potential and the refractory period. Approximately 90% of an administered dose of the drug is metabolized in the liver, and the remaining 10% is excreted unchanged via the kidneys. The action of lidocaine is more transient than that of procainamide, and the former penetrates the cardiac tissues more rapidly than does the latter drug.

**Indications:**

1. Lidocaine has been widely used, primarily for the treatment of ventricular tachyarrhythmias and VPCs associated with acute MI and cardiac surgery or cardiac catheterization.
2. In the past decade, lidocaine has gradually replaced procainamide because it is more effective and seldom produces hypotension when given properly.
3. Lidocaine is found to be the drug of choice in the treatment of various tachyarrhythmias, particularly AF with anomalous conduction in WPW syndrome, when urgent treatment is indicated (Chapter 13).

**Administration:**

1. For the initiation of therapy, direct injection of 75–100 mg of lidocaine (1–1.5 mg/kg) is done slowly, and the second dose may be repeated 5 minutes later.
2. In general, total doses should not exceed 750 mg, and it is advisable that no more than 300 mg should be administered during a 1-hour period.
3. When intravenous injection is not immediately feasible, alternatively, 200–300 mg of lidocaine may be given intramuscularly into the deltoid muscle. An additional intramuscular injection may be carried out 60–90 minutes later as needed.
4. It is recommended that lidocaine be administered under continuous electrocardiographic monitoring.
5. Following the termination of ventricular tachyarrhythmia, continuous intravenous infusion with a rate of 1–5 mg/min is needed for 24–72 hours in most cases in order to prevent recurrence of the arrhythmia.
6. When ventricular tachyarrhythmias do not recur, lidocaine may be replaced gradually with oral procainamide or quinidine.

**Side Effects and Toxicity:**

1. Toxicity of lidocaine is relatively uncommon.
2. The drug may produce dizziness, drowsiness, confusion, muscle twitching, disori-

entation, euphoria, cardiac and respiratory depression, convulsion, and hypotension.

3. Caution should be used in the repeated use of lidocaine in patients with severe liver or renal disease because accumulation may lead to toxicity.

## Propranolol (Inderal)

Propranolol is a beta-adrenergic receptor blocking agent that has been widely used for management of various tachyarrhythmias, including those induced by digitalis and those resistant to digitalis. Antiarrhythmic actions of propranolol are produced by 2 effects, inhibition of adrenergic stimulation of the heart and direct action on the electrophysiologic properties of cardiac tissue. The inhibition of adrenergic stimulation of the heart is needed for the treatment of catecholamine-induced arrhythmias. Direct membrane action on the electrophysiologic property is essential in the treatment of digitalis-induced arrhythmias. Thus, the overall effects of propranolol usually result in reduction of automaticity, including reduction of the sinus rate and prolongation of atrial and AV conduction time.

**Indications:**

1. Tachyarrhythmias associated with WPW syndrome: Propranolol is considered to be the drug of choice in the treatment of regular supraventricular (reciprocating) tachycardia with normal QRS complexes in this syndrome (Fig. 12–3).
2. Catecholamine-induced tachyarrhythmias: Propranolol is very effective in the treatment of tachyarrhythmias (of any origin) precipitated by physical exercise, emotional distress, or any other excessive sympathetic stimulation.
3. Arrhythmias associated with MVP syndrome (Barlow's syndrome).
4. Digitalis-induced tachyarrhythmias: Propranolol (Inderal) is used when potassium or phenytoin (Dilantin) is found to be ineffective or contraindicated (Chapter 17).
5. Atrial fibrillation or atrial flutter: Propranolol is used to reduce the ventricular rate in AF or atrial flutter when the rapid ventricular response is difficult to control by digitalis alone (Chapter 17).
6. Miscellaneous indications: Propranolol is found to be effective in terminating some cases of MAT. In addition, propranolol is useful when the arrhythmias are associated with IHSS, angina pectoris, or anesthesia.

**Contraindications:**

1. Bradyarrhythmias: Marked sinus bradycardia, sinus arrest, SA block, second or third degree AV block, SSS, and BTS
2. Congestive heart failure
3. Hypotension and cardiogenic shock
4. Bronchial asthma, bronchitis, and other chronic lung diseases
5. History of hypersensitive reaction to beta-blockers

**Administration and Dosage:**

1. Intravenous injection: Propranolol (Inderal) should be administered slowly under ECG monitoring. One to 2 milligrams is the usual dosage, and the second dose can be repeated 5–10 minutes later. Total dosage should not exceed 10 mg.
2. Oral administration when the clinical situation is not urgent. Propranolol may be given orally in doses ranging between 10 and 40 mg 3–4 times daily. The same dosage is recommended for long-term use or for prophylactic purposes.

**Side Effects and Toxicity:** Various side effects and toxicity of propranolol can be divided into 3 major categories: cardiovascular manifestations, respiratory manifestations, and miscellaneous manifestations.

Cardiovascular Manifestations:

1. Marked slowing of the heart rate, including sinus bradycardia, sinus arrest, SA block, AV JER, VER, ventricular standstill. Note that atropine should be used to counteract propranolol action.
2. Development or worsening of CHF. Proper digitalization and diuretic therapy are essential.

3. Development of hypotension. Isoproterenol (Isuprel) should be used.
4. Development of acute MI. Development of acute MI has been reported upon sudden discontinuation of propranolol. Thus, a gradual reduction of dosage is preferable whenever feasible.
5. Difficulty of cardiac resuscitation. When the patient on propranolol therapy develops cardiac arrest, especially during cardiac surgery, it is often difficult to resuscitate. Thus, it is recommended that propranolol be discontinued for 24–48 hours before cardiac surgery if possible.

Respiratory Manifestations: The development of asthmatic attacks has been reported in susceptible individuals, particularly in patients with a history of asthma or bronchitis, since Inderal increases airway resistance.

Miscellaneous Manifestations:

1. Hypoglycemia has been reported in patients under insulin therapy or recovering from anesthesia and in pediatric age groups during periods of restricted food intake.
2. Neurologic manifestations, such as lightheadedness, fatigue, lethargy, hallucination, mental depression, insomnia, and peripheral neuropathy.
3. Nonspecific or allergic manifestations include nausea, vomiting, diarrhea, constipation, fever, erythematous rashes, thrombocytopenia, granulocytosis, and alopecia.

## Procainamide (Pronestyl)

Procainamide was the traditional drug of choice in the treatment of VT until lidocaine was proven in the past decade to be a safer and more effective agent. Large amounts of procainamide (Pronestyl) had often been used in the treatment of VT, especially until DC cardioverters became readily available.

Procainamide has very similar electrophysiologic effects to quinidine. It slows electrical conduction, increases the refractory period, and depresses diastolic depolarization and automaticity. It has an indirect vagolytic action, and AV conduction may be facilitated when low doses are used. However, the direct effect of procainamide produces depression of AV conduction when a higher dose is used. The therapeutic levels are easily achieved by oral administration, since this drug is almost completely absorbed from the gastrointestinal tract. This drug should be administered with caution to patients with significant renal disease, because the drug is excreted primarily by the kidneys in unchanged form.

**Indications:**

1. Although procainamide has very similar electrophysiologic actions to quinidine, the former drug has been used primarily in the treatment of ventricular tachyarrhythmias.
2. At present, the primary indication for procainamide is to prevent the recurrence of ventricular tachyarrhythmias following their termination by DC shock and/or intravenous lidocaine.
3. Procainamide is also effective in the treatment of supraventricular tachycardia, although it is not the primary drug of choice. Procainamide has been used in place of quinidine when the patient is unable to take quinidine.
4. At present, large doses of parenteral procainamide are used only when a DC cardioverter is not available and lidocaine is found to be ineffective.
5. Procainamide is very effective for suppression of VPCs.

**Full Dosage:**

1. Intravenous administration: When intravenous procainamide must be used, 1–2 g of the drug diluted in 200 ml of 5% dextrose in water is administered by continuous intravenous drip at a rate of 100 mg every 2–4 minutes under continuous ECG monitor. A total intravenous dose should not exceed 2 g.
2. Oral administration: When the clinical situation is not urgent, procainamide may be given orally. Initially, 1 g of procainamide may be given by mouth, followed by

0.5 g every 2–3 hours as needed. A total oral dose should not exceed 3.5 g.

**Maintenance Dose:** The usual maintenance dose of procainamide is 0.25–0.5 g every 3 hours by mouth.

**Side Effects and Toxicity:**

1. Side effects and toxic manifestations of procainamide include nausea, vomiting, fever, leukopenia, lymphadenopathy, lupus erythematosus-like syndrome, convulsions, AV block, intraventricular block of varying degree, ventricular tachyarrhythmias, and hypotension.
2. In some patients who are sensitive to procainamide, such allergic manifestations as eosinophilia, urticaria, and agranulocytosis may be observed.
3. The major disadvantage of procainamide is that the drug has to be given every 3 hours (by mouth) because of its short half-life in order to maintain the therapeutic blood level.
4. Torsade de pointes is only occasionally observed during procainamide therapy because the Q-T interval prolongation induced by the drug is not as common as quinidine-induced Q-T interval prolongation (discussed previously in this chapter). In other words, procainamide commonly produces diffuse intraventricular block, whereas quinidine frequently causes Q-T interval prolongation leading to torsade de pointes (Fig. 7–5).

## Phenytoin (Dilantin)

The discovery of the antiarrhythmic properties of phenytoin (Dilantin) is another important addition to the management of various cardiac arrhythmias, particularly those induced by digitalis. Phenytoin has a similar structure to the barbiturates, but the electrophysiologic properties are different from those of other antiarrhythmic agents. The conduction velocity in the atria is accelerated by phenytoin, resulting from a faster depolarization of the atria, although the sinus rate is usually not influenced by this drug. Although the AV conduction may not be influenced by phenytoin, it may be accelerated. Intraventricular conduction is not altered significantly by this drug as a rule. One of the most important actions of phenytoin is that it counteracts the depressant effect on the AV conduction induced by digitalis or procainamide. In addition, phenytoin depresses diastolic depolarization and automaticity and shortens the duration of the action potential and the effective refractory period.

**Indications:**

1. At present, phenytoin is considered to be the drug of choice in the treatment of various tachyarrhythmias induced by digitalis. This is especially true in the management of digitalis-induced VT (Chapter 17).
2. For the secondary indications of phenytoin, the drug is also very useful in the place of procainamide or lidocaine when those drugs are found to be ineffective.
3. Phenytoin is a very useful drug in preventing various arrhythmias when it is administered intravenously (the usual dose: 100–250 mg) just a few minutes before DS shock is applied in patients who have been taking digitalis (any amount), especially when a possibility of DI is present (Chapter 17).
4. The efficacy of phenytoin in the treatment of tachyarrhythmias associated with the WPW syndrome is disappointing (Chapter 13).

**Full Dosage:**

1. Intravenous administration: The initial dose of phenytoin is between 125 and 250 mg intravenously for 1–3 minutes under ECG monitoring. Most patients respond within 3 seconds–5 minutes. The same dose may be repeated every 10–20 minutes as needed, but a total dose should not exceed 750 mg/hour. Continuous intravenous drip of phenytoin is not practical because the drug easily precipitates with various commonly used intravenous solutions.
2. Oral administration: When the situation is not urgent, 200 mg of phenytoin may be given orally as an initial dose, followed by 100 mg every 4–6 hours as needed.

**Maintenance Dosage:** Following the termination of the tachyarrhythmias, a maintenance dose of phenytoin 100 mg 3–4 times daily is often needed for varying periods depending upon the clinical situation. Oral phenytoin is often useful in place of procainamide or quinidine for long-term therapy.

**Side Effects and Toxicity:** Side effects and toxic manifestations of phenytoin (Dilantin) include respiratory and cardiac depression, such skin reactions as urticaria, and purpura, eosinophilia, drowsiness, ataxia, tremor, depression, nervousness, arthralgia, gingival hyperplasia, hypotension, and AV block of varying degree. Fortunately, these manifestations are usually rare.

## Disopyramide (Norpace)

Disopyramide (Norpace), which is a very similar antiarrhythmic oral agent to quinidine, has recently been approved for clinical use in the USA. Norpace is a local anesthetic that has a direct electrophysiologic effect on the heart, very similar to those of quinidine and procainamide. Norpace also possesses intense anticholinergic effects that may alter some of the drug's direct electrophysiologic properties.

It is important to remember that Norpace is considered to be one of the most potent negative inotropic agents available on the market among all antiarrhythmic drugs. Thus, the drug should not be administered in the presence of CHF or cardiogenic shock.

Approximately 85–90% of an orally administered Norpace is absorbed from the gastrointestinal tract, and peak plasma levels are reached within 2–3 hours. Renal excretion is the primary route of elimination, and about 50% of the drug is excreted unchanged in the urine. This is the reason that special caution must be used in the presence of renal impairment when using Norpace, and smaller than usual dosage is recommended under this circumstance.

In the normal heart, there is little or no effect on the sinus node recovery time or on the sinus rate by Norpace. In SSS, however, the abnormally prolonged sinus node recovery time is often further prolonged by Norpace. It can further prolong the H-V interval when there is a preexisting conduction disturbance, although the drug has little or no effect on the P-R interval, QRS interval, Q-T interval, A-H interval, or H-V interval in normal hearts. In addition, the effective refractory period of the anomalous pathway in the WPW syndrome is prolonged by Norpace, but the drug possesses variable effects on the effective refractory period in the AV node. The effective refractory period of the atria is usually prolonged by Norpace.

It is interesting to note that Norpace does not seem to affect the serum digoxin level, although the drug is very similar to quinidine in many other aspects.

**Indications:**

1. Indications for the use of Norpace are essentially the same as those for quinidine and procainamide.
2. The primary indications are for the prevention and treatment of ventricular tachyarrhythmias (e.g., frequent VPCs).
3. The secondary indications include the prevention of various supraventricular tachyarrhythmias, such as AF or atrial flutter.
4. Norpace may be used in the prevention and treatment of various tachyarrhythmias with anomalous AV conduction in the WPW syndrome because the drug prolongs the effective refractory period of the accessory pathway (Chapter 13).
5. The capability of Norpace to reduce the slope of phase 4 depolarization is important in the treatment of cardiac arrhythmias via enhanced automaticity.

**Contraindications:**

1. Congestive heart failure
2. Cardiogenic shock
3. Sick sinus syndrome
4. Renal insufficiency
5. Hypersensitivity to Norpace

**Administrations and Dosage:**

1. The usual recommended loading dosage (by mouth) is 300 mg.
2. The usual maintenance dosage is 100–200 mg every 6 hours following the loading dosage.

3. In some reports, 400 mg every 6 hours has been administered with varying degrees of success.
4. The therapeutic plasma levels of Norpace are 2–6 μg/ml, and the maximum effect is reached within 2–3 hours after oral administration.

**Side Effects and Toxicity:**
Cardiovascular Effects:

1. Norpace may cause multiform VT (torsade de pointe) initiated by VPCs with the R-on-T phenomenon as a result of prolonged Q-T interval, and it may lead to VF, syncope, and even sudden death.
2. Negative inotropic effect may cause CHF or aggravate the preexisting CHF and/or cardiogenic shock.
3. Sinus node recovery time is further prolonged by Norpace in SSS.
4. The H-V interval is further prolonged when there is a preexisting conduction abnormality, so that various intraventricular blocks may occur.
5. The drug may cause AV block of varying degrees (rare).

Anticholinergic Effects:

1. Dry mouth, nausea, or vomiting
2. Urinary hesitancy or retention
3. Blurred vision and precipitation of glaucoma
4. Constipation

Other Effects: Skin rash, jaundice, psychosis, hypoglycemia, and agranulocytosis have been reported in the medical literature.

## Bretylium

Bretylium tosylate (Bretylol) has been approved recently only for parenteral use for the treatment of life-threatening, drug-resistant, and/or DC shock-resistant VT and VF in the USA. The oral form of bretylium is still under investigation, primarily because the drug is poorly and erratically absorbed from the gastrointestinal tract.

The onset of antiarrhythmic effect is within a few minutes to 5–10 minutes following intravenous injection and 20 minutes following intramuscular injection. The primary route of elimination of bretylium is via the kidneys, and about 80–90% of the drug is excreted unchanged in the urine. Thus, the dosage should be reduced in patients with renal insufficiency.

The electrophysiologic effects of bretylium on the heart are via direct membrane effects on the myocardium and indirectly via the sympathetic innervation of the heart. The direct membrane effects on cardiac tissue prolong the action potential duration and effective refractory period of the Purkinje fibers and ventricular myocardium.

Bretylium possesses dual adrenergic effects. The initial sympathomimetic effect of the drug is releasing norepinephrine from adrenergic nerve endings. During this early stage, a new ventricular arrhythmia may be provoked or the preexisting ventricular arrhythmia may be aggravated by bretylium, leading to a more serious clinical outcome. When the transient sympathomimetic effect subsides, bretylium inhibits the release of norepinephrine from adrenergic nerve endings; thus, antiadrenergic effects of the drug are the important antiarrhythmic properties.

**Indications:**

1. Bretylium is used primarily for life-threatening VT or VF when these ventricular arrhythmias are refractory to more commonly used drugs, such as lidocaine or procainamide, and DC shock.
2. Bretylium may be capable of terminating VF (chemical defibrillation).
3. Direct current shock is often effective to terminate VF following administration of bretylium even when the initial DC shock was ineffective.
4. Bretylium may be effective to prevent VF by raising the ventricular fibrillatory threshold.

**Administration and Dosage:**

1. Bretylium is given by intravenous injection, intravenous infusion, or intramuscular injection.
2. Oral use is not approved for clinical use.

3. The initial dose of intravenous injection is 5–10 mg/kg (i.e., 350–500 mg), slowly over 10–20 minutes.
4. When VF or life-threatening VT continues or recurs, the same dosage may be repeated and DC shock may be repeated every 15 minutes, until the total dose of 30 mg/kg is reached.
5. For maintenance dose, 5–10 mg/kg may be given slowly by intravenous injection every 6–8 hours, or, alternatively, the drug can be given by continuous intravenous infusion at 1–2 mg/ minute.
6. When the intravenous route is not immediately feasible, bretylium may be given intramuscularly, 5–10 mg/kg every 6–8 hours.
7. The onset of the antifibrillatory effect occurs within a few minutes to 5–10 minutes following intravenous injection, and the therapeutic plasma levels are found to be 1.33 $\mu$g/ml.

**Side Effects and Toxicity:**

1. Hypotension, particularly postural hypotension, is a serious side effect.
2. Vertigo, dizziness, and syncope may occur.
3. During acute therapy, nausea and vomiting are common.
4. During long-term therapy, severe parotid pain may be observed.
5. The most undesirable effect of bretylium is its transient sympathomimetic effect soon after administration. During this stage, bretylium may provoke a new ventricular arrhythmia or may aggravate the preexisting ventricular arrhythmia.

## Verapamil

Verapamil, which is a papaverine derivative with unique electropharmacologic properties, is one of the newest FDA-approved antiarrhythmic agents in the USA. Initially, verapamil was introduced during the 1960s as an antianginal agent, but the drug is now considered to be one of the most important antiarrhythmic agents in the treatment of various supraventricular tachyarrhythmias, including those associated with WPW syndrome (Chapter 13).

Verapamil is a calcium-blocking agent, and it blocks the influx of calcium and possible sodium ions through the slow channels of cardiac tissue. Verapamil produces slowing of the sinus rate, and it prolongs the A-H interval and the functional as well as effective refractory periods of the AV node. The H-V interval and the QRS duration are not altered by the drug.

Orally administered verapamil is almost completely (90–100%) absorbed from the gastrointestinal tract, but bioavailability is not more than 10–20% as a result of extensive first-pass metabolism through the liver. Hepatic metabolism is the major route of elimination, and only 7% of the drug is excreted in the urine unchanged. Oral doses of verapamil are about 8–10 times larger than intravenous doses because of the above-mentioned first-pass hepatic effect. Orally administered verapamil is not as effective as intravenous verapamil either in terminating a variety of supraventricular tachyarrhythmias or in reducing the ventricular rate in AF or atrial flutter.

**Indications:**

1. For termination of various supraventricular tachyarrhythmias, particularly those generated by reentry mechanism.
2. Conversion of AF or atrial flutter to sinus rhythm by verapamil has been reported, but the primary role of the drug is to reduce the ventricular rate in these atrial arrhythmias.
3. For termination of reciprocating tachycardia with normal QRS complexes in WPW syndrome (Fig. 12–3).
4. Verapamil is found to be not effective for ventricular arrhythmias.

**Contraindications:**

1. Advanced or complete AV block
2. Sick sinus syndrome and bradytachyarrhythmia

**Administration and Dosage:**

1. The recommended dosage for intravenous injection is 0.075–0.15 mg/kg slowly over 1–3 minutes, followed by intravenous in-

fusion of 0.005 mg/kg/min or 5–10 mg over 1–3 minutes, repeated at 30 minutes.
2. For children, the same dosage (0.075–0.15 mg/kg) regimen has been recommended.
3. For oral administration, the usual recommended dosage is 40–80 mg every 8 hours, and the maximum doses should be not more than 240 mg every 8 hours.

**Side Effects and Toxicity:**

1. For cardiovascular effects, verapamil may cause hypotension, AV block of varying degrees, marked sinus bradycardia, and sinus arrest.
2. Sick sinus syndrome and the preexisting AV block are often worsened by verapamil.
3. Noncardiac adverse effects of verapamil may include nausea, headache, constipation, dizziness, rash, flushing, urinary retention, and ankle edema.

## Antiarrhythmic Agents Under Investigation

Various antiarrhythmic agents under investigation will be briefly discussed here. They include amiodarone, aprindine, mexiletine, tocainide, encainide, acecainide, metoprolol, acebutolol, ethmozin, and nifedipine.

**Amiodarone:**

1. Amiodarone, which is a benzofuran derivative initially introduced as an antianginal drug, is now widely used as one of the most popular antiarrhythmic agents in Europe, Asia, and South America.
2. Amiodarone is found to be effective for acute and chronic treatment of various supraventricular as well as ventricular tachyarrhythmias.
3. Amiodarone is under active clinical investigation in the USA in view of the drug's long half-life and low toxic:therapeutic ratio, in addition to the excellent therapeutic results reported as an antiarrhythmic agent elsewhere in the world.
4. Amiodarone prolongs the duration of the action potential in the atria as well as in the ventricles, and it possesses antiadrenergic action.
5. Amiodarone slows the sinus rate by virtue of prolonging sinus node recovery time and prolongs the A-H interval as well as the P-R interval. The H-V interval is, however, not altered by the drug. Amiodarone prolongs the effective and functional refractory periods of the AV node and the relative refractory period of the His Purkinje system.
6. Since amiodarone is capable of prolonging the effective refractory period in the anomalous pathway, the drug has been widely used in Europe and South America as the agent of choice for a variety of tachyarrhythmias associated with the WPW syndrome. Remember that the conduction through the normal AV conduction system as well as the anomalous pathway will be slowed by amiodarone. Thus, amiodarone is probably the most ideal antiarrhythmic agent for all types of tachyarrhythmias in the WPW syndrome (Table 13–1).
7. Amiodarone may be injected intravenously to terminate or slow the ventricular response in various tachyarrhythmias when the treatment is urgently indicated. The oral drug is also effective prophylactically for a variety of tachyarrhythmias, including those associated with the WPW syndrome (Figs. 10–3 and 12–3).
8. The recommended intravenous dosage is 5–10 mg/kg, and the oral dosage is 200–800 mg/day. The onset of action following intravenous injection is 5–10 minutes, while the onset of action following oral amiodarone is 4–6 hours. The half-life of the drug is reported to be at least 2 weeks.
9. Amiodarone is contraindicated for patients with SSS and advanced or complete AV block. The drug should be given with caution when there is intraventricular block.
10. Amiodarone may cause nausea, vomiting, gastrointestinal discomfort, slate-gray skin discoloration, and micro-

deposits in the cornea. In addition, thyroid metabolism may be disturbed by amiodarone because the drug resembles thyroxine chemically, and various symptoms of hyperthyroidism or, more commonly, hypothyroidism may be observed.

**Aprindine:**

1. Aprindine, which was originally developed in Belgium, has been relatively popular in many European countries in the treatment and prevention of various supraventricular and ventricular tachyarrhythmias. The drug is available for oral and parenteral use.
2. The initial enthusiasm regarding its clinical use has been tempered by an extremely narrow toxic:therapeutic ratio with serious adverse effects, such as agranulocytosis that may be fatal unless detected early. The drug has been under clinical investigation in the USA for several years.
3. Aprindine has a potent local anesthetic effect and a terminal amine structure very similar to lidocaine. The electrophysiologic properties of aprindine are similar to quinidine and procainamide.
4. The effect of aprindine on the sinus rate is variable, but it slows the conduction diffusely at almost all levels of the heart. The drug prolongs the A-H interval, P-R interval, QRS interval, and H-V interval. The effective refractory period of the atria, AV node, and His Purkinje system are prolonged by aprindine.
5. Aprindine has been widely used in Europe in the prevention and treatment of various tachyarrhythmias associated with the WPW syndrome, since the drug slows the conduction in the anomalous pathway. In addition, aprindine is found to be especially useful in the treatment of various arrhythmias associated with the MVP syndrome.
6. Aprindine is shown to be easily absorbed from the gastrointestinal tract, and about 65% of the drug and its metabolites are excreted in the urine.
7. The onset of action following intravenous injection and oral administration is 5–10 minutes and 2 hours, respectively. The maximum antiarrhythmic effect following oral administration is usually observed within several days because the half-life is very long (20–30 hours).
8. The recommended intravenous dose is 200 mg at a rate of 2 mg/min, followed by 100 mg over 30 minutes, and then 100 mg over 6 hours. The oral loading dose is 200–300 mg, and it is followed by 100–150 mg daily in 2–3 doses. The therapeutic plasma levels of aprindine are reported to be 1–2 $\mu$g/ml.
9. Common side effects are dose-related neurologic symptoms, including ataxia, dizziness, nervousness, tremors, seizures, and impairment of memory. The most serious adverse effects of aprindine are agranulocytosis and cholestatic jaundice. Since the drug possesses a moderate negative inotropic effect, it may cause slight ventricular dysfunction even with therapeutic doses.

**Mexiletine:**

1. Mexiletine is a local anesthetic agent with anticonvulsant properties, and its pharmacoelectrophysiologic effects are similar to those of lidocaine. The drug is available for parenteral as well as oral use, and it is an antiarrhythmic agent for ventricular arrhythmias.
2. Although orally administered mexiletine is almost completely (80–90%) absorbed from the gastrointestinal tract in healthy subjects, the drug is found to be absorbed much less in cardiac patients, especially those suffering from acute MI. Metabolism through the liver is the main route of elimination, and 10% of the drug is excreted unchanged in the urine.
3. The recommended oral dose of mexiletine is 200–300 mg every 6–12 hours, and the intravenous loading dose is 1,200 mg given over a 12-hour period. The intravenous maintenance dose is 250–500 mg every 12 hours. The half-life of mexiletine is 10–14 hours, but it tends to be more prolonged in serious cardiac patients with

acute MI. The therapeutic plasma levels are reported to be 1–2 μg/ml.

4. Intravenous injection of mexiletine is shown to be very effective in treating acute ventricular arrhythmias, but its toxic effect is much more frequent than is that of lidocaine. Thus, the usefulness of mexiletine for acute ventricular arrhythmias is considerably limited. Consequently, the major role of mexiletine is probably to control chronic ventricular arrhythmias, particularly VPCs, with long-term oral administration.
5. Since the toxic:therapeutic ratio is relatively narrow, mexiletine frequently produces adverse effects that are mostly dose-related. Cardiovascular side effects and toxicity include hypotension, myocardial dysfunction, intraventricular blocks, and bradyarrhythmias, and these problems are commonly encountered following intravenous mexiletine. Even with a low therapeutic dose, mexiletine often causes neurologic symptoms, including blurred vision, tremors, nystagmus, dizziness, dysarthria, paresthesia, and alteration of mental state.

**Tocainide:**

1. Tocainide is the primary amine analog of lidocaine with a slightly different chemical structure suitable for oral use. The electrophysiologic properties of tocainide are almost identical to those of lidocaine.
2. Tocainide is shown to be well absorbed from the gastrointestinal tract, and the maximum serum levels are reached within 60–90 minutes following oral administration. Approximately 60% of the drug is metabolized by the liver, whereas 40% is excreted unchanged in the urine.
3. The recommended oral dose of tocainide is 400–600 mg every 8–12 hours, and the therapeutic plasma levels are reported to be 6–12 μg/ml. The half-life is 10–17 hours.
4. The major role of tocainide is for the suppression of ventricular tachyarrhythmias, particularly VPCs on a long-term basis.
5. The major cardiovascular adverse effect of tocainide is production of hypertension secondary to an increase in peripheral vascular resistance. Gastrointestinal side effects include anorexia, nausea, vomiting, constipation, and abdominal discomfort. Neurologic adverse effects may include tremors, headache, dizziness, paresthesia, and visual disturbances. Production of antinuclear antibodies has been reported during tocainide therapy.

**Encainide:**

1. Encainide was developed in the USA and released recently as a new investigational antiarrhythmic agent for ventricular arrhythmias, particularly VPCs.
2. Encainide possesses local anesthetic properties, and the chemical structure resembles that of procainamide. The drug is reported to be extremely active at low blood concentrations.
3. The usual oral dose of encainide is 100–300 mg per day in 4–6 divided doses. The therapeutic plasma half-life is reported to be 3–4 hours.
4. Orally administered encainide is reported to prolong significantly the atrial and ventricular effective refractory periods, AV nodal conduction, conduction via anomalous pathways in the WPW syndrome, and conduction through the His-Purkinje system. Thus, the drug commonly produces the prolongation of the P-R interval, QRS duration, and the Q-T interval. These ECG changes do not appear to indicate toxicity of encainide, however.
5. Adverse effects of encainide are reported to be mild and infrequent. They may include leg cramps, metallic taste in the mouth, dizziness, vertigo, paresthesia, and diplopia.

**Ethmozin:**

1. Ethmozin, which is a phenothiazine derivative, was synthesized in the Soviet Union about 15 years ago as an antiarrhythmic agent for supraventricular arrhythmias.
2. Alterations in the excitability threshold and an increase in the refractory period of

the atrial as well as ventricular myocardium appear to play important roles.

3. Although the precise therapeutic dosage schedule has not been fully established, intravenous injection of ethmozin in doses of 1–3 mg/kg was reported to bring about the onset of therapeutic effect within 5 minutes. The suggested oral maintenance dose is 75–150 mg every 6 hours.
4. Adverse effects are reported to be relatively uncommon, but ethmozin may produce nausea, vomiting, gastrointestinal discomfort, dizziness, vertigo, blurred vision, and mild hypotension.

**Acebutolol:**

1. Acebutolol is a cardioselective beta-adrenergic blocking agent, and it possesses the usual beta-blocking effects, including prolongation of AV nodal as well as SA conduction. In addition, His-Purkinje conduction may be slowed at high plasma concentrations.
2. Acebutolol is reported to reduce the ventricular response in AF or atrial flutter, and the drug may convert these atrial tachyarrhythmias to sinus rhythm. It has been shown that acebutolol is very effective in treating VPCs in various clinical circumstances, including MI. In addition, the potential role of acebutolol in treating a variety of cardiac arrhythmias associated with chronic obstructive pulmonary disease, including MAT, has been reported.
3. The recommended intravenous dose of acebutolol is 10–20 mg every 4 hours, and the oral dosage is 300 mg every 8 hours.
4. Side effects of acebutolol include marked sinus bradycardia, AV block of varying degrees, and depression of myocardial contractility.

**Nifedipine:** Nifedipine is a calcium antagonist that was originally developed as an antianginal drug, particularly for coronary artery spasm. It has been shown that nifedipine is a very effective antiarrhythmic agent for various cardiac arrhythmias, including life-threatening VT and VF associated with coronary artery spasm.

## ANTIBRADYARRHYTHMIC AGENTS

Because of the ready availability of artificial pacemakers, various antibradyarrhythmic agents (Table 18–3) have been used much less commonly in the past decade. Nevertheless, these agents are valuable for the management of such milder forms of slow rhythms as marked but transient sinus bradycardia. In addition, antibradyarrhythmic agents are extremely useful for urgent situations, such as Adams-Stokes syndrome, when artificial pacemakers are not immediately available. Atropine sulfate and isoproterenol are probably the most commonly used drugs.

### Atropine Sulfate

**Indications:**

1. Atropine is primarily used to accelerate the sinus rate by vagal inhibition. Thus, this is the drug of choice for marked symptomatic sinus bradycardia, sinus arrest, or SA block, usually associated with acute diaphragmatic MI or DI.
2. Secondary indication for atropine is Wenckebach AV block due to DI or acute diaphragmatic MI when the patient is symptomatic from the arrhythmia itself. However, in most cases, Wenckebach AV block does not require treatment.

**Administration:**

1. Atropine is best administered intravenously in a dosage between 0.3 and 1 mg (up to 2.0 mg), and a similar dosage may be repeated every 4–6 hours as needed. The total dosage of atropine should not exceed 4 mg. The effect of the drug is usually prompt.
2. Atropine may be given subcutaneously if the intravenous route is not feasible immediately.

TABLE 18–3. Antibradyarrhythmic agents, including dosage, action, indications, and toxicity

| Drugs | Dosage | Onset of Action | Maximum Effect | Duration of Action | Indications | Side Effects and Toxicity |
|---|---|---|---|---|---|---|
| Atropine sulfate | 0.3–2 mg $\bar{q}$ 4–6 h IV inj. as needed or the same dose may be given by SC inj. (total: 4 mg) or 0.4–0.8 mg $\bar{q}$ 4–6 h PO for mild form | 1–5 min | Few min–30 min | 4–6 h | Primary: Sinus bradycardia, sinus arrest, SA block<br>Secondary: First degree and occasionally second degree AV block | Dry mouth, urinary retention, exacerbation of glaucoma, hallucinations, hyperpyrexia, postural hypotension, sinus tachycardia, VPC, ventricular tachycardia |
| Isoproterenol (Isuprel) | 0.02–0.05 mg (up to 0.1 mg) IC or IV inj., or 0.1–0.4 mg SC or IM inj. $\bar{q}$ 2–6 h as needed or 1 mg/200 cc 5% D/W IV infusion, 1–4 μg/min initially and may increase to 5–10 μg/min as needed. | At once | At once | Minutes | Ventricular standstill, severe AS syndrome<br>Primary: High degree or complete AV block<br>Secondary: Sinus bradycardia, sinus arrest, and SA block | Tremor, nausea, nervousness, sweating, weakness, dizziness, headache, palpitation, VPC, ventricular tachycardia and fibrillation, hypotension |
| | 10–30 mg sublingually $\bar{q}$ 1–6 h (for mild cases) | Irregular | Irregular | Irregular | | |
| Epinephrine hydrochloride (Adrenalin) | 0.3–0.6 ml of 1:1000 solution IV, IM, SC, or IC inj., or 0.5–1 mg/250 ml 5% D/W IV infusion, 1–4 μg/min initially and may increase to 4–8 μg/min as needed. | At once | At once | Very short | High degree or complete AV block and ventricular standstill | Trembling, pallor, nervousness, hypertension, VPC, ventricular tachycardia and fibrillation |
| Ephedrine | 30–60 mg PO $\bar{q}$ 2–4 h | — | — | — | High degree or complete AV block | Urinary retention, nervousness, vertigo, insomnia, hypertension, ventricular tachyarrhythmias |
| Corticosteroids | Hydrocortisone IV inj. 200–600 mg for 24 h or Solu-Medrol 80 mg daily by IM inj. or Prednisone 40–60 mg daily PO | — | — | — | Primary: AV block with acute onset<br>Secondary: Chronic AV block | Prolonged steroid therapy may induce sodium retention<br>Cushing's syndrome, dissemination of TB, aggravation of diabetes mellitus, glaucoma, and psychosis |
| Molar sodium lactate | 5–7 ml/kg IV infusion over periods of hours. If urgent, 25–50 ml rapid IV drip initially | — | — | — | AV block in the presence of acidosis or hyperkalemia | Precipitation of CHF, alkalosis, hypokalemia, ventricular tachyarrhythmias |
| Chlorothiazide | 0.5–2 g daily (PO) for 6–8 weeks | — | — | — | Sinus rhythm with intermittent AV block | Hypokalemia, precipitation of gout, predispose to digitalis toxicity |

$\bar{q}$, every; IV, intravenous; SC, subcutaneous; IC, intracardiac; IM, intramuscular; D/W, dextrose in water; PO, by mouth; h, hours; AS syndrome, Adams-Stokes syndrome; TB, tuberculosis.

Reproduced with permission from Chung: Principles of Cardiac Arrhythmias, 3rd ed. Baltimore, Williams & Wilkins, 1983.

3. Oral administration of atropine has been used, but its effectiveness is less predictable.

**Side Effects and Toxicity:**

1. Serious toxic effects of atropine are uncommon, but VPCs or ventricular tachyarrhythmias may be induced.
2. Common side effects or mild toxicity include a dry mouth, urinary retention, exacerbation of glaucoma, hallucinations, hyperpyrexia, and marked sinus tachycardia.

## Isoproterenol (Isuprel)

Before artificial pacemakers were available for clinical use, the treatment of choice for complete AV block was the administration of isoproterenol. The drug is still very useful in the treatment of Adams-Stokes syndrome during an emergency or temporarily until an artificial pacemaker can be inserted. Thus, isoproterenol is at present still the drug of choice in the treatment of Adams-Stokes syndrome due to bradyarrhythmias, primarily complete AV block. Isoproterenol is capable of accelerating both the supraventricular and the ventricular pacemakers and of improving AV conduction. The drug possesses a potent inotropic action leading to an increment in the stroke volume, amplitude of myocardial contraction, and coronary blood flow.

**Indications:**

1. The primary indication for isoproterenol is in the treatment of Adams-Stokes syndrome due to complete AV block or ventricular standstill until an artificial pacemaker is inserted.
2. As secondary indications, isoproterenol may be used, in place of atropine, in the treatment of symptomatic sinus bradycardia, sinus arrest, and SA block.

**Administration:**

1. Isoproterenol can be given by direct intracardiac (IC), intravenous (IV), intramuscular(IM), or subcutaneous injection (SC), or it may be given by intravenous infusion.
2. In emergency situations, such as in severe Adams-Stokes syndrome or ventricular standstill, isoproterenol can be given by intracardiac or intravenous injection.
3. The usual dosage is between 0.02 and 0.05 mg, but up to 0.1 mg may be administered. Otherwise, the drug can be given subcutaneously or intramuscularly in a dosage of 0.1–0.4 mg every 2–6 hours as needed.
4. Continuous intravenous infusion of isoproterenol is indicated in severe cases in order to maintain the ventricular rate around 50–60 beats/min until an artificial pacemaker can be inserted. The usual method is to dilute 0.1 mg of isoproterenol in 200 ml of 5% dextrose in water, and the initial infusion rate is 1–4 μg/min. The infusion rate may be increased to 5–10 μg/min, and, occasionally, up to 40 μg/min may be required to maintain an ideal ventricular rate.
5. The most popular route for this drug is sublingually, and the usual dosage is 10–30 mg every 1–6 hours. Occasionally, the drug can be given as often as every 30 minutes as needed.

**Side Effects and Toxicity:**

1. Side effects or mild toxicity of isoproterenol include tremor, nervousness, sweating, nausea, weakness, headache, dizziness, palpitation, and hypotension.
2. A serious toxic effect is the production of ventricular tachyarrhythmias, which may occur equally with small or large doses.

## Epinephrine (Adrenalin)

Epinephrine has been almost as popular as isoproterenol in the treatment of Adams-Stokes syndrome. However, epinephrine is considered to be definitely inferior to isoproterenol because it produces significant hypertension and is prone to provoke ventricular irritability, particularly VF.

Epinephrine is capable of accelerating the atrial rate as well as the ventricular rate. The degree of acceleration of the atrial rate has no relationship to the initial atrial rate, whereas the degree of acceleration of the idioventricular rate is closely related to the initial ventricular rate. The degree of acceleration of the idioventricular rate is the greatest when the initial ventricular rate is very slow, while the enhancement of the ventricular rate is insignificant when the initial ventricular rate is relatively rapid.

**Indications:**

1. The primary indication for epinephrine is in the treatment of ventricular standstill, particularly associated with acute MI.
2. The secondary indication for epinephrine is in the treatment of Adams-Stokes syndrome due to high degree or complete AV block until an artificial pacemaker is inserted.

**Administration:**

1. In urgent situations, as in ventricular standstill, epinephrine 0.3–0.6 ml of 1:1000 solution may be given by intravenous, intramuscular, subcutaneous, or even intracardiac injection. Slow injection over a period of several minutes is recommended under ECG monitoring, and the rate of injection should be regulated according to the patient's response.
2. For long-term therapy, 0.5–1 mg 1:1000 solution of epinephrine diluted in 250 ml of 5% dextrose in water can be given by a continuous infusion. The initial rate of the intravenous drip is usually 1–4 $\mu$g/min, and the rate may be increased to 4–8 $\mu$g/min, according to the patient's response.

**Side Effects and Toxicity:**

1. Side effects or mild toxicity of epinephrine include nervousness, trembling, pallor, and hypertension.
2. A serious toxic effect is the production of VT and VF.

## MANAGEMENT OF TACHYARRHYTHMIAS ASSOCIATED WITH WPW SYNDROME (CHAPTER 13)

When tachyarrhythmias occur only transiently and with a short duration in the patient with the WPW syndrome, treatment is usually not indicated. However, WPW syndrome characteristically produces recurrent supraventricular tachyarrhythmias in many patients. Therefore, every physician should be fully familiar with the diagnostic criteria (Chapter 13) as well as the management of the WPW syndrome.

There are several ways to approach the management of WPW syndrome-related tachyarrhythmias (Table 13–1).

1. The first step is to apply CSS when the tachycardia is regular regardless of the QRS configuration (Fig. 12–3).
2. When CSS is ineffective, propranolol (Inderal) is the drug of choice in the treatment of regular supraventricular (reciprocating) tachycardia with narrow (normal) QRS complexes. The drug can be given either intravenously or orally, depending upon the clinical circumstance. Propranolol is extremely effective in young individuals.
3. Digitalis is equally effective for the above-mentioned situation if propranolol is found to be ineffective. It is very important to remember that digitalis should be avoided when the tachyarrhythmia (particularly AF) shows anomalous AV conduction in the WPW syndrome (Fig. 10–3). The reason for this is that the anomalous AV conduction may be enhanced by digitalis, leading to an extremely rapid rate. Sudden death has been reported under this circumstance when the patient developed VF secondary to extremely rapid supraventricular tachyarrhythmias.
4. Lidocaine (Xylocaine) is the drug of choice in the treatment of AF or atrial flutter with anomalous conduction (resembles VT) in WPW syndrome (Fig. 10–3).

5. For regular supraventricular (reciprocating) tachycardia with anomalous conduction, lidocaine should be used first. When the clinical situation is not urgent, quinidine or procainamide may be tried orally.
6. In extremely urgent situations, especially in AF or atrial flutter with anomalous conduction and very rapid ventricular rate (Fig. 10–3), DC shock should be applied immediately.
7. At times, an artificial pacemaker with overdriving pacing is indicated in refractory cases.
8. Various surgical approaches, such as ligation of anomalous pathways, have been tried in the treatment of refractory tachyarrhythmias associated with WPW syndrome, but the surgical result is not always promising.
9. For prophylactic purposes, propranolol (small dosage) is most commonly used, and digitalis or verapamil is the second drug of choice for reciprocating tachycardia.
10. For the prevention of AF or atrial flutter with anomalous AV conduction, quinidine or Pronestyl is recommended.
11. Sedatives or mild tranquilizers are often beneficial in many cases.
12. Amiodarone appears to be the most effective agent in the treatment as well as the prevention of various tachyarrhythmias in the WPW syndrome, but the drug is not available for routine clinical use in the USA.

# Chapter 19

# Artificial Cardiac Pacing

It has been well documented that artificial cardiac pacing is one of the most important and reliable ways to manage various cardiac arrhythmias, particularly bradyarrhythmias. Until a decade ago, the primary indication for permanent artificial pacing had been in the treatment of complete AV block. However, the most common indication for permanent artificial pacemakers at present is in the treatment of the SSS. In addition, artificial pacing with overdriving pacing rate (faster than usual pacing rate) is often a life-saving measure for refractory tachyarrhythmias. Bradytachyarrhythmia (BTS) exists when the abnormal heart rhythms consist of a component of rapid rhythm and one of slow rhythm. In this case, artificial cardiac pacing has a very important role because drug therapy alone is usually ineffective. Bradytachyarrhythmia syndrome is usually a late manifestation of SSS (Chapter 14).

The artificial cardiac pacemaker functions in a very similar manner to the natural pacemaker to initiate the electrical impulses generated by small batteries. The electrical impulses travel through the pacing electrodes to the heart from the pulse generator. The artificial pacemaker is timed to produce the electrical impulses (usually about 70–72 beats/min) just like the cardiac impulses initiated by the natural pacemaker (sinus node). In most cases, the heart is capable of pumping adequate amounts of blood under the control of an artificial pacemaker.

Approximately 250,000 people (500,000 according to some reports) live with artificial cardiac pacemakers in America alone, and 25,000–40,000 (100,000–110,000 according to some medical reports) new patients will require an artificial pacemaker implantation annually. Although it is difficult to know exactly how many people worldwide live with an artificial pacemaker at the present time, it is estimated to be at least 500,000 people (750,000–1,000,000 according to some reports). The total number of artificial pacemakers sold within the last 20 years is estimated to be approximately at least 1.5–2 million, possibly more. It is clearly evident that artificial cardiac pacing can provide not only the prolongation of human life, but also a significant improvement in the quality of life. Long-term administration of various drugs (e.g., isoproterenol, atropine, epinephrine) for bradyarrhythmias is no longer necessary because of the ready availability of artificial pacemakers in most civilized countries.

The fundamental principles for the utilization of an artificial pacemaker were established as early as 1932, and external cardiac pacing was introduced into clinical medicine in 1952. In 1957, temporary direct myocardial stimulation in the treatment of complete AV block was introduced, and a transistorized, self-contained, implantable pacemaker for long-term correction of chronic complete AV block was established in 1960. Mercury zinc cells had been used for the energy source until 10–15 years ago, and a lithium battery has replaced the mercury zinc battery entirely for all types of artificial pacemakers in recent years. In general, a lithium battery lasts 10–12 years in most clinical circumstances. The earlier pacemakers lasted only 15–18 months, and therefore frequent replacement of the pulse generator was required at that time. The nuclear-powered pacemaker was introduced about 20 years ago in clinical medicine, but it is not commonly used because there is no particular advantage over the lithium-powered pacemaker.

There are many types of artificial pacemakers on the market, but the most commonly used model is a demand ventricular pacemaker. The demand pacemaker has a sensing device that cuts the pacemaker off if the natural heart rhythm is faster than the preset pacing rate.

When the patient's own rhythm becomes slower than the preset pacing rate, the sensing device turns the artificial pacemaker on again. This is the reason the term "demand" or "standby" pacemaker is used. In other words, the demand artificial pacemaker works only when it is needed. In the past few years, multiprogrammable pacemakers have been introduced in clinical medicine. In this new type of artificial pacemaker, various functions (e.g., pacing rate, energy output, sensitivity) of the pacemaker can easily be controlled and adjusted noninvasively after implantation in order to provide the best pacing for a given individual. The multiprogrammable pacemakers will eventually replace all nonprogrammable pacemakers.

Following implantation of an artificial pacemaker, every patient should have periodic check-ups and should carry out the necessary daily care because the artificial pacemaker needs care as does any mechanical device, and complications or malfunctions may occasionally occur.

## INDICATIONS FOR ARTIFICIAL PACEMAKERS

The precise criteria for the use of a temporary or a permanent pacemaker vary slightly from institution to institution, but the following conditions are generally accepted.

### Short-term Pacing (Temporary Pacing)

1. Symptomatic second degree or third degree AV block, especially during acute MI, requires temporary pacing. It should be noted that AV block per se does not require artificial pacing.
2. Symptomatic and drug-resistant sinus arrhythmias, including sinus bradycardia, sinus arrest, SA block, and AV junctional bradyarrhythmias (often manifestations of SSS).
3. Bifascicular block and incomplete TFB associated with acute anterior MI (Fig. 9–3) usually require short-term pacing (prophylactic pacing) because these findings are often followed by a slow VER due to complete AV block (infranodal AV block or complete BBBB).
4. Emergency treatment for Adams-Stokes syndrome, symptomatic BBBB, and SSS.
5. Before or during implantation of a permanent pacemaker when the patient is symptomatic (e.g., syncope or near-syncope).
6. Prophylactic pacing during major surgery when Adams-Stokes syndrome and/or marked bradyarrhythmias are anticipated.
7. Drug-resistant tachyarrhythmias by overdriving pacing rate.

At present, the most commonly used pacemaker for short-term pacing is the temporary transvenous type. In almost all situations, a demand unit is preferable to a fixed-rate unit. This is because normal AV conduction may be present during the insertion of a pacemaker (especially when it is being used prophylactically) and because it is not uncommon to observe normal AV conduction occurring intermittently following the development of complete AV block. A bipolar or unipolar catheter electrode is inserted, via a jugular or arm vein, into the right ventricle, preferably in the apical region, under direct vision utilizing fluoroscopy, with an image intensifier. Otherwise, the blind float technique may be used in certain cases. In this method, the catheter electrode is advanced gently into position as the location of the tip is monitored by ECG. The usual pacing rate is around 70–72 beats/min.

When a physiologic pacing is desired, of course, AV sequential (bifocal) pacing mode is preferable. One of the important benefits of atrial pacing is its ability to suppress a variety of ectopic tachyarrhythmias, particularly those of supraventricular origin. Thus, atrial pacing, coronary sinus pacing, and AV sequential pacing are advantageous in the treatment of BTS or drug-resistant tachyarrhythmias. When there is significant AV conduction disturbance under these circumstances, AV sequential pacing (bifocal pacing) must be carried out.

## Long-term Pacing (Permanent Pacing)

The decision as to whether long-term pacing is indicated or not is very serious because the patient must live with an artificial pacemaker all his life and must observe various necessary cautions and daily care. The pulse generator should be changed every 8–12 years in most cases (every 3–6 years in older models), depending upon the model. One of the most serious problems following permanent pacemaker implantation is malfunction of the unit, which may be fatal. At times, it is difficult to judge whether a permanent artificial pacemaker is definitely required because there is some controversy among physicians in certain clinical circumstances. In general, in the following situations, long-term pacing is indicated.

1. Symptomatic and/or advanced SSS (Figs. 5–19, 14–1, 14–2, and 14–3)
2. Symptomatic, chronic second degree (usually Mobitz type II) or third degree (infranodal) AV block (Figs. 8–3 and 19–1)
3. Complete AV block in acute MI (regardless of the location of MI) lasting more than 2–3 weeks.
4. Congenital complete AV block.
5. Symptomatic BBBB (Table 9–2)
6. Recurrent Adams-Stokes syndrome (usually due to Mobitz type II, advanced or complete AV block and SSS)
7. Recurrent drug-resistant tachyarrhythmias benefited by temporary pacing.
8. Carotid sinus syncope (Fig. 12–4) (may or may not be due to SSS)

When the indication for a permanent pacemaker has been determined, the type of pacemaker suitable for the patient must be determined in view of the patient's age, general condition, and underlying disease. When physiologic pacing is desired, AV sequential (bifocal) pacing is preferable because the artificial pacing can provide almost identical hemodynamic consequences to the natural sinus rhythm, and the maximal cardiac output can be maintained. This is the reason that bifocal pacing has become the most commonly used method of artificial pacing in most clinical circumstances today. One of the major advantages of atrial pacing is its capability to suppress various ectopic tachyarrhythmias, particularly those of supraventricular origin. Drug-resistant tachyarrhythmias or bradytachyarrhythmias are often best treated with atrial pacing, coronary sinus pacing, or AV sequential pacing. Of course, AV sequential pacing has to be used when there is significant AV conduction disturbance under these circumstances. Fixed-rate ventricular pacemaker is seldom used today because various complications occur frequently. Most pacemaker manufacturers continuously produce the fixed-rate ventricular pacemakers primarily for foreign countries. Ordinary demand ventricular pacing is adequate in the treatment of complete AV block when physiologic artificial pacing is considered to be not essential.

## Artificial Pacemakers in Acute Myocardial Infarction

A special comment is in order regarding the use and abuse of artificial pacemakers in acute MI because there is significant controversy among physicians on this topic.

**Indications for Temporary Pacing in Acute Myocardial Infarction, Regardless of Location:**

1. Symptomatic and drug resistant bradyarrhythmias of any origin or mechanism
   a. Sinus bradycardia, sinus arrest, SA block
   b. Atrioventricular block (second degree, high degree, and complete)
   c. Atrioventricular JER and VER
   d. Bilateral bundle branch block (Table 9–2)
2. Sick sinus syndrome and BTS
3. Drug-resistant tachyarrhythmias
4. Direct current shock-resistant tachyarrhythmias
5. Ventricular standstill

**Indications for Temporary Pacing in Acute Diaphragmatic Myocardial Infarction:**

1. Drug-resistant symptomatic, second degree, high degree, or complete AV block,

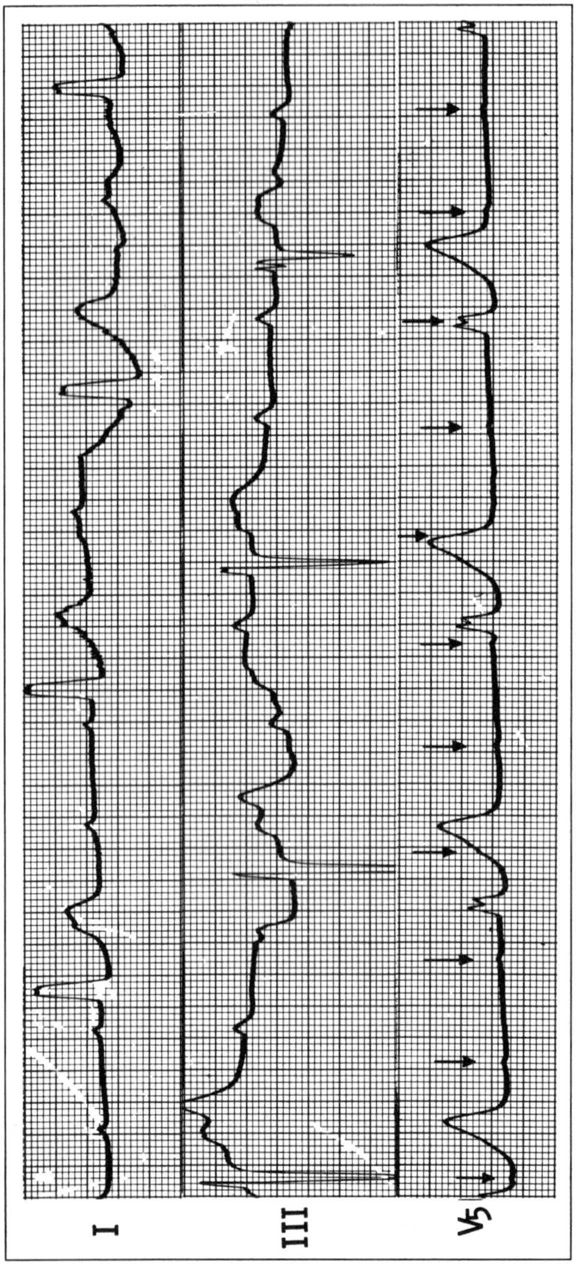


Fig. 19–1. Arrows indicate sinus P waves. The tracing reveals sinus rhythm (indicated by arrows) and VER (idioventricular rhythm, ventricular rate: 32 beats/min) due to complete AV (infranodal) block as a result of complete TFB (complete BBBB).

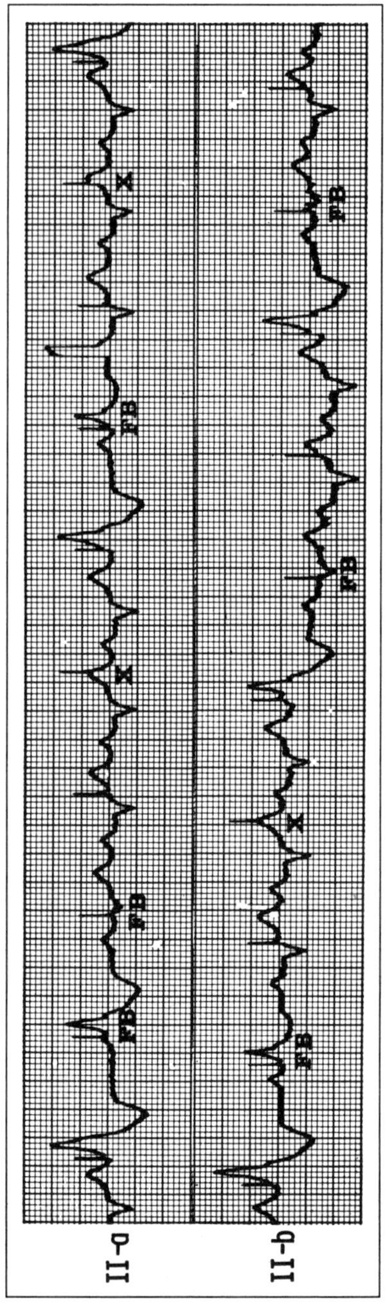


Fig. 19–2. Sinus rhythm with first degree AV block and intermittent fixed-rate ventricular pacemaker rhythm. Note frequent fusion beats (FB) and R-on-T phenomena (X). Leads II-a and II-b are not continuous.

sinus bradycardia, sinus arrest, SA block, and AV JER
2. Extremely slow ventricular rate (below 40 beats/min) due to any mechanism (even when the exact underlying mechanism is uncertain)
3. SSS and BTS
4. Refractory ectopic tachyarrhythmias
5. Ventricular standstill

**Indications for Temporary Pacing in Acute Anterior Myocardial Infarction:**

1. Complete AV block—pacing (often permanent) is indicated in every case regardless of symptoms
2. Mobitz type II AV block (usually permanent pacing is indicated)
3. Drug-resistant symptomatic sinus bradycardia, sinus arrest, SA block, slow escape rhythm with or without AV block
4. Sick sinus syndrome and BTS
5. Various forms of BBBB (BFB and TFB) with acute onset (Table 9–2)
6. Refractory ectopic tachyarrhythmias
7. Ventricular standstill

**Indications for Permanent Pacing in Acute Myocardial Infarction:**

1. Mobitz type II AV block, regardless of symptoms
2. Complete AV block (complete TFB) in acute anterior MI regardless of symptoms
3. Symptomatic and/or advanced SSS and BTS regardless of location of MI
4. Symptomatic and drug-resistant bradyarrhythmias with slow ventricular rate (less than 40 beats/min) in acute diaphragmatic MI lasting more than 2–3 weeks
5. Recurrent or persisting drug-resistant and/or DC shock-resistant ectopic tachyarrhythmias benefited by temporary pacing
6. Acute BFB with intermittent complete AV block in acute anterior MI regardless of symptoms

**No Value of Artificial Pacing in Acute Myocardial Infarction:**

1. First degree AV block alone (acute or preexisting)
2. Asymptomatic Wenckebach AV block (acute or preexisting)
3. Asymptomatic or transient sinus or AV junctional bradyarrhythmias
4. Nonparoxysmal AV JT or VT and ventricular parasystolic tachycardia
5. Left anterior hemiblock alone (acute or preexisting)
6. Preexisting RBBB or LBBB alone or left posterior hemiblock alone

**Equivocal or Questionable Value of Artificial Pacing in Myocardial Infarction:**

1. Acute RBBB alone
2. Acute LBBB alone
3. Acute left posterior hemiblock alone
4. Transient acute BFB (asymptomatic)
5. Acute LBBB or RBBB, or left anterior or posterior hemiblock with first degree AV block and/or prolonged H-V interval
6. Late (more than 1 week after the onset of acute episode) development of acute BFB (asymptomatic)
7. Preexisting bifascicular or incomplete TFB (asymptomatic)

## TYPES OF ARTIFICIAL PACEMAKERS

### Fixed-Rate Ventricular Pacemakers

1. The fixed-rate pacemaker is designed to function regardless of the patient's own natural rhythm (Fig. 19–2).
2. A fixed-rate ventricular pacemaker can be used with relative safety in patients with established chronic complete AV block when normal AV conduction is unlikely to occur, even temporarily.
3. In addition, older patients with relatively good cardiac function, using a fixed-rate pacemaker are able to carry out their ordinary activities adequately, since a maximum cardiac output is not important to sustain their limited physical requirements.
4. In approximately 25% of patients who

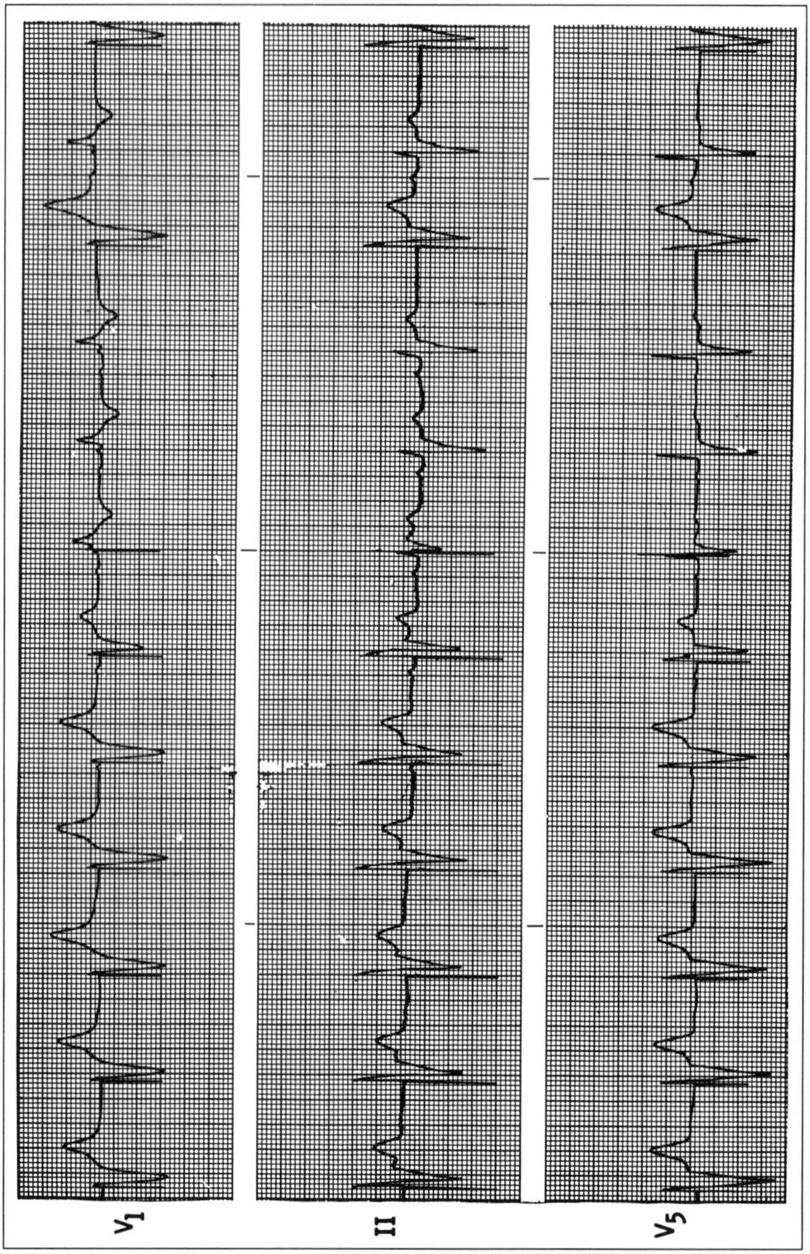


Fig. 19–3. Sinus rhythm with intermittent demand ventricular pacemaker rhythm. Right BBB with left anterior hemiblock is indicative of BFB.

require permanent pacing for Adams-Stokes syndrome, normal AV conduction (either normal sinus rhythm or second degree AV block) may return either temporarily or even for long periods of time. In this case, the patient's own rhythm competes with the pacemaker rhythm so that the patient may develop VF as a result of the R-on-T phenomenon. Primarily because of this, a demand pacemaker is preferable in many patients in whom normal AV conduction may return even momentarily.

5. A fixed-rate pacemaker is often used when overdriving pacing is indicated for treatment of drug-resistant ectopic tachyarrhythmias.
6. A fixed-rate pacemaker is seldom used today because other newer pacemakers possess various superior aspects.

## Demand (Standby) Ventricular Pacemaker

1. In the past 10–15 years, demand pacemakers have gradually replaced fixed-rate pacemakers because of a definite superiority in the former in avoiding competition between the natural rhythm and the artificial pacemaker rhythm.
2. The demand ventricular pacemaker functions only when the R-R intervals of the natural rhythm exceed a preset limit (Fig. 19–3). Therefore, a demand pacemaker is particularly ideal for temporary pacing when bradyarrhythmias are transient or intermittent.
3. It is important to recognize hysteresis (the interval from the natural beat to the immediately following paced beat is longer than the consecutively occurring pacing interval) in some models of demand units (Fig. 19–4). Otherwise, the finding may be misdiagnosed as malfunction.
4. There are some disadvantages in using transvenous catheter electrodes, including perforation of the ventricles, failure of pacing due to migration or exit block, infection, and fracture.

**Atrial Synchronized Pacemaker:**

1. A more physiologic type of artificial pacemaker is the atrial synchronized pacemaker.
2. In this type of pacemaker, the pulse generator is triggered by the natural P wave of atrial depolarization, and ventricular stimulation follows after an optimal delay corresponding to the P-R interval (Fig. 19–5). In other words, an atrial synchronized pacemaker functions as an electronic bundle of His.
3. The major advantage of this type of pacemaker is its ability to provide maximum augmentation of the cardiac output at changing atrial rates in order to meet varying physiologic requirements.
4. Another benefit is its utilization of the atrial contribution to ventricular filling to further augment cardiac output.
5. Thus, the atrial synchronized pacemaker becomes extremely valuable in younger or more active patients.
6. When AT or atrial flutter occurs, the pacemaker induces AV block of varying degree so that an optimum ventricular rate is maintained.
7. Although the advantages of an atrial synchronized pacemaker are definitely known, electronic failure is frequent, and thoracotomy takes longer because of the complexity of the device.
8. An atrial synchronized pacemaker is contraindicated in AF, marked sinus bradycardia, and unstable atrial activity, such as SA block, sinus arrest, and atrial standstill.

## Bifocal (Atrioventricular Sequential) Demand Pacemaker

1. The bifocal (AV sequential) demand pacemaker consists of 2 demand units, a conventional QRS-inhibited ventricular pacemaker, and a QRS-inhibited atrial pacemaker (Fig. 19–6).
2. In this model, the escape interval of the atrial pacemaker is designed to be shorter

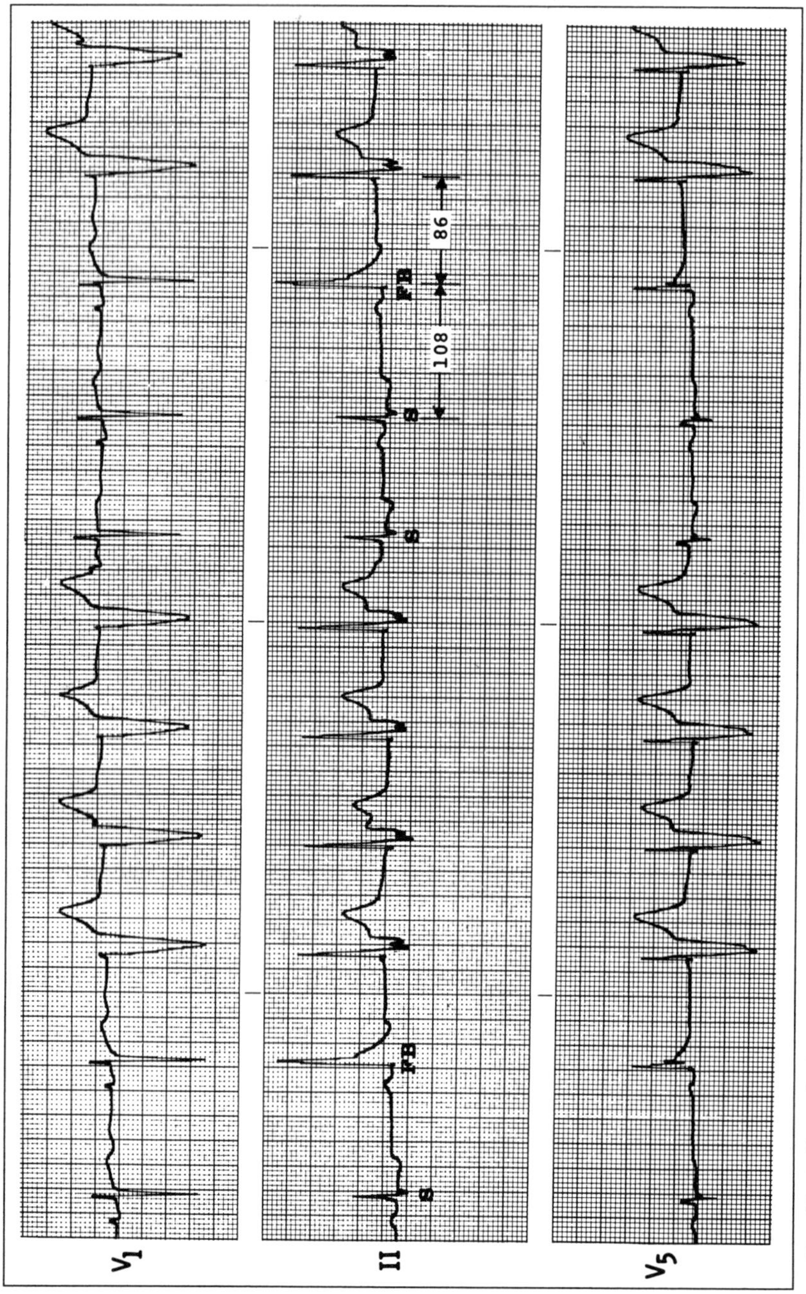


**Fig. 19–4.** Sinus rhythm (S) with intermittent demand ventricular pacemaker rhythm and pacemaker hysteresis. Note that the R-R interval from the sinus beat to the next pacing beat is longer than the consecutively occurring pacing cycle—called "pacemaker hysteresis." There are occasional ventricular fusion beats (FB). (The numbers represent hundredths of second.)

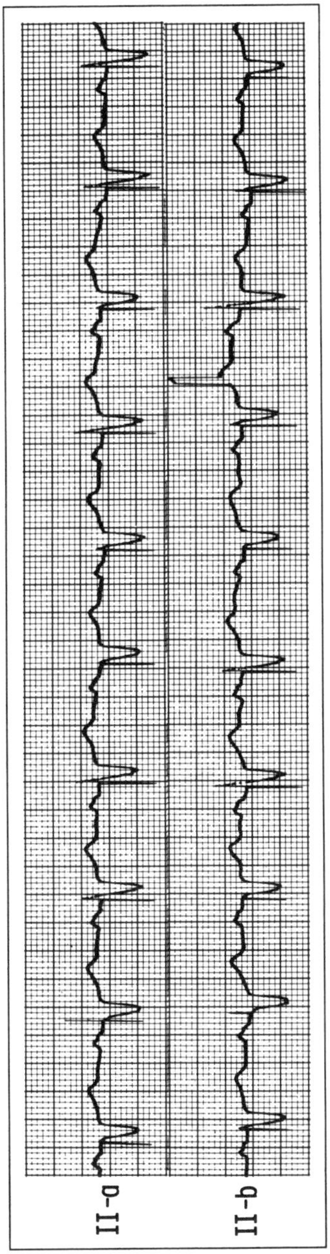


**Fig. 19–5.** Atrial synchronized pacemaker rhythm. Leads II-a and II-b are not continuous.

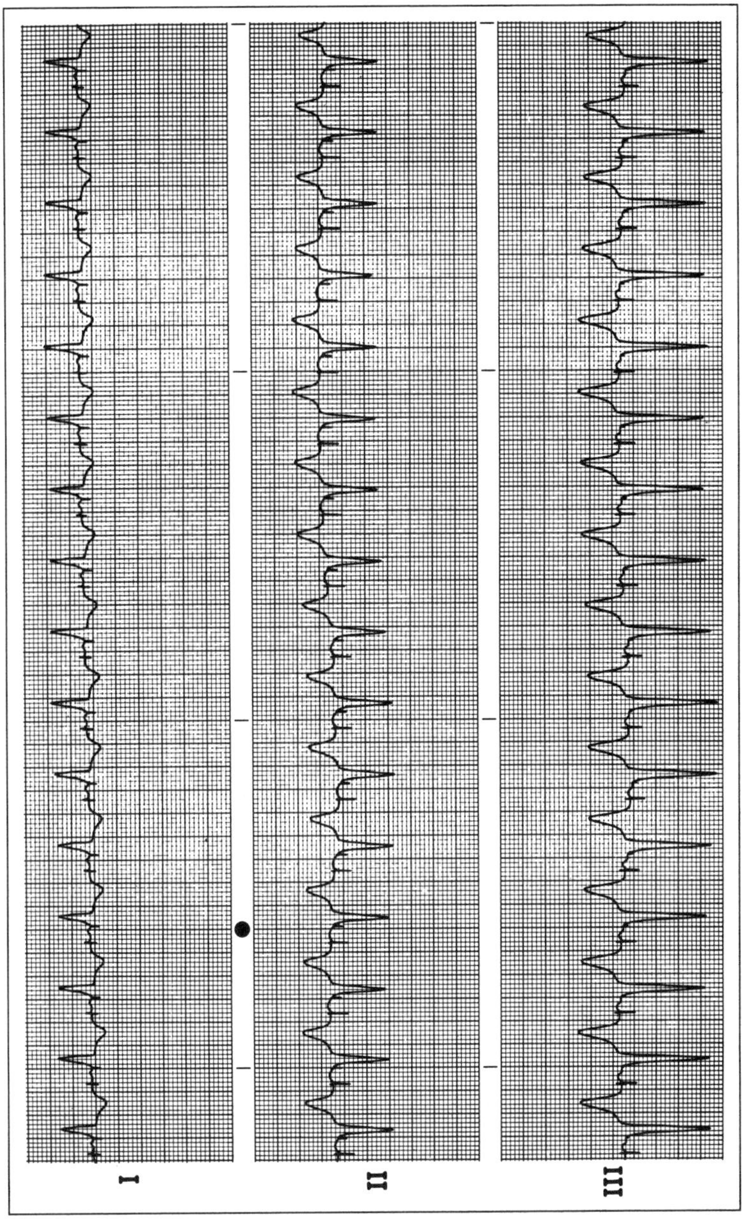


**Fig. 19–6.** Bifocal (AV sequential) pacemaker rhythm.

than that of the ventricular pacemaker. Thus, the difference between these 2 escape intervals is a determining factor for the AV sequential delay.

3. The bifocal demand pacemaker can stimulate both atria and ventricles in sequence, or it may stimulate the atria alone or remain totally dormant. Thus, the pacemaker functions automatically according to the individual patient's needs.
4. In general, the bifocal demand pacemaker is considered to be indicated in SSS, significant atrial bradyarrhythmias associated with intermittent high degree or complete AV block (symptomatic), and high degree or complete AV block (symptomatic), in that atrial contribution to the ventricular output is essential.
5. The bifocal demand pacemaker does not compete with spontaneous ventricular contractions.

## Multiprogrammable Pacemaker

1. The purpose of multiprogrammability of artificial pacing is to provide the optimal cardiac function to an individual with a specific clinical circumstance by modifying and controlling various pacemaker parameters (functions) noninvasively after pacemaker implantation.
2. The primitive idea of the programmability of artificial pacing was introduced as early as 1960, but modern programmable pacemakers had been introduced in early 1973 for the first time. Initially, only 2 pacemaker functions (pacing rate and energy output) were programmed.
3. Newer multiprogrammable pacemakers are capable of modifying many parameters including:
   a. Pacing rate
   b. Energy output (pulse amplitude or duration)
   c. Sensitivity (sensing threshold)
   d. Refractory period
   e. Hysteresis
   f. Pacing mode
   g. Atrioventricular delay
4. Nine of fourteen pacemaker manufacturers in the USA provide models that possess multiprogrammability.
5. The pacing rate can be adjusted from 30–120 beats/min (up to 400 beats/min in some temporary pacing models).
6. The programmable pacemaker is very useful in patients with SSS and BTS (Figs. 14–1 and 14–3) by selecting the optimal pacing rate for the patient's exact needs.
7. In elderly individuals and patients with angina pectoris, a relatively slow pacing rate is desirable. Depending upon the patient's cardiac status, the pacing rate may have to be increased or reduced.
8. For refractory tachyarrhythmias, overdrive pacing is indicated. In this case, the most effective pacing rate may be selected exactly for the patient's need noninvasively.
9. The energy source for the multiprogrammable pacemaker is lithium, which usually lasts 10–12 years.
10. Disadvantages of the programmable pacemaker may include the following:
    a. Higher probability of malfunction because of complexity
    b. Higher cost
    c. Greater educational burdens for physicians, technicians, and all involved personnel because of complex design
    d. Increased reluctance of cardiac patients with programmable pacemakers to travel overseas or to small towns where sophisticated medical facilities and highly trained cardiologists or cardiac surgeons are not readily available

## Miscellaneous Remarks

The pacing site may be in the atria or coronary sinus region in order to utilize the atrial contribution and normal activation of the entire heart. In coronary sinus pacemaker rhythm, the retrograde P wave is initiated by the pacing

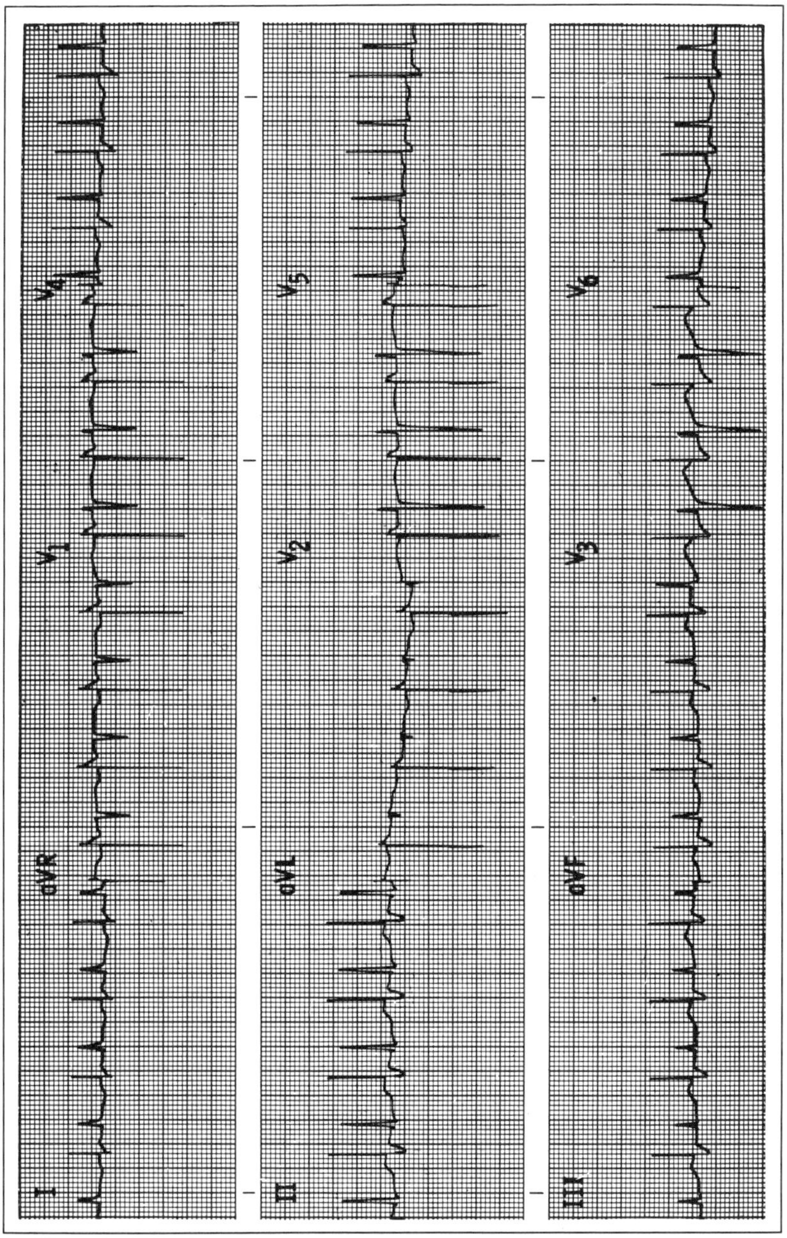


**Fig. 19–7.** Coronary sinus pacemaker rhythm.

spike and followed by the optimal P-R interval and normal QRS complex (Fig. 19–7).

Nuclear-powered artificial pacemakers were introduced more than a decade ago into clinical medicine, particularly in many European countries, but they are not frequently used today because there is no clear advantage to the nuclear-powered pacemaker over pacemakers powered with lithium. In addition, the usual problems associated with the nuclear-powered pacemaker prevent its usage in clinical medicine.

## COMPLICATIONS OF ARTIFICIAL PACING

During the insertion or implantation of an artificial pacemaker, the danger of inducing VF is always possible, and, therefore, a cardioverter must be readily available. In addition, various commonly used antiarrhythmic agents (Chapter 18) also should be available immediately. Common complications are as follows.

### Malfunctioning Artificial Pacemakers

A malfunctioning unit may be manifested in the following ways.

**Acceleration of Pacing Rate (Runaway Pacemaker):**

1. Runaway pacemaker is common when a fixed-rate pacemaker is used (Fig. 19–8).
2. When the runaway pacemaker runs extremely fast, the preexisting bradyarrhythmia reappears.
3. In advanced cases of runaway pacemaker, VF may occur. On the other hand, VF can occur even in a normally functioning pacemaker.
4. Runaway pacemaker is a medical emergency. In this case, the malfunctioning unit should be disconnected from the heart promptly. This can be done by cutting the electrode wires near their attachments to the pacer. Replacement with a temporary pacemaker connected to the bare electrode ends usually results in a prompt recovery.
5. Antitachyarrhythmic agents are ineffective for runaway pacemaker.

**Slowing of Pacing Rate:**

1. Slowing of pacing rate is a common form of malfunction when a demand unit is used.
2. Slowing of pacing may be associated with irregular pacing (Fig. 19–9).

**Irregular Pacing:**

1. Irregular pacing is usually observed in an advanced or late state of malfunction (Fig. 19–9).
2. Irregular pacing may be associated with slowing or acceleration of the pacing rate.

**Failure of Cardiac Capture:**

1. Failure of cardiac capture is a very common problem (Fig. 19–10).
2. Failure of cardiac capture may be associated with runaway pacemaker or slowing of pacing rate.
3. Failure of capture may occur in a normally functioning pacemaker because of various causes (e.g., quinidine or procainamide toxicity, hyperkalemia, advanced underlying heart disease).

**Failure of Sensing:**

1. Failure of sensing may occur alone, but it often coexists with failure of cardiac capture (Fig. 19–10).
2. Failure of sensing may be associated with other manifestations of malfunction.
3. Failure of sensing may, of course, occur in normally functioning pacemakers for various reasons (e.g., low amplitude of QRS complex of the natural beats).

### Perforation of the Ventricles

1. Perforation of the ventricles can occur when a transverse catheter electrode is used.

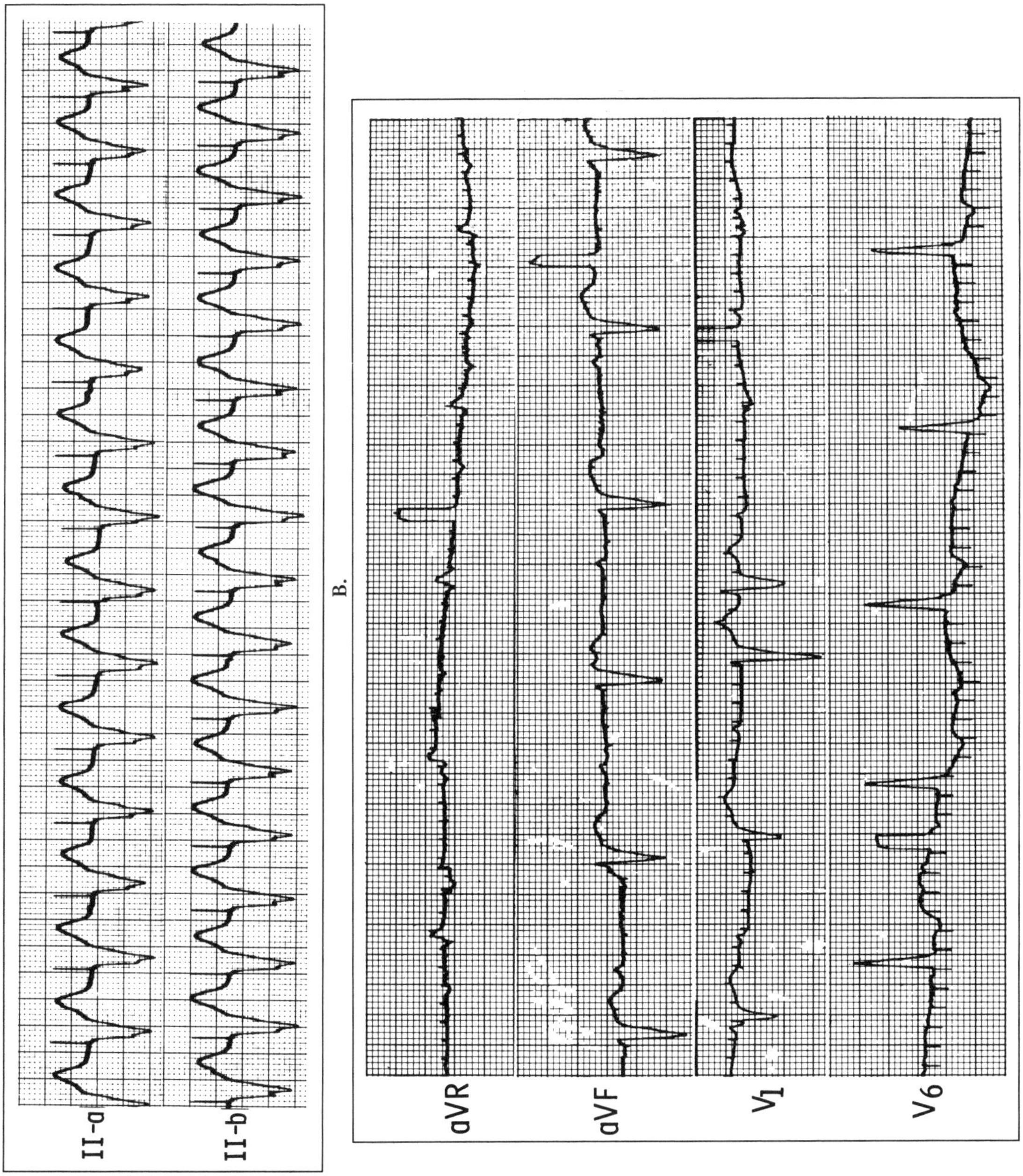


**Fig. 19–8. A.** Malfunctioning pacemaker is manifested by acceleration of the pacing rate (rate: 100–130 beats/min), a “runaway pacemaker.” **B.** Far-advanced runaway pacemaker shows extremely rapid pacing rate (rate: 430/min) with the preexisting complete AV block and a VPC (in lead $V_1$).

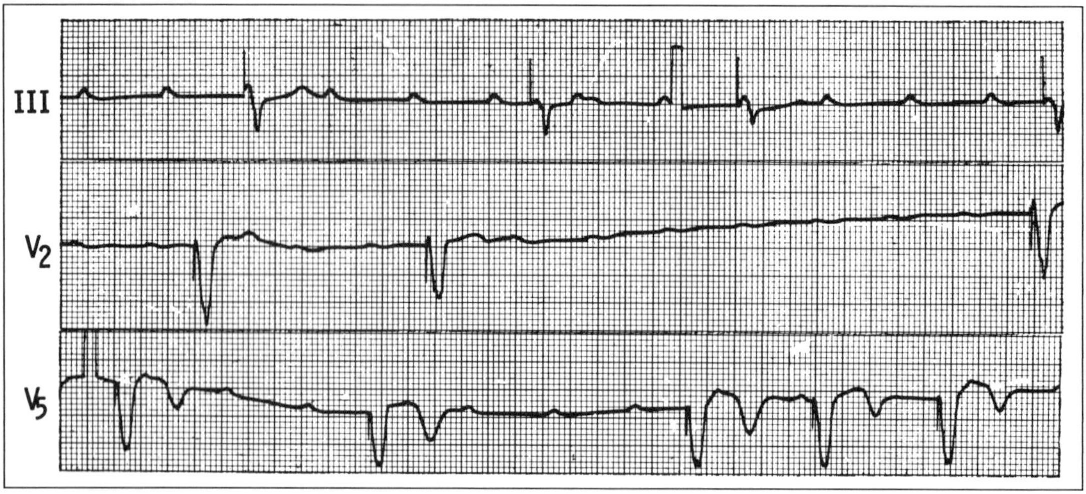


**Fig. 19–9.** Malfunctioning pacemaker is manifested by slow and markedly irregular pacing.

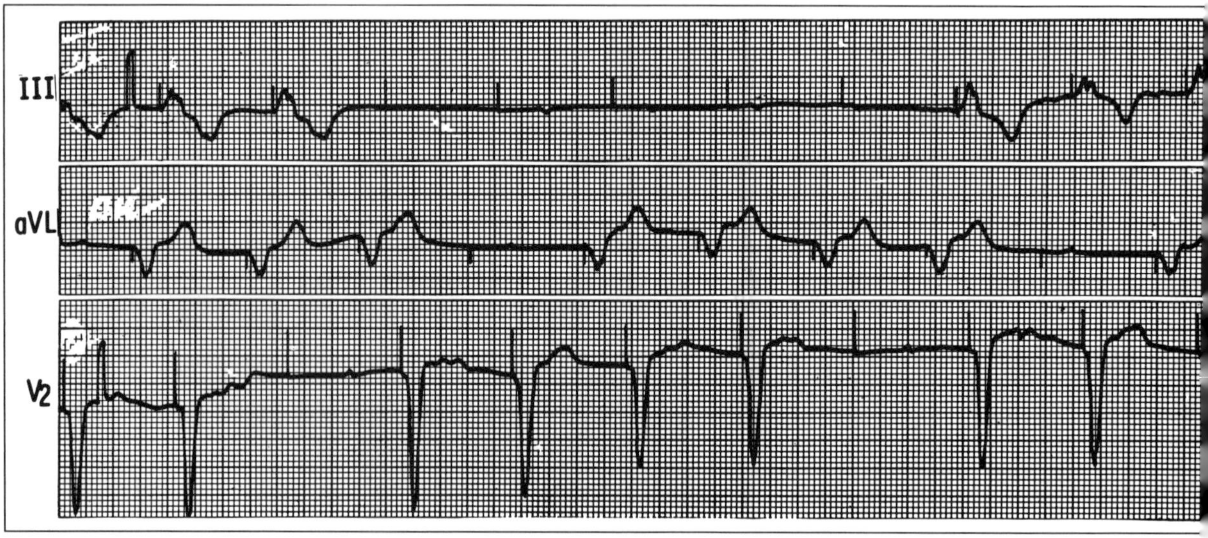


**Fig. 19–10.** Malfunctioning pacemaker is manifested by frequent occurrences of failure of the ventricular capture.

2. Perforation of the ventricles may be suspected when the following findings occur unexpectedly:
   a. Right bundle branch block
   b. Recurrent diaphragmatic contraction
   c. Pericarditis or pericardial effusions
   d. A pansystolic murmur (due to rupture of the ventricular septum)

## Other Findings

1. Electrode fracture
2. Infection
3. Thrombosis or embolism
4. Knotting of the wire
5. Various cardiac arrhythmias, which may be due to malfunction of the unit or which

may simply coexist with the normally functioning pacemaker rhythm.

## POSSIBLE INTERFERENCE WITH ARTIFICIAL PACEMAKER FUNCTION

The following may interfere with artificial pacemaker function:

1. Electric shavers
2. Automobile motors
3. Motorcycles
4. Malfunctioning TV sets
5. Direct contact with an ungrounded electrical appliance
6. Indirectly by proximity to equipment producing strong, rapidly fluctuating magnetic fields
7. Muscle stimulator for home use
8. Electric motors fitted with brushes and commutators
9. Motor-operated hospital beds
10. Electrosurgical and physical therapy equipment
11. Direct current shock

## FACTORS MODIFYING PACEMAKER FUNCTION

There are various factors that may modify the artificial pacemaker function:

1. Sympathomimetic amines may increase myocardial irritability.
2. Hyperkalemia may cause failure of cardiac capture.
3. Fibrosis around a pacemaker electrode may cause failure of cardiac capture.
4. Advancement of underlying heart disease may cause failure of cardiac capture.
5. Quinidine or procainamide toxicity may cause failure of cardiac capture.

## AFTERCARE OF PATIENTS WITH ARTIFICIAL PACEMAKERS

### What the Patient Has To Do

1. Every patient with a permanent pacemaker should check the pulse 1 or 2 times daily in order to be certain that the pacemaker's preset rate remains constant.
2. In case of alteration of the pulse rate (either slowing or increasing), a physician should be notified immediately, since this may be indicative of malfunction of the pacemaker.
3. When any new symptoms or signs, such as chest pain, syncopal episode, dizziness, or wound infection, occur, a physician should be notified immediately.

### What the Physician Has To Do

1. The patient should be fully instructed regarding the usual daily care, including common signs of a malfunctioning pacemaker, following the pacemaker implantation and before discharge.
2. The patient should be given an identification card indicating the name of the patient, date of pacemaker implantation, the name of the surgeon who performed the pacemaker implantation and/or the physician who will follow the pacemaker care after discharge, the name of the institution where the pacemaker was implanted, the type and model number of the the pacemaker and manufacturer's name, and a medical summary, including medications (optional).

**Pacemaker Follow-up Care:**

1. First visit (1 month after discharge)
   a. Check surgical wound.
   b. Detect gross evidence of malfunction.
   c. Ask usual pulse rate and any complaint, such as chest pain or syncopal episode.

2. Routine visit (every 3–6 months). Perform such procedures as ECG analysis.
3. Elective hospitalization: For pulse generator change.
4. Emergency hospitalization: For replacing malfunctioning unit.

**Pacemaker Follow-up Procedure for Each Visit:**

1. Complete check-up of patient's cardiac status and status of pacemaker implantation site and the pacemaker function.
2. Long rhythm strips (leads II and $V_1$) to check the pacing rate and to compare with preset rate.
3. A 12-lead ECG (at least once or twice per year) to detect any unexpected or new ECG abnormality.
4. When the patient's own sinus rhythm returns following implantation of a demand pacemaker, certain maneuvers, such as reducing the patient's own heart rate by CSS, by edrophonium chloride (Tensilon) injection, or by accelerating the artificial pacemaker rate by using a magnet, should enable one to check the function of the pacemaker.
5. Ask about any unusual or new complaint, such as chest pain or fainting episodes.
6. Arrange elective or emergency surgery as needed.

**Electrocardiographic Analysis of Pacemaker Function:**

1. Long rhythm strip (lead II) and preferably 6-lead ECG at each visit.
2. A 12-lead ECG every 12 months (routine check-up), when malfunction is suspected and when the patient has unusual or new symptoms.
3. Measure pacing rate to compare with preset rate.
4. Measure pacemaker artifact amplitude to compare with preset amplitude (often special equipment is needed).
5. Detect cardiac arrhythmias.

**Radiographic Analysis of Pacemaker Function:**

1. Chest radiographs (sometimes of abdomen) are taken before discharge, 6–9 months after discharge, and yearly thereafter. In addition, films should be taken immediately when a malfunction is suspected.
2. Check the position of the pacemaker and lead system. Malposition, twisting, angulation, and rotation of electrode or pulse generator should be checked.

**Pacemaker Clinic:**

1. When the pacemaker clinic with a specially designed pacemaker follow-up device is available, various pacemaker functions can be tested.
2. This can be done upon each patient's visit to the clinic, but the follow-up care can be provided through a long-distance telephone (a specially designed trans-telephonic monitoring system).
3. Various pacemaker functions (e.g., pacing rate, energy output) can be adjusted as needed when the pacemaker has multiprogrammable capability.

# Chapter 20

# Direct Current Shock

Direct current (DC) shock has been widely used to terminate supraventricular as well as ventricular tachyarrhythmias in various clinical circumstances. Direct current shock is often a lifesaving measure in terminating VT or VF. Because of the ready availability of DC cardioverters, the use of large dosages of various antiarrhythmic drugs (Chapter 18), especially quinidine and procainamide, is no longer necessary in most clinical situations. It has been shown that about 90% of the cases of AF are successfully converted to sinus rhythm, and 95–97% of cases of VT can be terminated by the procedure. It has also been shown that 90 of 100 patients with AF refractory to large doses of quinidine could be converted to sinus rhythm by DC shock. Electrical cardioversion has been found to be much safer than various antiarrhythmic drugs when the procedure is applied properly.

For successful cardioversion, it is very important to apply the procedure properly, and all possible contraindications should be eliminated. It should be emphasized that DC shock not only may be ineffective for digitalis-induced tachyarrhythmias but also may be fatal, since ventricular tachyarrhythmias or ventricular standstill may be induced. In general, when treating digitalis-induced tachyarrhythmias, DC shock should be attempted only as a last resort after all available measures have been exhausted (Chapter 17).

An automatic implantable minidefibrillator has been tried in humans in recent years with favorable results (discussed later in this chapter).

The use of the DC cardioverter may be divided into 2 major categories: (1) the treatment of acute tachyarrhythmias and (2) elective cardioversion for chronic AF and atrial flutter.

## TECHNICAL CONSIDERATIONS, PREPARATIONS, AND PRECAUTIONS

Specific maintenance care is necessary to be certain that DC shock equipment is in good working condition.

1. In general, the electrical integrity of the equipment should be checked every month by the biomedical engineering personnel.
2. Paddles must be large enough to stimulate most of the heart muscle fibers simultaneously. Otherwise, small paddles may deliver high electric current density in a localized pathway and cause myocardial damage.
3. For external DC shock, anterior and posterior paddles are ideal, but 2 anterior paddles are an alternative choice. Anterior and posterior paddles are preferable because the patient lies on the flat posterior paddle and only the anterior one needs to be held by the operator (a physician or nurse). This method is an important safety measure, particularly with the equipment in which one paddle is grounded. The anterior–posterior paddle position is said to lower the amount of electrical energy necessary for electrical shock treatment considerably.
4. As a rule, food should be withheld for at least several hours before applying DC shock (except for emergency treatment) in order to avoid vomiting.
5. Induced transient amnesia is necessary during application of DC shock (except for emergency treatment), and the amnesia can be easily produced by intrave-

nous injection of diazepam (Valium) in a dosage of 5–10 mg. General anesthesia or premedication is unnecessary. The duration of action of the Valium is only 3–4 minutes, and additional doses may be given, if necessary, within a few minutes after the first injection.

6. The treatment room where DC shock will be applied should be fully equipped for continuous cardiac monitoring and full CPR facilities, including all cardiac emergency medications and artificial cardiac pacemaker.
7. Recording of specific ECG leads should be possible as needed before, during, and after the electrical shock treatment. Before DC shock treatment, a short heart rhythm strip (lead $V_1$ or II) should be recorded in order to confirm the underlying heart rhythm so that it will be obvious when normal sinus rhythm is restored after DC shock treatment.
8. Paste (ECG paste is commonly used) should be applied liberally to the patient and rubbed well into his/her skin to reduce electrical resistance.
9. It should be certain that no part of the patient's skin is in direct contact with the metal of the trolley of the bed on which he/she is lying. No one should touch the patient, the bed, or any equipment to which the patient is attached at the moment of applying DC shock.
10. For elective cardioversion, all types of digitalis preparations should be withheld for at least 24–48 hours before the electrical shock treatment.
11. If the shock treatment cannot be postponed in patients who are taking digitalis, 100–250 mg of Dilantin should be given by intravenous injection before DC shock. Alternatively, 50–75 mg of lidocaine (Xylocaine) or 50–100 mg of procainamide (Pronestyl) may be injected intravenously in place of Dilantin. These medications may reduce the incidence of serious arrhythmias considerably.
12. Since the thromboembolic phenomenon is relatively high in certain high-risk groups, anticoagulants may be beneficial before and after DC shock. Anticoagulant therapy is highly recommended for patients with recent MI, cardiomyopathies, rheumatic heart disease (RHD), artificial heart valves, previous history of thromboembolic phenomenon, and for elderly people. Many physicians recommend anticoagulant therapy at least a few days to 1 week before DC shock and 3–4 weeks after the shock treatment under these circumstances. The true efficacy of the routine use of anticoagulant therapy for DC shock treatment is not certain.
13. After the termination of the tachyarrhythmia by DC shock, the 12-lead ECG should be recorded. The ECG should be monitored for at least the next 24 hours.
14. In addition, blood pressure (BP) should be measured every half-hour until it becomes stable and reaches the control value before the shock treatment.
15. A chest x-ray film may be taken within 24 hours to exclude the possibility of pulmonary edema, especially when a high-energy level shock was applied.
16. Even when normal heart rhythm is restored by DC shock, various medications may be needed thereafter.

## DIRECT CURRENT CARDIOVERSION FOR ACUTE TACHYARRHYTHMIAS

1. For the treatment of various supraventricular and ventricular tachyarrhythmias with acute onset, DC cardioversion is often a life-saving measure.
2. When a clinical situation is extremely urgent, such as in the treatment of life-threatening VT or VF, premedication for transient amnesia or anesthesia is not needed. Thus, 100–200 watt seconds of DC shock can be applied directly. If the arrhythmias persist, DC shock with increased energy (200–400 watt seconds) should be applied immediately following the first shock.
3. If the clinical situation is not extremely urgent, small amounts of thiopental so-

dium (Pentothal) or diazepam (Valium) may be administered in order to induce a transient anesthesia or amnesia immediately before the application of DC shock.
4. Premedication may not be indicated when only a small energy discharge is required, particularly in the treatment of atrial flutter.
5. Following termination of ventricular tachyarrhythmias, continuous intravenous infusion of lidocaine (Xylocaine) or, less commonly, procainamide is usually indicated, followed by oral maintenance therapy with procainamide (Pronestyl), quinidine, or disopyramide (Norpace).
6. When AF or atrial flutter is terminated by DC shock, maintenance doses of oral quinidine and digitalis are needed in most instances.
7. Various tachyarrhythmias associated with WPW syndrome can be terminated successfully by DC shock (Chapter 13).

## CONTRAINDICATIONS OR NONINDICATIONS FOR DIRECT CURRENT SHOCK

One of the most important aspects in considering the indications for DC cardioversion is the probability of restoration of sinus rhythm and of its maintenance for a reasonable period of time. In general, a heart that is difficult to convert to sinus rhythm is also difficult to maintain in sinus rhythm. It has been shown that the success of conversion is not directly influenced by the type of heart disease, prior resistance to quinidine therapy, age or sex of the patient, presence or absence of CHF, occurrence of thromboembolism, or degree of ventricular chamber enlargement.

In the following situations, DC shock is either contraindicated or not indicated:

1. Digitalis toxicity and/or hypokalemia (Chapter 17)
2. Severe mitral insufficiency and/or marked left atrial hypertrophy
3. Atrial fibrillation or atrial flutter with advanced or complete AV block (often a manifestation of SSS)
4. Chronic AF with duration of 5 years or longer
5. Imminent valvular surgery
6. Lone AF with slow ventricular rate (often a manifestation of SSS)
7. Marked first degree AV block (P-R interval of more than 0.28 second) before the onset of AF
8. Recurrence of AF or atrial flutter during adequate digitalis and quinidine therapy
9. Sick sinus syndrome

In general, chronic AF with advanced or complete AV block is a manifestation of advanced SSS (Chapter 14).

## COMPLICATIONS OF DIRECT CURRENT SHOCK

Complications can be reduced to a minimum or even avoided in most instances when the patient is properly selected and the procedure is properly applied. In general, complications of DC cardioversion are directly related to technical errors during the procedure, severity of the atrial damage, and improper use or overdosage of antiarrhythmic drugs. Technical errors in using a DC cardioverter include failure to synchronize the discharge, disregard for ECG artifacts that may trigger electrical discharge during the vulnerable period and lead to the development of VF, and excessive energy settings. In addition, excessive dosage of digitalis and/or various antiarrhythmic agents produces various and sometimes more serious postcardioversion arrhythmias.

1. Direct current shock may unmask digitalis-induced arrhythmias (Chapter 17).
2. Ventricular tachyarrhythmias may develop following DC shock, particularly during digitalis therapy (Chapter 17).
3. Preexisting advanced or complete AV block or ventricular standstill may occur following DC shock. When there is markedly prolonged ventricular standstill after termination of any ectopic tachyarrhyth-

mia, the diagnosis of SSS is strongly suspected, providing that the arrhythmia is not drug induced (e.g., DI). When any bradyarrhythmia (marked sinus bradycardia, advanced or complete AV block, ventricular standstill, AV JER or VER) is observed following termination of any tachyarrhythmia, these arrhythmias represent bradytachyarrhythmias in which an artificial pacemaker is indicated in most cases (Chapter 19).

4. When the stable sinus rhythm fails to appear following termination of any ectopic tachyarrhythmia (particularly AF or atrial flutter) by DC shock, the finding indicates marked sinus node dysfunction (SSS, Chapter 14) or marked sinus node depression from digitalis or antiarrhythmic agents (e.g., quinidine).
5. Direct current cardioversion may induce new atrial tachyarrhythmias. This is considered to occur when the electrical discharge is given during the atrial vulnerable period. Cardioversion-induced atrial tachyarrhythmias can be terminated by an additional DC shock in most cases.
6. The occurrence of thromboembolism, particularly cerebrovascular accidents in elderly individuals, within 24–48 hours following DC shock is not uncommon.
7. Intense and repeated DC shocks in dogs produce myocardial damage associated with increased serum MB creatine phosphokinase (CPK), but conventional DC shock does not cause such change in humans.
8. Superficial burn of the skin under the paddle may be induced by repetitive applications of DC shock, especially when insufficient jelly is applied.

## CARDIAC ARRHYTHMIAS RELATED TO DIRECT CURRENT SHOCK

Although DC shock is indispensable in terminating various supraventricular as well as ventricular tachyarrhythmias in many patients, certain cardiac arrhythmias may develop following the procedure. Some cardiac arrhythmias may be observed immediately following DC shock, even during ideal situations. Serious arrhythmias tend to develop from the procedure when there is DI or electrolyte imbalance (especially hypokalemia), when the patient is elderly with advanced heart disease and/or preexisting conduction defect, and when the procedure is improperly performed.

1. It is very common to observe atrial or AV JPCs following the termination of supraventricular tachyarrhythmias (AF, atrial flutter, or AT and AV JT), and in some cases, ventricular tachyarrhythmias.
2. Similarly, occasional appearances of AV JEBs or a period of AV JER with or without AV dissociation are not uncommon during the first 1–3 seconds (sometimes longer) following cardioversion.
3. Sinus bradycardia and sinus arrhythmia preceded by a short period of sinus arrest are also not infrequently encountered 1 or 2 seconds after the termination of a tachyarrhythmia. Irregular and slow sinus activity in this circumstance is simply due to the sinus node's requiring a warm-up period following a depression by a rapid ectopic impulse discharge. However, a failure of the sinus node to take over cardiac activity for a long period of time, such as is seen in AV JER without discernible P waves, or with extremely slow and irregular sinus activity, indicates that the sinus node is diseased (SSS, Chapter 17) or markedly depressed by digitalis or antiarrhythmic agents.
4. When the heart is severely damaged and the sinus node as well as ectopic escape pacemakers are unable to produce impulses following cardioversion, atrial as well as ventricular standstill is produced.
5. Varying degrees of AV block may be observed following DC shock when there is a preexisting AV conduction defect. First degree AV block is extremely common following the termination of chronic AF or atrial flutter. In this case, recurrence of the AF or atrial flutter is very common, and repeated cardioversion has little value.
6. It has been reported that cardioversion

may change a preexisting AF to atrial flutter or AT, or vice versa, instead of a sinus rhythm. The reason for the development of new atrial tachyarrhythmias following DC shock is probably the fact that the electrical discharge may fire during the vulnerable period of the atria. This is particularly true when the P-R intervals are long and the AV conduction ratios vary. Cardioversion-induced atrial tachyarrhythmias can be terminated by an additional DC shock in most cases.

7. The appearance of occasional VPCs immediately following DC shock is relatively common and is insignificant clinically.
8. However, frequent VPCs and runs of VT or VF are serious problems.
9. The most common cause of VF that develops immediately following DC shock is improper synchronization, that is, the electrical discharge falls during the vulnerable period of the ventricles (the R-on-T phenomenon).
10. The development of ventricular tachyarrhythmias immediately after DC shock is often attributed to digitalis and/or quinidine intoxication, even in the presence of proper synchronization.
11. Frequent VPCs or even short runs of VT may be provoked when DC shock is applied to a patient with hypoventilation during deep anesthesia.
12. In general, unnecessarily high energy discharges are prone to induce various cardiac arrhythmias.

## ELECTIVE CARDIOVERSION

1. Elective cardioversion is indicated for the treatment of chronic tachyarrhythmias, primarily AF or atrial flutter, when restoration of sinus rhythm is considered to be beneficial.
2. Less commonly, elective cardioversion is applied to terminate other tachyarrhythmias, such as atrial or AV JT.

**Purpose of Elective Cardioversion:** Elective cardioversion is indicated when a restoration of sinus rhythm is considered to be beneficial. In general, cardioversion is expected to provide:

1. An increment of cardiac output leading to improvement of CHF and increase in exercise tolerance
2. Better control of the ventricular rate
3. Reduction of thromboembolic phenomenon

**Preparation for Elective Cardioversion:**

1. Before DC cardioversion is attempted, all possible contraindications and nonindications must be carefully avoided.
2. Every patient with chronic AF or atrial flutter must be digitalized, and quinidized 24 hours to 1 week prior to DC cardioversion. At least 15% of cases of chronic AF can be converted to sinus rhythm by digitalis alone or a combination of digitalis and quinidine (oral maintenance dose).
3. It is important to remember that short-acting digitalis preparations, such as digoxin, should be withheld for 24–48 hours immediately before DC shock is applied.
4. If a long-acting digitalis preparation, such as digitoxin, has been used, the drug should be discontinued for 3–5 days prior to cardioversion.
5. The use of an anticoagulant 1–2 weeks before and after DC cardioversion has been emphasized by many investigators in order to prevent thromboembolism, but its practical value is uncertain. However, anticoagulation is recommended in patients with prior or recent systemic emboli.
6. Pentothal or diazepam (Valium) may be used prior to cardioversion, especially when high energy discharge is required.

## AUTOMATIC IMPLANTABLE DEFIBRILLATOR

There has been a remarkable new development by a team of physicians and scientists at Johns Hopkins University Hospital in Baltimore, and favorable therapeutic achievements have been demonstrated after in-depth experimental studies in the past 15 years.

1. The new implantable device, called a "minidefibrillator" or "automatic implantable defibrillator," is implanted under the skin of the abdomen and attached to the heart by 2 electrodes, 1 through the veins to the right atrium and the other to the apex of the right ventricle.
2. This minidefibrillator senses the onset of VF and automatically delivers the electrical shocks (700 volts) to the heart to terminate the arrhythmia and restore sinus rhythm.
3. The size of the new device is comparable to that of a cigarette pack, and it weighs about 250 g (9 ounces).
4. The electrical shocks can be delivered in 15–20 seconds after the initiation of VF, and a conscious patient feels a sharp tingling sensation from the shock.
5. When VF persists and normal heart rhythm is not restored by the first electrical shock, the minidefibrillator commands up to 3 more shocks.
6. The device has a capacity of delivering as many as 100 electrical shocks during the 3-year life of its lithium batteries.
7. The expected cost of this minidefibrillator is approximately $5,000.
8. The way in which the automatic minidefibrillator works is somewhat comparable to that of an artificial cardiac pacemaker.
9. If this new electronic device is found to be effective and safe and it becomes available in clinical practice, many cardiac patients, particularly those recovered from MIs, can have protection against VF outside the hospital so that sudden death may be prevented.

# Chapter 21

# Cardiopulmonary Resuscitation

Cardiopulmonary resuscitation (CPR) may be required when the cardiopulmonary system fails to provide adequate and effective function. It is indicated when the heart and/or lungs stop their functions suddenly and unexpectedly. The purpose of CPR is to restore the normal functions of the heart and lungs so that the delivery of adequate oxygen to vital organs is reestablished and maintained. Cardiac arrest most commonly occurs during the first few hours of acute MI, and permanent brain damage is a common end result when CPR is not applied within 4 minutes, even if the cardiac function is restored.

All medical as well as paramedical personnel must be capable of performing CPR. In addition, it is highly advisable for the general public to learn the proper technique of CPR simply because cardiovascular collapse is totally unpredictable. Full understanding of CPR is most urgently needed for family members of MI victims because the chance of developing cardiovascular collapse among these cardiac patients is much greater than in healthy individuals. The technique of CPR is relatively easy to learn even for a layperson, and CPR courses are given frequently by the local heart association and many other medical organizations.

## INDICATIONS FOR CPR

Cardiopulmonary resuscitation should be performed immediately when there is a sudden cessation of effective cardiopulmonary performance. In most medical institutions, particularly in the USA, Code Blue is commonly used to designate cardiopulmonary arrest. Cardiopulmonary arrest is usually manifested by:

1. Loss of consciousness
2. Loss of pulses
3. Loss of respiration
4. Loss of heart tones
5. Loss of BP

For whom should CPR be performed? Obviously, the answer is not simple, because different philosophical views may be involved. For example, CPR would seem to be inappropriate for patients with incurable or terminal illness, such as terminal cancer, and for elderly patients with irreversible and terminal strokes. Thus, CPR should be aimed primarily at patients in whom restoration of cardiopulmonary function will result in the potential for continuous productive life.

## TEAM AND EQUIPMENT FOR CPR

Cardiopulmonary resuscitation can be performed by 1 person, but it is preferable to have a team, especially in the hospital. There must be a standardized and well-organized team for CPR at every medical institution, and the team should be available instantly when cardiovascular collapse occurs. Each member of the team should be clearly aware of his/her duty for CPR.

1. Senior physician or director of CPR team assumes overall responsibilities and directs all necessary procedures and drug therapy.
2. Junior physician (or nurse) performs closed-chest cardiac resuscitation (massage) and artificial ventilation (respiration).
3. Junior physician starts the intravenous line for administration of various drugs.
4. Nurse has access to and prepares the required drugs, administers intravenous medications, and monitors cardiac rhythm and BP.

**TABLE 21–1. Drugs commonly used in cardiopulmonary resuscitation**

| Indication | Drug | Dosage |
|---|---|---|
| Asystole | Isoproterenol | 200–1,000 mg IV or IC infusion of 2–12 mg/min |
| | Epinephrine | 200–1,000 mg IV or IC infusion of 2–12 mg/min |
| | Calcium chloride | 10 ml (10% solution) IV to a total of 30 ml |
| Bradycardia | Atropine | 0.3–1.2 mg IV bolus |
| | Isoproterenol | IV infusion of 2–6 mg/min |
| Ventricular tachycardia/fibrillation | Lidocaine | 50–100 mg bolus to a total of less than or equal to 300 mg IV infusion 2–4 mg/min |
| | Pronestyl | 100 mg bolus to a total of less than 1,000 mg IV infusion of 2–4 mg/min |
| | Dilantin | 100 mg over 5 minutes Repeated to a total of less than 500 mg |
| | Propranolol | 1 mg IV $\bar{q}$ 5–10 min to a total of 5–10 mg |

Reproduced with permission from Chung: Principles of Cardiac Arrhythmias, 3rd ed. Baltimore, Williams & Wilkins, 1983.

5. Laboratory technician may be available to perform all necessary laboratory tests ordered by physicians.

Of course, organized teamwork for CPR cannot be expected if the cardiopulmonary collapse occurs outside the hospital. Under this circumstance, 1 or 2 persons or whoever is available should initiate the necessary CPR until a more experienced medical or paramedical team arrives at the scene. In the hospital, certain equipment and various drugs (Tables 18–1, 18–3, and 21–1) are necessary for CPR. For example, a cardioverter for DC shock is the most important equipment to terminate tachyarrhythmias, particularly VF (Chapter 20). An artificial cardiac pacemaker should also be available for the treatment of various bradyarrhythmias, particularly complete AV block (Chapter 19). It is preferable to have equipment for artificial respiration. A tracheal tube is, of course, essential for establishment of an airway when cardiopulmonary arrest occurs in the hospital.

## TECHNIQUES AND INITIAL MEASURES

The purpose of the initial measures for CPR is to initiate and maintain ventilation of the lungs so that adequate amounts of oxygenated blood can be delivered to all organs. Thus, the initial measures should include clearing the airway, initiating and maintaining respiration, and restoring blood circulation. A forceful blow to the sternum can terminate VF and may restore normal sinus rhythm. If the maneuver is not successful, however, one should immediately proceed to the next step as follows.

The patient should be placed in a supine position. One hand is placed behind the neck, and the other hand is placed on the forehead (Fig. 21–1). When the head is tilted back, this maneuver lifts the tongue from the back of the throat so that the airway will be fully open. During this maneuver, any obvious foreign

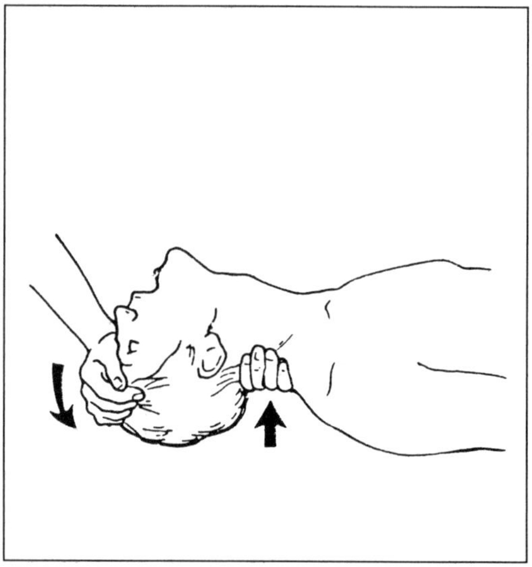

Fig. 21–1. Head-tilt method of opening the airway (see text).

body in the mouth and in the remaining airway should be removed promptly. In many patients, this maneuver alone may be adequate to restore breathing and to recover from cardiopulmonary arrest.

## Mouth-to-Mouth Resuscitation

1. While maintaining the backward tilt of the head with one hand, one should pinch the nostrils closed with the other hand.
2. Then, one should place his/her mouth over the patient's mouth, completely sealing the patient's mouth so that there is no leak of air (Fig. 21–2).
3. At the end of inspiration, one should exhale a larger than normal breath into the patient's mouth.
4. If the technique is correct, a rise should be noted in the patients' chest.
5. There should be no loss of air through the nose or mouth as the lungs are inflated.
6. After inflation of the lungs, one should remove his/her mouth from the patient's mouth, allowing the patient's lungs to deflate.
7. Air should be heard escaping from the lungs during this period.

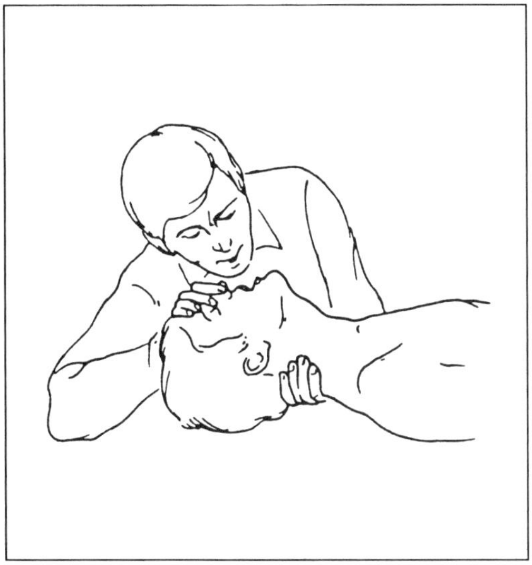

**Fig. 21–2.** Mouth-to-mouth resuscitation (see text).

## Mouth-to-Nose Resuscitation

1. The principle of mouth-to-nose resuscitation is essentially the same as that of mouth-to-mouth resuscitation.
2. In this technique, while maintaining the backward tilt with one hand, one should close the patient's jaw and seal the patient's mouth with the other hand.
3. Then one should place his/her mouth over the patient's nose, and after inhaling deeply, again exhale through the patient's nose.
4. Artificial respiration should be performed at a rate of 12 times/min.

## Problems with Artificial Respiration

1. If there is resistance to inflation of the lungs, a foreign body in the airway should be suspected.
2. One should roll the patient onto his/her side and deliver a firm blow between the shoulder blades in order to dislodge the foreign body (e.g., a piece of meat).
3. The patient's mouth and the remaining airway should then be explored for a foreign body.
4. Another maneuver that has been popularized recently for the removal of a foreign body is the Heimlich maneuver, which can be performed with the patient upright or supine. When the patient is upright, grasp him/her from behind below the rib cage, with the operator's fist against his/her abdomen. If the patient is supine, place the operator's hands one on top of the other on the patient's abdomen, between the rib cage and the navel. In both maneuvers, the hand is thrust quickly into the patient's abdomen. The thrust increases the pressure within the large airways and thus pops out the foreign body.
5. As can be expected, vomiting may occur during CPR. Suction equipment should be readily available for that purpose.
6. Gastric distention is best handled by inserting an indwelling nasogastric tube.

Recurrence of gastric distention may be prevented by intermittent epigastric pressure.

## Closed-chest Cardiac Massage

1. The next step of the initial resuscitative measures is the application of cardiac massage. Closed-chest cardiac massage is recommended in almost all clinical circumstances except when the patient is already in the operating room or when chest wounds preclude closed-chest massage.
2. For closed-cardiac massage, the patient's back must be placed on a firm surface.
3. When the patient is on a soft surface, such as a bed, a hard board should be placed under the patient's back.
4. The operator should be alongside the patient.
5. Place the heel of one hand over the lower third of the patient's sternum.
6. The hand of the operator should not touch the patient's chest, except for the heel of the hand.
7. The other hand may rest on the first hand (Fig. 21–3).
8. The patient's chest should be depressed 1.5–2 inches, and the pressure should be smooth and uninterrupted.
9. Following compression, release the sternum and ready the hand for the next compression.
10. The duration of the chest compression should be similar to that of relaxation.
11. The chest compression should be about 60 times/min and should be coordinated with artificial respirations.
12. If only one operator is present, it is recommended that 15 chest compressions be performed, followed by 2 quick artificial respirations.
13. When 2 or more operators are available, every fifth chest compression should be followed by a ventilation.
14. In order to assess the efficacy of the closed-chest cardiac massage, peripheral pulses should be palpated periodically.

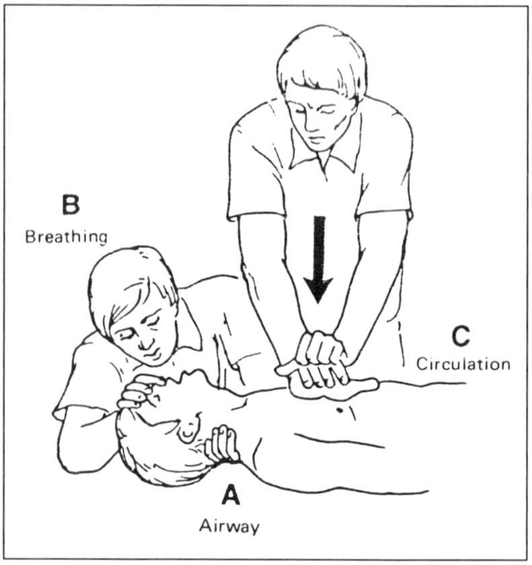


**Fig. 21–3.** Two-rescuer resuscitation with mouth-to-mouth resuscitation and external cardiac massage (see text).

15. When an indwelling arterial line is in place, the contour of the pressure pulse obtained will be of value in assessing the efficiency of cardiac massage.
16. Although closed-chest cardiac massage is a safe procedure, one must not be overly vigorous in chest compression, particularly in children. Various complications may include fractures of the ribs and sternum, hemothorax, hemopericardium, pneumothorax, bone marrow emboli, rupture of the stomach, lacerations of the liver and spleen, and rupture of the aorta. These complications usually occur because of inappropriate application of cardiac massage.
17. Various types of mechanical devices (some manual, others automatic) are available for closed-chest cardiac massage. In the hands of trained persons, these devices make cardiac massage easier and facilitate resuscitative efforts. However, these devices should never be used by inexperienced persons. Misapplication of these devices may result in not only ineffective resuscitation but also further injury to the patient.

### Evaluation of Efficacy of Initial Measures

1. During the initial measures of CPR, one must check for the presence or absence of several signs that indicate the success or failure of the resuscitative efforts.
2. Important signs include pulses in the femoral or carotid arteries, heart tones, spontaneous respiratory efforts, and palpable or recordable BP.
3. Of course, one should also be alert to any change in the patient's neurologic status and state of consciousness.
4. When there is any evidence that the resuscitative efforts have been sucessful, one may stop and observe the patient for several seconds.
5. If the cardiovascular collapse has been reversed, the patient should continue to be observed very closely, and the cause of the collapse should be investigated by a physician.
6. When the resuscitative efforts have been successful outside the hospital setting, the patient should be transported promptly to the nearby ER by ambulance or similar vehicle equipped with cardiovascular emergency care and a continuous monitoring system.
7. If, however, there is no change in the patient's status, artificial respiration and cardiac massage must be continued. CPR should not be stopped for longer than 5 seconds.
8. It is difficult to indicate when to stop the CPR because many medicolegal as well as philosophical factors are involved.

## SECONDARY MEASURES

In the hospital, if there is no response to the initial measures, a physician must perform the following while CPR is continued.

1. Quickly review the patient's chart to extract any pertinent information.
2. Obtain an ECG to assess the cardiac rhythm and to evaluate any abnormal finding, such as acute MI or pulmonary embolism.
3. Obtain an arterial blood gas analysis to assess the acid-base balance and the adequacy of artificial respiration.
4. Obtain a blood sample for the determination of serum electrolytes (e.g., potassium, sodium, calcium, and chloride).
5. If an intravenous infusion site is not already available, one should be established.

When these steps have been taken, further emergency treatment should be administered as indicated. For various cardiac arrhythmias, proper medication(s), DC shock, and artificial pacemakers may be required (Chapters 16, 18, and 19). Medications commonly used in CPR are summarized in Table 21–1.

## TERMINATION OF CARDIOPULMONARY RESUSCITATION

There are 2 major reasons to terminate CPR: (1) failure to restore an appropriate cardiac rhythm and adequate pumping action of the heart and (2) evidence of severe and irreversible brain damage. Cardiopulmonary resuscitation, of course, is terminated when the cardiopulmonary functions are fully established. Otherwise, it should be continued. Determination of the severity of brain damage is often difficult even for experienced physicians, and it can have medicolegal ramifications. By and large, severe brain damage is suggested by unconsciousness, lack of spontaneous movement, lack of spontaneous respiration, and dilatation of pupils without response to light. It is wise for lay people to continue CPR until medical personnel determine whether CPR should be terminated or not.

## CARE AFTER CARDIOPULMONARY RESUSCITATION

1. Following successful CPR, assessment of the underlying cause of the cardiopulmonary collapse is essential.
2. Thus, every individual who recovers from cardiopulmonary arrest must be closely

observed and treated in the CCU for at least several days.

3. When there is any significant arrhythmia, it should be treated with proper medications, DC shock, and/or artificial pacemaker (Chapters 16, 18, 19, and 20).
4. Likewise, the underlying heart diseases (e.g., acute MI) should be treated accordingly.
5. A careful and complete assessment of the degree of recovery should be part of post-CPR care.
6. Particular attention should be directed to the patient's neurologic status. If there is any evidence of significant brain damage, neurologic consultation is required.
7. As a rule, all patients who recover from cardopulmonary collapse by CPR should be observed for several weeks (at least 2–3 days in the CCU) to insure their stability.
8. During the observation period, emergency resuscitative facilities should be immediately available because cardiopulmonary collapse may recur, particularly in patients with acute MI or unstable angina.

# Chapter 22

# Uncommon Cardiac Arrhythmias

In this chapter, relatively uncommon cardiac arrhythmias with related topics are discussed briefly. They include parasystole, atrial dissociation, coronary sinus rhythm, coronary nodal rhythm, left atrial rhythm, electrical alternans, and aberrant atrial conduction (Chung's phenomenon).

## PARASYSTOLE

Parasystolic rhythm is of special interest since its mechanism of ectopic impulse formation is different from that of other ectopic rhythms.

Parasystole consists of the simultaneous activity of 2 (rarely more) independent impulse-forming centers, 1 of which is protected from the other, each competing to activate the atria or ventricles or both. The parasystolic pacemaker may be located anywhere in the heart but is commonly located in the ventricles (Fig. 22–1), less commonly in the AV junction (Fig. 22–2), and rarely in the atria (Fig. 22–3).

The incidence of parasystole varies at different institutions. This depends upon the degree of interest and knowledge of physicians and electrocardiographers regarding the interpretation of cardiac arrhythmias. This author found 105 instance (0.13%) of parasystole in a total of 80,000 ECGs.

Various studies regarding parasystole indicate that this arrhythmia is frequently encountered in elderly individuals, especially in those with diseased hearts, but parasystole is considered to be relatively benign arrhythmia. There is no age preferential regarding the location of ectopic foci. The peak incidence is between the fifth and seventh decades. Ventricular parasystole has been encountered much more frequently than has the supraventricular entity.

### Mechanism

Protection block (entrance block) and exit block are forms of unidirectional block in the heart. It is generally agreed that the parasystolic center, regardless of location, is protected by a unidirectional block from the transmission of impulses originating from any basic rhythm (protection block). If a continuous protection block ensues, the parasystolic pacemaker will act as the dominant pacemaker and produce a continuous parasystolic rhythm or even a parasystolic tachycardia. The exit block, which is in the opposite direction of the protection block, prevents outward transmission of the parasystolic impulses. If there is an occasional exit block, the parasystolic beats appear intermittently; if the exit block is continuous, the parasystolic rhythm will disappear. Exit block must be assumed to occur when the parasystolic rhythm is calculated to be rapid and the ectopic heart action that it causes is slow in spite of the nonrefractory phase of the basic rhythm.

### Diagnosis

The diagnosis of parasystole is made by proving the independence of the ectopic rhythm from the basic rhythm. The following diagnostic criteria are used: (1) varying coupling intervals, (2) constant shortest interectopic intervals, and (3) frequent appearance of fusion beats.

**Varying Coupling Intervals:** The coupling intervals of ordinary premature beats (extrasystoles) are usually constant because the ectopic beats are dependent upon the basic rhythm. Parasystole should be suspected whenever coupling intervals show considerable variability

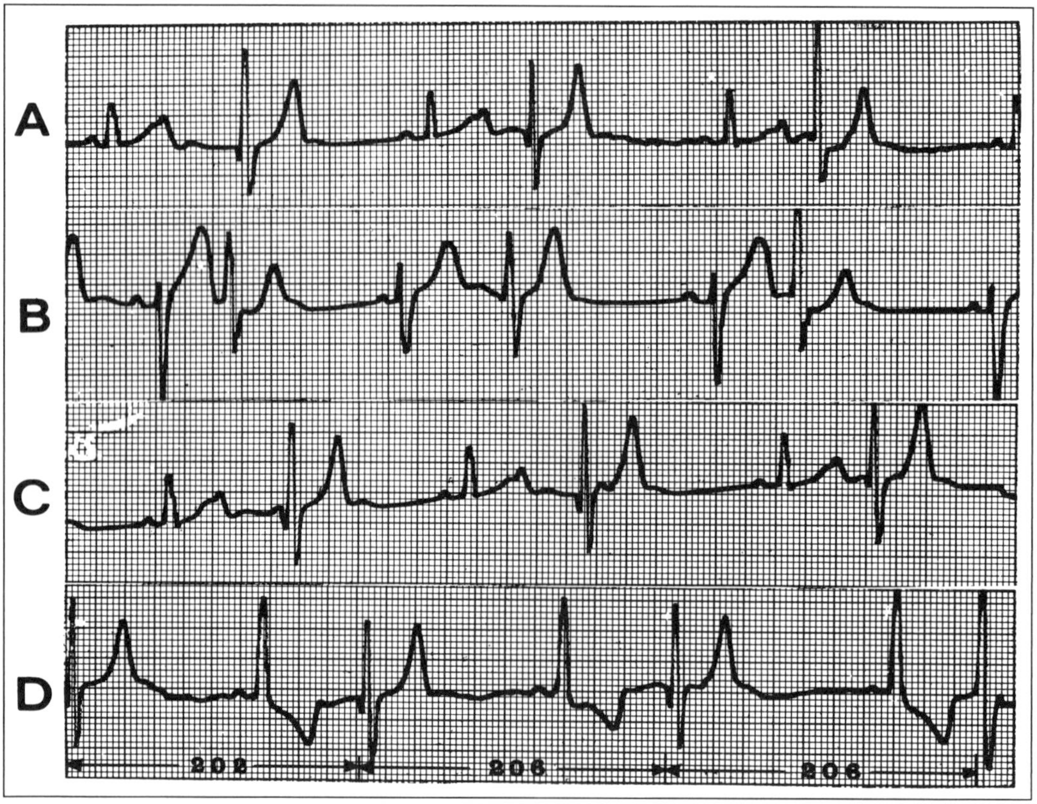


**Fig. 22–1.** Sinus rhythm with ventricular parasystole. Note that coupling intervals vary, and the shortest interectopic intervals are constant. The Holter monitor ECG rhythm strips A, B, C, and D are not continuous. (The numbers represent hundredths of a second.)

(generally 0.06 second or more). Parasystolic beats may appear very early or late in the cycle of the basic rhythm. It should be noted that the coupling intervals may vary to a lesser degree if the sinus node is prematurely activated by the parasystolic impulse. This phenomenon is common in atrial parasystole, but it may be found also in AV junctional or in rare instances of ventricular parasystole.

**Constant Shortest Interectopic Intervals:** Constant interectopic intervals indicate that the ectopic focus produces impulses regularly and independently from the basic rhythm if the above-mentioned criterion is present. The basic rhythm is almost always sinus and less commonly AF or atrial flutter.

If the interectopic intervals are long, they should be a multiple of the shortest interectopic interval. However, occasionally, direct measurement of the parasystolic cycle is not possible. This is the case when only every other or third parasystolic beat appears on the electrocardiogram, particularly in the presence of a long interectopic interval. In this circumstance, a common denominator should be detected, although an erroneous interpretation is possible because a long interectopic interval can be a multiple of many different cycle lengths.

**Rate:** Parasystolic rates may range between 20 and 400/min, but in most cases, the parasystolic rates range from 30–50 beats/min (Figs. 22–1, 22–2, and 22–3). The rapidity of discharge of the parasystolic impulse is considered to be outside the limit of physiologic automaticity of the usual impulse formation. Parasystolic tachycardia (the usual rate: 70–130 beats/min) nearly always originates from a ventricular focus (Fig. 7–12), but, rarely, atrial or AV junc-

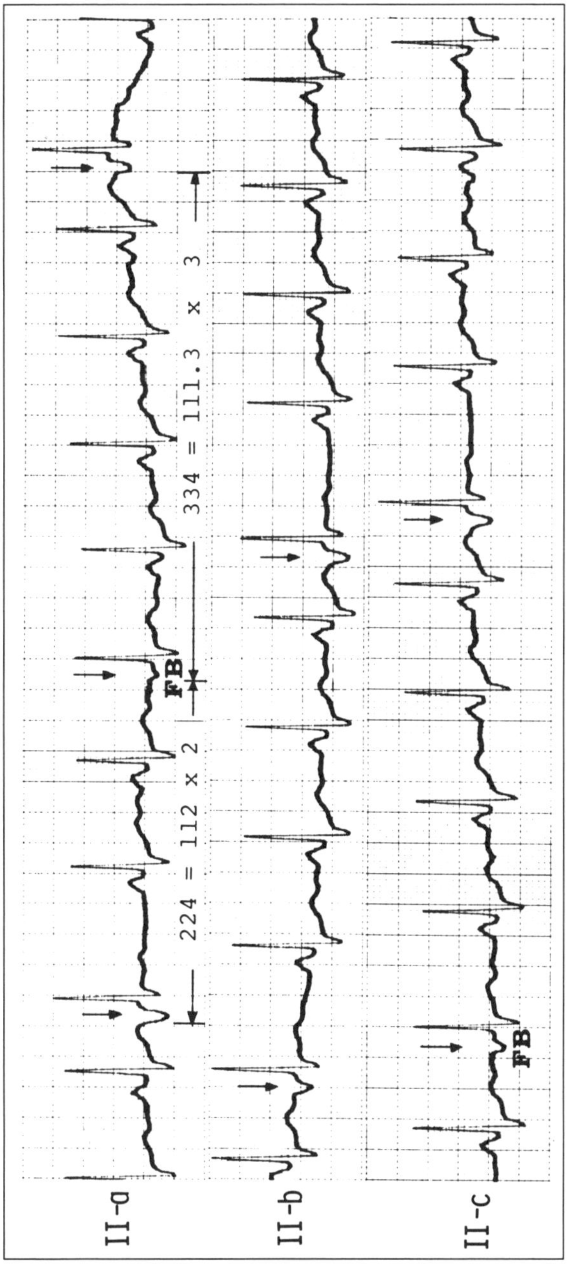


**Fig. 22–2.** Sinus rhythm with AV junctional parasystole (indicated by arrows). Note that the direct parasystolic cycle is not shown in this tracing because of exit block of varying degree. There are occasional atrial fusion beats (FB). Leads II-a, II-b, and II-c are not continuous. (The numbers represent hundredths of a second.)

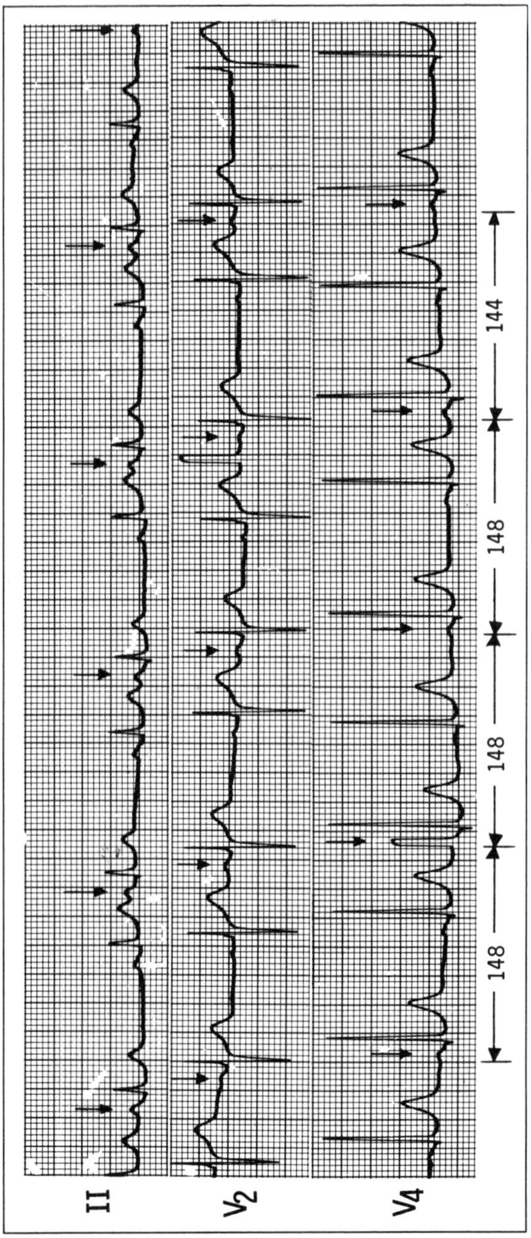


Fig. 22–3. Sinus rhythm with atrial parasystole (indicated by arrows). (The numbers represent hundredths of a second.)

tional parasystolic tachycardia may be observed.

**Fusion Beats:** If 2 impulses from different foci arrive more or less simultaneously in the heart, each impulse activates a part of the chamber involved, producing the appearance of an intermediate or mixed complex. Ventricular fusion beats are very common in ventricular parasystole (Fig. 22–1), especially when the rate of the basic rhythm is rapid, as in sinus tachycardia, or irregular, as in AF. When one sees this in the absence of other arrhythmic forms, such as incomplete AV dissociation, the possibility of ventricular parasystole should be strongly considered.

Atrial fusion beats are not as common as ventricular fusion beats and occur if impulses from 2 different foci simultaneously stimulate the atria. In atrial parasystole, atrial fusion beats may occur when the ectopic beat appears very late in the cycle of basic rhythm. In this circumstance, the sinus node fires the impulse just before the ectopic impulse reaches it. In AV junctional parasystole and rarely in ventricular parasystole (in the presence of sinus rhythm), 1 part of the atrial chamber may be activated in a retrograde fashion, resulting in P waves that are intermediate in contour between sinus and ectopic P waves. The contour of atrial or ventricular fusion beats may vary from beat to beat depending upon the portion of the chamber activated by the 2 different foci.

## Clinical Significance

Parasystole has been frequently encountered in elderly persons and in those with diseased hearts, although, occasionally, the arrhythmia has been found in apparently healthy hearts. Parasystolic VT is relatively common during the first 72 hours of acute MI, but the arrhythmia is benign and self-limited in most cases. It can be said that the most important clinical significance of parasystole is that VPCs are frequently digitalis induced, whereas ventricular parasystole is not due to DI (Chapter 17).

# ATRIAL DISSOCIATION

Atrial dissociation, characterized by 2 sets of independent P waves, has been produced experimentally and has also been found in human hearts. Although some investigators are skeptical about the existance of atrial dissociation in human hearts, various clinical studies have documented many cases showing this arrhythmia without doubt. It should be pointed out, however, that various artifacts must be excluded when the diagnosis of atrial dissociation is entertained. Atrial dissociation is commonly due to unilateral slow atrial rhythm, but it may be due to unilateral AF, atrial flutter, or AT.

## Diagnostic Criteria

Atrial dissociation is characterized by the presence of a unilateral ectopic atrial rhythm independent of the basic rhythm (sinus or ectopic). In addition, none of the impulses of the unilateral atrial rhythm is conducted to the ventricles. The unilateral atrial rhythm is commonly a slow rhythm, but occasionally it may be a tachycardia, flutter, or fibrillation. Rarely, unilateral atrial rhythm may be sinus in the presence of coronary sinus artificial pacemaker rhythm.

**Unilateral Slow Atrial Rhythm:** The most common form of atrial dissociation is a slow unilateral ectopic atrial rhythm (Fig. 22–4). Nearly always, the basic rhythm is sinus, and it may be ectopic, such as AV junctional rhythm or tachycardia, or even AF, atrial flutter, or AT. None of the unilateral atrial impulses is conducted to the ventricles, regardless of the basic rhythm, because the ectopic atrial rhythm is always limited to a portion or all of 1 atrium. In other words, the impulses of the basic rhythm and the ectopic atrial rhythm do not interfere with each other. Thus, the P-P or R-R cycles of the basic rhythm are undisturbed by the ectopic atrial rhythm. It is common to observe that bizarre and larger P waves occur intermittently when the ectopic P wave is superimposed on the P wave of the basic rhythm. The rate of the uni-

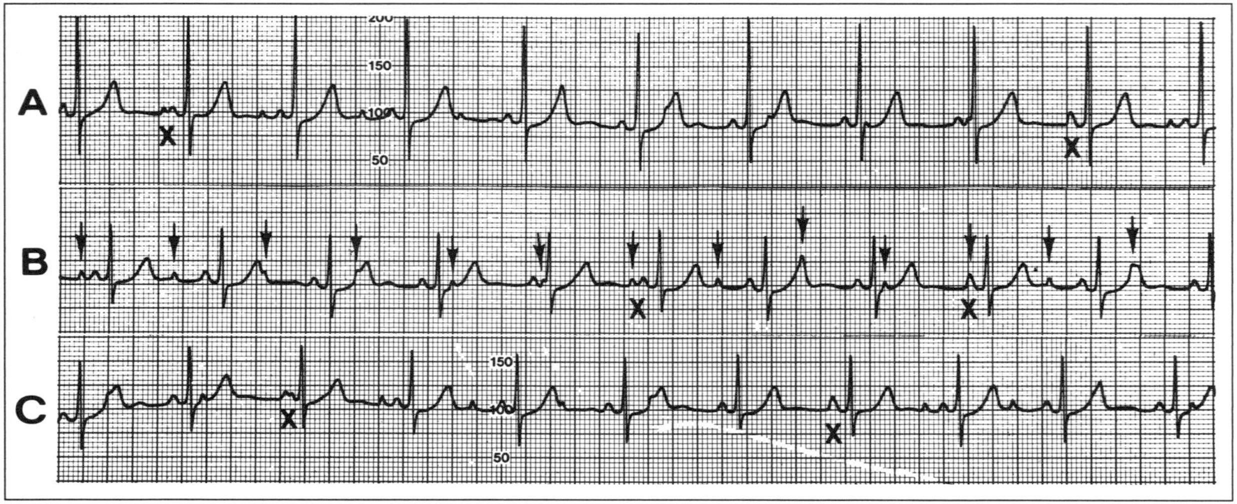


**Fig. 22–4.** Sinus rhythm with unilateral atrial rhythm (indicated by arrows) producing atrial dissociation. Note that the sinus and ectopic P waves are superimposed in many areas (X).

lateral atrial rhythm is usually between 30 and 50/min (Fig. 22–4).

In general, the P-P intervals of the ectopic atrial rhythm are not precisely regular, and the variation of the interectopic intervals is greater than that of atrial parasystole. The configuration of the ectopic P wave in atrial dissociation is bizarre but is smaller than that of the sinus P wave. The small ectopic P wave in this circumstance is attributed to depolarization of a small area of the atria. At times, unilateral ectopic atrial focus may produce a very unstable and irregular slow rhythm.

**Unilateral Atrial Tachycardia:** Unilateral AT occurs extremely rarely in atrial dissociation. The basic rhythm is commonly sinus, but it may be ectopic. Unilateral AT may persist for a long period of time, even when the sinus node ceases to produce an impulse. In this case, ventricular standstill may be observed unless a subsidiary pacemaker takes over ventricular activity. The P-P cycles in unilateral AT usually vary markedly in comparison to ordinary AT. It is difficult to ascertain the usual rate range in this arrhythmia because only a few cases have been reported. However, the usual rate seems to be much slower than that of ordinary AT.

**Unilateral Atrial Fibrillation:** It is not uncommon to observe unilateral AF in the presence of any basic rhythm. The basic rhythm is frequently sinus but an ectopic atrial rhythm has been reported. For instance, AT or atrial flutter or AV junctional rhythm may be present as the underlying rhythm and may coexist with an independent, unilateral AF. However, a diagnosis of atrial dissociation becomes extremely difficult when 2 ectopic rhythms coexist. When the basic rhythm is a regular sinus rhythm, the P-P or R-R cycles are regular in spite of the coexistence of AF because the sinus and ectopic impulses do not interfere with each other. On rare occasions, transitional ECG changes from normal sinus rhythm to unilateral AF (atrial dissociation), followed by uncomplicated AF, can be recorded in the same patient.

**Unilateral Atrial Flutter:** Less commonly than unilateral AF, atrial dissociation may be due to unilateral atrial flutter. The flutter cycles in atrial dissociation are usually irregular compared with ordinary atrial flutter. As in unilateral slow atrial rhythm, the atrial flutter wave in atrial dissociation is often smaller than that of ordinary atrial flutter.

**Unilateral Sinus Rhythm:** On rare occasions, sinus rhythm may be present in the atria as a unilateral atrial rhythm in the presence of coronary sinus pacemaker rhythm producing atrial dissociation. Under this circumstance, the sinus P waves are not followed by the QRS complexes and are independent of the artificial pacemaker-induced atrial rhythm.

## Differential Diagnosis

Atrial dissociation should be distinguished from atrial parasystole, regularly occurring APCs, postcardiac transplantation ECG, and various artifacts.

In both atrial parasystole and atrial dissociation (unilateral slow atrial rhythm or tachycardia), the ECG shows 2 independent atrial rhythms, 1 of which is activated by the sinus node and the other by an ectopic focus anywhere in the atria. In parasystole, in most cases, the impulse can be conducted to the atria and ventricles whenever the myocardium or conduction system is in the nonrefractory phase (Fig. 22–3). In contrast to this, the ectopic atrial impulse in atrial dissociation is never conducted to the ventricles and is always limited to a small or large area of 1 atrium (Fig. 22–4). In addition, the configuration of the ectopic P wave in parasystole is similar to or larger than the sinus P wave, while the P wave in atrial dissociation is small and more bizarre or has a fibrillating or fluttering character. The interectopic interval in atrial dissociation is more variable than in atrial parasystole.

When nonconducted APCs occur regularly, the ECG may resemble atrial dissociation. However, the constant coupling intervals (the interval from the ectopic P wave to the preceding P waves of the basic rhythm) definitely exclude atrial dissociation. Other characteristic features of APCs enable one to differentiate them without much difficulty.

The ECG obtained from a patient with a cardiac transplantation shows a tracing identical to atrial dissociation. This is observed because 2 independent pacemakers, 1 from the recipient's and the other from the donor's heart, control the cardiac activity. In this case, the rhythm originating from the donor's heart is the basic and dominant rhythm, whereas the rhythm of the recipient's own heart is unilateral rhythm that is localized in a very limited area of the atrium. The postcardiac transplantation ECG may show a basic sinus rhythm of the donor's heart with another independent sinus rhythm from the recipient's heart. On the other hand, the donor's sinus rhythm may coexist with the unilateral ectopic atrial rhythm (e.g., AF) of the recipient heart. Differential diagnosis from atrial dissociation may be impossible without knowing the history of cardiac transplantation. Atrial dissociation must be differentiated from various artifacts, including loose contact of the electrodes, rhythmic tick, rhythmic contraction of the diaphragm as in hiccough or diaphragmatic flutter, rhythmic movement of other somatic muscles such as in parkinsonism, interference from a dial telephone, and the heartbeats of another person who touches the patient when the ECG is taken.

### Mechanisms

With regard to a possible mechanism of atrial dissociation, we may assume that an ectopic atrial focus controls either a part or all of the atrium, probably because of intraatrial block, so that none of the sinus beats interferes with the ectopic atrial rhythm and also so that the ectopic atrial rhythm does not disturb the basic rhythm. None of the ectopic P waves is conducted to the ventricles, indicating that the blocked zone is located in the supranodal area, rather than assuming that the ectopic P waves are not strong enough to produce conduction to the ventricles. The phenomenon of atrial dissociation has recently been attributed to dissociation of a part of the atrial myocardium with ectopic impulse formation and protective entrance and exit block or dynamic bidirectional block. If there is no block, the ectopic P wave should conduct to the ventricles whenever the AV junctional tissues are nonrefractory.

### Clinical Significance

Atrial dissociation is almost always found in patients with intractable CHF. Atrial dissociation has been observed in critically ill patients and occurs most commonly a few hours before death.

## ELECTRICAL ALTERNANS

Electrical alternans is a relatively rare ECG phenomenon, the presence of which almost always is considered indicative of organic heart disease. However, very rarely it has been found in the absence of cardiac disease when the heart rate was rapid.

Electrical alternans is defined as alternating P, QRS, or T complexes or any combination of these occurring with regular rhythmicity and with constant intervals between the complexes. The complexes should originate from 1 pacemaker and should not have any relationship to respiration or any other periodic extracardiac phenomena. On rare occasions, electrical alternans may be observed in AF, and, in this case, the R-R intervals naturally vary. In addition, electrical alternans may be observed in atrial flutter or AT and AV JT.

The incidence of electrical alternans varies at different institutions depending upon the interest and the knowledge of the physicians who interpret the ECGs. However, approximately 5 instances of electrical alternans can be observed in 10,000 ECGs obtained from general hospitals. The most common form of electrical alternans involves QRS complexes alone and is termed "ventricular electrical alternans." The occurrence of total (atrial and ventricular) electrical alternans is much less frequent. Extremely rarely, electrical alternans may involve only the ST segment, T waves, or U waves. Isolated atrial electrical alternans is equally rare.

A 2:1 electrical alternans is a common alternating ratio, and a 3:1 alternating ratio is a rare occurrence. Extremely rarely, 4:1, 4:2, 5:3, 5:2, 5:1, and so on alternating ratios may be observed.

## Diagnosis

Electrical alternans is diagnosed when the configuration of the P, QRS, ST, T, or U complexes, or any combination of these, alternates with regular rhythmicity, provided that the complexes originate from 1 pacemaker. Electrical alternans commonly involves QRS complexes (ventricular electrical alternans), but rarely it may involve the P waves as well as the QRS complexes (total electrical alternans). Electrical alternans involving only the ST segment, T wave or U wave is extremely rare.

**Ventricular Electrical Alternans:** This is the most common form of electrical alternans, and it involves the QRS complexes alone. Among this group, a 2:1 electrical alternans is the most common alternating ratio (Fig. 22–5), and a 3:1 alternating ratio is a rare occurrence. In these cases, electrical alternans may occur during a rapid or a slow rate. Ventricular electrical alternans may persist, but more commonly its occurrence is transient or intermittent. The underlying rhythm is commonly sinus in ventricular electrical alternans, and occasionally it is an ectopic rhythm, such as AF, atrial flutter, AT, or AV JT. Extremely rarely, unusual alternating ratios, such as 4:2, 4:1, 5:3, 5:2, 5:1, ventricular electrical alternans may occur. It should be noted that ratios in electrical alternans are expressed in the following manner: 2:1 ventricular electrical alternans indicates that every other QRS complex alternates its configuration, whereas 3:1 ventricular electrical alternans designates that alternation of the QRS complexes occurs at every third beat.

**Atrial Electrical Alternans:** The term "atrial electrical alternans" is used when the alternation involves only the P waves (Fig. 22–6). As seen in ventricular electrical alternans, the most common alternation ratio is 2:1 (Fig. 22–6), and a 3:1 or higher ratio is unusual. Atrial electrical alternans is much less common than ventricular electrical alternans.

**Total Electrical Alternans:** The term "total electrical alternans" is used when the alternation involves the P waves and QRS complexes simultaneously. Total electrical alternans, like ventricular electrical alternans, may show 2:1 or 3:1 ratios. Alternation of the P waves is usu-

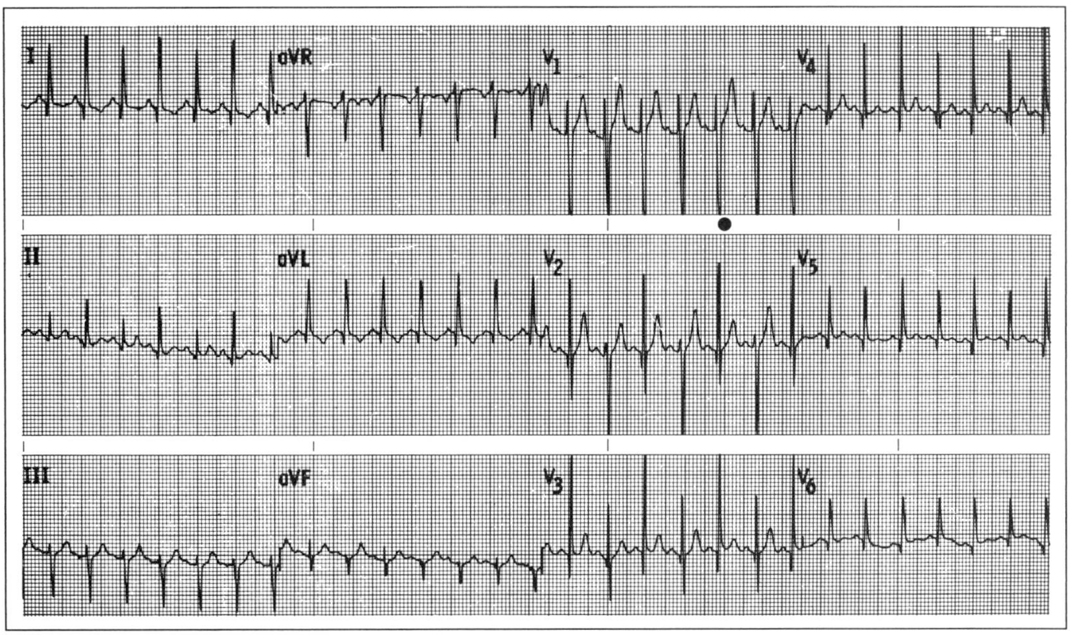


**Fig. 22–5.** Marked sinus tachycardia with 2:1 ventricular electrical alternans.

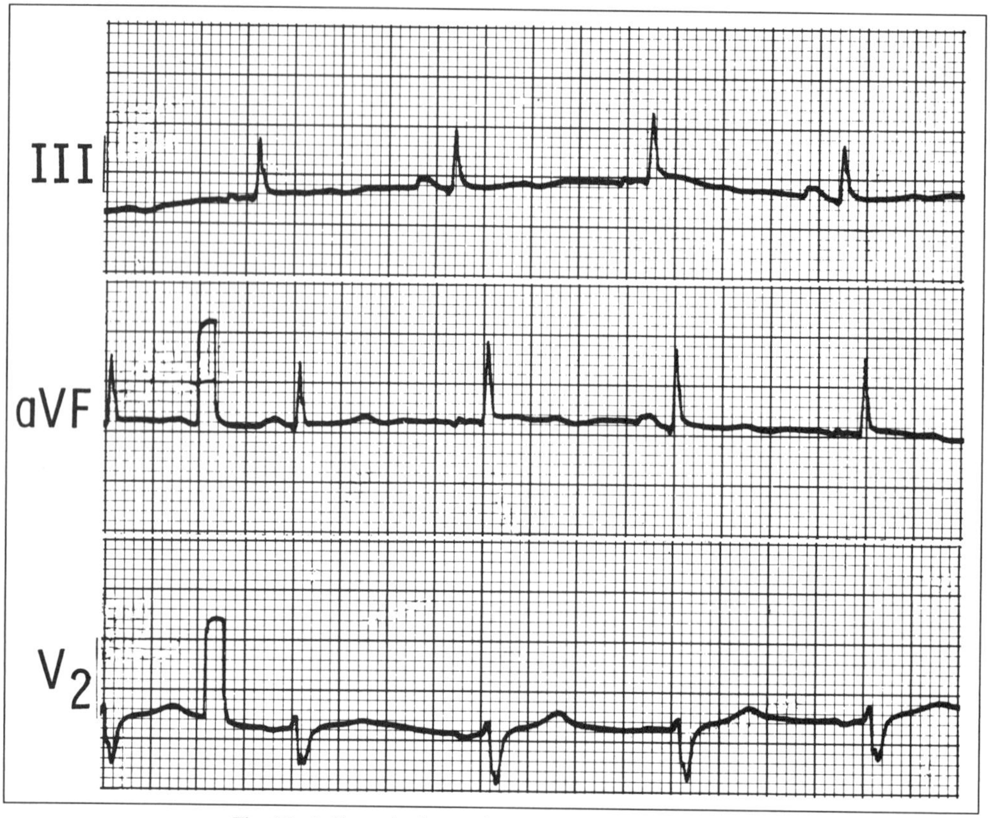


**Fig. 22–6.** Sinus rhythm with 2:1 atrial electrical alternans.

ally much less evident than that of the QRS complexes in total electrical alternans because of the smaller complex in the former.

**Electrical Alternans Involving ST Segment, T waves, or U Waves:** Extremely rarely, electrical alternans may involve only the ST segment and/or the T wave (Fig. 22–7). Electrical alternans involving only U waves is extremely rare. In these circumstances, artifacts due to various periodic extracardiac phenomena should be excluded.

**Electrical Alternans in Artificial Pacemaker-induced Ventricular Rhythm:** Very recently, extremely unusual ventricular electrical alternans was observed in artificial pacemaker-induced ventricular rhythm in a patient with acute MI.

## Mechanism

The exact mechanism of electrical alternans is not yet clearly understood. However, various hypotheses have been presented, such as anatomic alternation of the cardiac position, alternation of cardiac output, and alternating prolongation of the refractory phase of some part of the heart.

This author is inclined to favor the last hypothesis of alternating prolongation of the refractory phase of the heart as the mechanism of production of electrical alternans.

## Clinical Significance

Electrical alternans per se is purely an electrocardiographic diagnosis, but it is frequently accompanied by pulsus alternans. Interestingly, pulsus alternans, which is mechanical alternation in the force of ventricular contraction, is only rarely accompanied by electrical alternans. Furthermore, pulsus alternans is a relatively common phenomenon, whereas electrical alter-

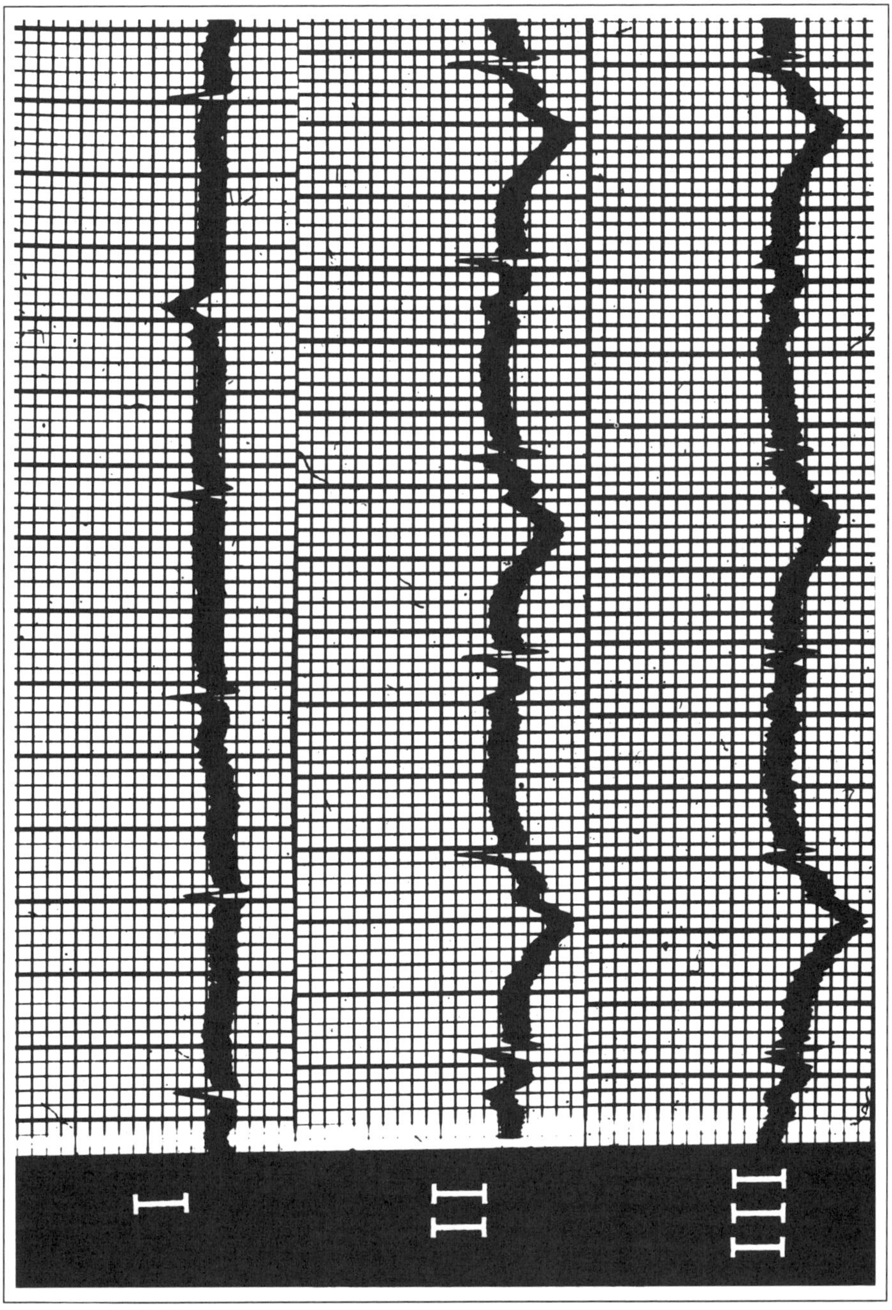


Fig. 22–7. Sinus rhythm with electrical alternans involving ST segment and T wave.

nans is a rare occurrence. Both electrical and pulsus alternans per se do not produce any symptoms.

Electrical alternans that occurs in rapid sinus tachycardia, especially during cardiac surgery, is usually insignificant clinically. In contrast to this, electrical alternans occurring at a relatively slow rate is usually pathologic. The most common underlying disorders that produce electrical alternans include severe CHF and massive pericardial effusion.

## ABERRANT ATRIAL CONDUCTION (CHUNG'S PHENOMENON)

Occasionally, the P wave of the sinus beat immediately following an APC may have a bizarre configuration that is different from the P wave of an APC or of sinus origin (Fig. 5–6). This is termed "aberrant atrial conduction" (Chung's phenomenon) and is analogous to aberrant ventricular conduction. Less commonly, aberrant atrial conduction may also be observed immediately following AV JPCs or VPCs. In addition, aberrant atrial conduction rarely occurs immediately following atrial, AV junctional, or even ventricular parasystolic beats.

Aberrant atrial conduction usually involves the P wave of only 1 sinus beat immediately following an ectopic beat. However, on rare occasions, aberrant atrial conduction may occur in 2 or more consecutive sinus beats. When this occurs, aberrant atrial conduction is much more marked in the first sinus P wave than in the second sinus P wave.

The exact mechanism involved in the production of aberrant atrial conduction (Chung's phenomenon) is not clearly understood, but it probably occurs because the refractory period of the atria is altered immediately following an ectopic impulse.

Aberrant atrial conduction must be differentiated from wandering atrial pacemaker, an AV JEB following a postectopic pause, coexisting multifocal premature contractions, and various artifacts.

The clinical significance of aberrant atrial conduction (Chung's phenomenon) is again uncertain because of its rare occurrence. However, all cases of aberrant atrial conduction observed by this author were found in patients with diseased hearts.

## CORONARY SINUS RHYTHM

Coronary sinus rhythm is defined as the cardiac rhythm with retrograde P waves that precede the QRS complexes, with the P-R interval longer than 0.12 second (Fig. 22–8). Thus, the ECG finding of coronary sinus rhythm closely simulates the AV junctional tachycardia or rhythm with prolonged P-R interval, and it is impossible to distinguish between coronary sinus rhythm and AV junctional tachycardia or rhythm with slight antegrade conduction delay. The P wave axis of coronary sinus rhythm is between −60 and −90° (the same as that of AV junctional tachycardia or rhythm).

Clinically, coronary sinus rhythm is considered to be a benign arrhythmia that is usually self-limited.

## CORONARY NODAL RHYTHM

The term "coronary nodal rhythm" is seldom used today, and it probably has only a historical recognition. The reason for this is that the P-R interval is shorter than 0.12 second in many circumstances, and the finding is considered to be a normal variant as long as the P wave is upright in lead II and inverted in lead aVR (the usual sinus P wave axis). Most cardiologists interpret this ECG finding as sinus rhythm with a short P-R interval without any further explanation.

The traditional criteria of coronary nodal rhythm are cardiac rhythm with a short P-R interval (shorter than 0.12 second) and normal P axis (same as normal sinus rhythm) with constant P-R interval (Fig. 22–9). Clinically, the P-R interval is often short during various stressful situations and during physical exercise. However, the diagnosis of WPW syndrome should be suspected when dealing with an ex-

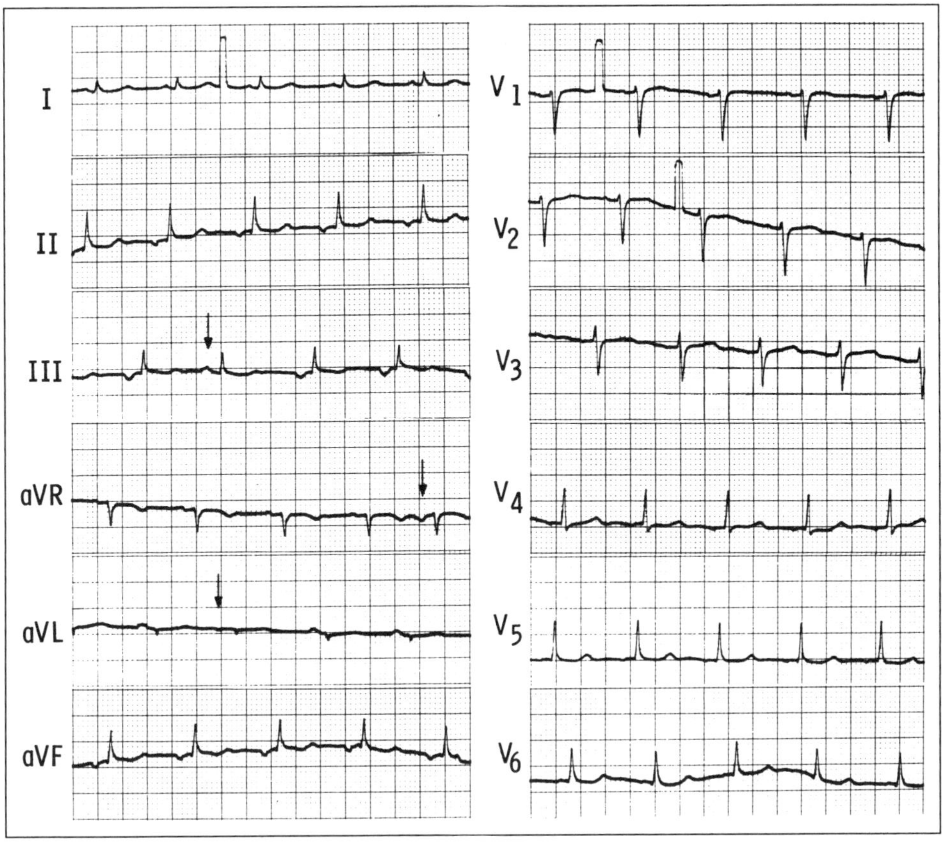


**Fig. 22–8.** Coronary sinus rhythm with occasional APCs (indicated by arrows).

tremely short P-R interval (Chapter 13). Lown-Ganong-Levine (LGL) syndrome, which is considered to be a variant of WPW syndrome, has a short P-R interval with no clear delta-wave (Chapter 13). Otherwise, AV junctional tachycardia or rhythm with isorhythmic AV dissociation may produce the ECG finding that superficially resembles so-called coronary nodal rhythm when the sinus P waves preceding the QRS complexes (AV junctional origin) march through with very similar heart rates (Chapter 6).

## LEFT ATRIAL RHYTHM

Left atrial rhythm is a relatively ill defined cardiac arrhythmia that is considered to be clinically insignificant by most cardiologists. In fact, some cardiologists are skeptical about the diagnosis of left atrial rhythm.

Traditionally, the diagnosis of left atrial rhythm is established when the following findings (Fig. 22–10) are present:

1. Regular cardiac rhythm with the P-R intervals 0.12 second or more
2. Inverted P waves in leads II, III, and aVF (the P axis: −60 to −90°)
3. Isoelectric or inverted P wave in lead I
4. Upright P wave (no negative component) in lead $V_1$ and inverted P waves in leads $V_{4-6}$
5. Heart rate: 60–100 beats/min (sometimes slower than 60 and faster than 100 beats/min)

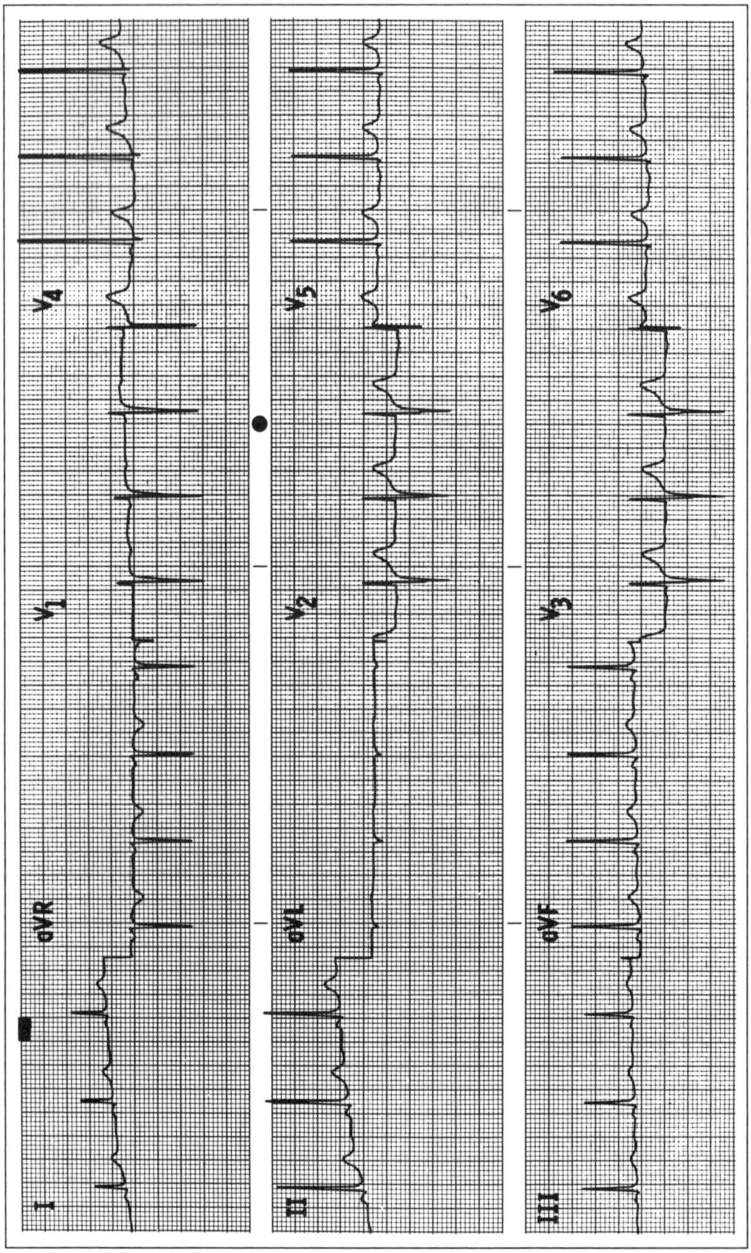


**Fig. 22–9.** So-called coronary nodal rhythm (see text).

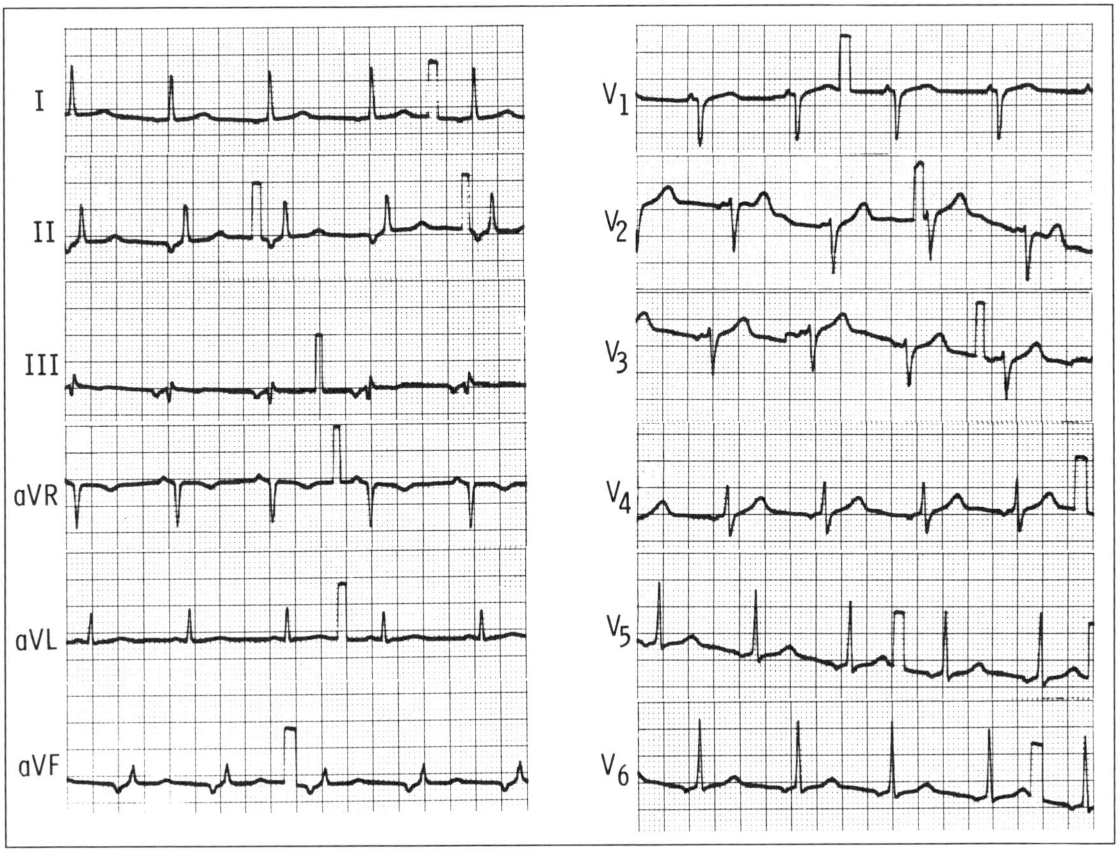


**Fig. 22–10.** Left atrial rhythm (see text).

## CARDIAC TRANSPLANTATION

Electrocardiographic findings following cardiac transplantation have been described in experimental animal studies as well as in clinical medicine. As can be expected, 2 independent atrial rhythms, 1 from the recipient's heart and the other from the donor's heart, will be produced. The 2 atrial pacemakers are separated by the suture line, and they produce 2 independent atrial rhythms, superficially resembling atrial parasystole and closely simulating or even being identical to atrial dissociation. In fact, the 2 atrial rhythms produced by cardiac transplantation comprise an iatrogenically induced atrial dissociation. Different combinations of the 2 atrial mechanisms may be observed following cardiac transplantation. The atrial rhythm originating from the donor's heart is frequently a sinus mechanism, but occasionally a heart with an ectopic atrial rhythm has been used as the donor's heart, while the recipient's heart is frequently in AF or atrial flutter. When the atrial mechanism is ectopic in origin in either the donor's or the recipient's heart, the identification of 2 atrial activities becomes extremely difficult because AF or atrial flutter waves will be superimposed on other waves. Occasionally, P waves of both the recipient's and the donor's hearts may have synchronization, but this phenomenon is merely coincidental.

The atrial impulses originating from the recipient's heart are localized in the small area of the atrial stump and are never conducted to the ventricles. Thus, the atrial rhythm, in this case, is analogous to unilateral atrial rhythm in atrial dissociation. Conversely, the atrial rhythm of the donor's heart is conducted to the ventricles to produce the dominant rhythm. When a history of cardiac transplantation is not available for the ECG interpretation, the differential diagnosis from atrial dissociation is very difficult or even impossible.

The exercise response in patients following cardiac transplantation is of special interest. It has been demonstrated that during mild or moderate exercise the donor's atrial rate did not change significantly, whereas the atrial rate of the recipient's heart was consistently accelerated, and it returned to the resting rate upon termination of the exercise. The donor's heart rate was significantly accelerated, however, when vigorous exercise was performed. These exercise responses in human cardiac transplants were similar to those in experimental animal studies. Similarly, the donor's heart rate was unchanged by a Valsalva maneuver, whereas the recipient's atrial rate was accelerated by the procedure.

Electrocardiographic changes may be observed when the rejection phenomenon occurs following cardiac transplantation. The most common and earliest finding of the rejection is a decrease in the QRS voltage. This is more clearly demonstrable when a myocardial lead is utilized. In addition, a right axis deviation of the QRS complex, prolonged intraventricular conduction, and subendocardial injury or ischemia are also common findings resulting from rejection. Various arrhythmias, including atrial tachyarrhythmias, supraventricular tachycardia, AV JT, and sinus bradycardia following cardiac transplantation, have been reported.

## HOLIDAY HEART SYNDROME

The term "holiday heart syndrome" has become popular among physicians recently. It describes a group of healthy individuals who develop a variety of cardiac arrhythmias after brief drinking sprees. Since this particular alcohol-induced event occurs more frequently during holidays and weekends, such medical terminology seems to be appropriate.

Extra heartbeats (premature beats) and AT are the most common cardiac arrhythmias. A variety of abnormal heart rhythms is most likely to be provoked by the release of epinephrine-like substances. Abnormal heartbeats and rhythms often disappear when drinking stops. Otherwise, digitalis and/or antiarrhythmic agents may be required for a short duration.

The heart is found to be normal in most individuals with the holiday heart syndrome. A chance of developing various and more serious cardiac arrhythmias is greater in cardiac patients when they drink alcohol excessively.

## CONGENITAL Q-T SYNDROME

Congenital Q-T syndrome is a familiar disorder characterized by Q-T interval prolongation associated with ventricular arrhythmias, syncope, or even sudden death. Some individuals with this syndrome are deaf.

Jervell and Lange-Nielson syndrome occurs as an autosomal recessive inheritance with Q-T interval prolongation and associated deaf-mutism. In 1 study, 4 of 6 siblings had this disorder, and 3 experienced sudden death. Ramano-Ward syndrome occurs as an autosomal dominant with Q-T interval prolongation and without associated deafness.

The cause of the Q-T prolongation is not known. Syncopal episodes often occur during physical exercise. It has been well documented that syncope or sudden death occurs as a result of VF due to the R-on-T phenomenon.

Prophylactic antiarrhythmic therapy is indicated, but the means of defining its efficacy are yet to be determined. Long-term antiarrhythmic therapy is indicated primarily for prevention of ventricular tachyarrhythmias.

## LIQUID PROTEIN DIETS

It has been well demonstrated that liquid protein diets are frequently associated with life-threatening cardiac arrhythmias. Sudden death has been reported during or soon after taking liquid protein diets. Death under this circumstance is usually due to VF, which is initiated by VPCs with the R-on-T phenomenon secondary to markedly prolonged Q-T interval with broad T wave. Therefore, the ECG finding produced by liquid protein diets is very similar to quinidine-induced Q-T interval prolongation with broad T wave. The mode of sudden death resulting from the liquid protein diet is comparable to that resulting from quinidine or quinidine-like drugs (e.g., procainamide or disopyramide).

Thus, ventricular tachyarrhythmia induced by low protein diets is multiform (polymorphous) VT (a form of torsade de pointes), which is often a precursor of VF and sudden death. Torsade de pointes is described fully in Chapter 7.

Liquid protein diets are not recommended because of the above-mentioned life-threatening complications, including sudden death. In most cases, the victims are young to middle-aged women who try to lose weight very rapidly without any medical supervision by taking liquid protein diets that are extremely low in calories and lack various essential nutrients, especially protein.

# Index

t indicates table